Basics of
MEDICAL
PHYSIOLOGY

Basics of MEDICAL PHYSIOLOGY

Second Edition

D. Venkatesh | H.H. Sudhakar

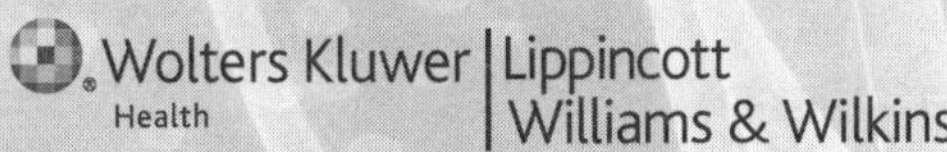

Wolters Kluwer Health | Lippincott Williams & Wilkins

New Delhi • Philadelphia • Baltimore • New York
London • Buenos Aires • Hong Kong • Sydney • Tokyo

Commissioning Editor: Ms. P. Sangeetha
Development Editor: Dr. Munish Khanna
Production Editor: Ms. Honey Pal
Compositor: Nutech Digital
Assistant Manager Manufacturing: Mr. Anil Kumar Gauniyal

Copyright © 2010 by Wolters Kluwer Health (India)

10th Floor, Tower C,
Building No. 10
Phase – II, DLF Cyber City,
Gurgaon, Haryana (India)

First Impression, 2010
Second Impression, 2011
Third Impression, 2012

ISBN-13: 978-81-8473-223-8

Published by Wolters Kluwer (India) Pvt Ltd

Printed and bound at Sanat Printers, Haryana

For product enquiry, please contact – Marketing Department (marketing@wolterskluwerindia.co.in)

Preface to the Second Edition

We express our sincere thanks to our beloved students and faculties for patronizing and popularizing this book. We have great pleasure in presenting the second edition. The book has been thoroughly revised and updated, and the presentation has been further enhanced. However, its student-friendly features, namely clarity and simplicity of presentation, have been kept intact.

Recognizing the value of the book and its usefulness for students, our well wishers pressurized us to make it available for larger groups of students, both domestically and internationally. In this endeavor, we found Wolters Kluwer to be suitable partners as their policies matched very well with our principles. We are confident that they will do a good job in introducing the book to all students.

While the book would be useful to all undergraduates in reviewing and revising the subject before examinations, it would be particularly useful to students from dentistry and allied health streams.

We hope that students and faculties find this edition as useful as the previous one and they continue to use and recommend it as before. We would welcome comments and suggestions for the further improvement of the book and would gratefully acknowledge any constructive feedback.

D. Venkatesh

H.H. Sudhakar

Preface to the First Edition

We placed our first book *Basics of Medical Physiology* (level 2) in the hands of our beloved students and colleagues last year with an apprehension about its acceptability. Response to the book has been encouraging and the experience satisfying. With the patronage of our well wishers, we could bring out second edition of the book in less than a year with a lot of value additions. We express our sincere thanks to all those who made our maiden effort a great success.

It was our desire to present a book to bridge the gap between the ocean of information available and little knowledge about the subject for a beginner. The readers have opined that the contents in the book are balanced and presentation lucid. In short, it is student friendly. Although we have made a humble beginning, we feel that lot more needs to be accomplished.

Encouraged by the response for the earlier book, honoring our commitment to provide useful information to our students, we have decided to bring out this book *Basics of Medical Physiology* (level 3).

We have maintained the student-friendly features of the earlier book but made it richer in relevant content. Emphasis is laid on the applied physiology. Simple illustrative diagrams have been included. To help the students to prepare for examination, an extensive question bank and multiple choice questions have been provided.

We are confident that our students and colleagues will appreciate our effort and give all the support and encouragement for this book also.

We thank our editorial team, artists, and the printer for doing a neat job to bring out this book within a short time.

D. Venkatesh

H.H. Sudhakar

Table of Contents

6   Gastrointestinal System   129

7   Excretory System   156

8   Central Nervous System   178

9 Special Senses — 223

10 Endocrinology — 248

11 Reproductive System — 276

Introduction

Physiology is the branch of science dealing with the study of the functions of living beings. It is a dynamic study of life describing the vital functions of the living organisms at organ, cellular, and molecular levels. The term physiology is a combination of Greek word *physis*, meaning "nature," and *logos*, meaning "science" or "study." Physiology is closely associated with medicine. Alteration in the normal physiology leads to causation of disease and pathology. Restoring the normal physiology is the essence of medical management.

Medical physiology deals with the functioning of the human body. It takes a global and holistic view of the human body, requiring an integrated understanding of events at the cellular and organ level. Physiology is the mother of several biological sciences responsible for the development of disciplines like biochemistry, biophysics, and neurosciences. Hence, the boundaries of physiology are not sharply defined.

Physiologists have attempted to understand the intricate control systems and regulatory mechanisms that influence the body to function, survive, and maintain stability in the ever-changing external environment. Ability of the body to maintain constancy of the internal environment is termed **homeostasis**. The concept of homeostasis was developed by a French physiologist, Claude Bernard. The term homeostasis (*homoios*, meaning "the same," and *stasis*, meaning "standing") was suggested by an American physiologist, Walter B. Cannon, in the year 1932.

Cannon suggested that every regulatory mechanism of the body is aimed at maintaining constancy of the internal environment. The internal environment is not static. Even under constantly changing external environment, the internal environment is dynamically changing and is maintained relatively constant.

A wide range of fluctuation in the environmental temperature does not significantly alter the core temperature which is kept constant at about 37°C. This ability of the body to regulate its own function and return to normal condition forms the basis for understanding the mechanism of the disease.

The study of physiology is done by understanding the functions of the specific organ system. It is done at different levels: at organ system, organelle, tissue, and cellular levels. More complex and intricate physiological basis is understood at the molecular level. Later, an attempt is made to evaluate the integration of the organ system for smooth functioning of the body.

An important character of life is to respond to changes in the external environment. This property is termed **responsiveness**. Withdrawal of the limb from a painful stimulus is a classical example for this property. The living tissues transmit a wave of excitation from one region of the body to another region. This is **conduction of impulse**. Responsiveness and conduction are very well developed in the excitable tissues like muscle and nerve.

The functions of the body are regulated by the nervous system and endocrine system. The endocrine glands produce specialized chemical messengers called **hormones**. These hormones modify the function of another organ, termed the **target organ**.

The tissues require energy to carry out their metabolic activities. The source of energy and a constant supply of oxygen are required for the generation of energy. The complex food products ingested by animals are broken down into simpler substances, absorbed and assimilated by the digestive system. The simpler food substances like glucose, fatty acids, and amino acids are used by individual cells to satisfy their energy requirement.

Every individual cell needs oxygen to varying extent to produce energy. The cells are drawn away from the environment because of the complex structure of the organ system. The oxygen requirement of each cell is satisfied by a well-established transport system—cardiovascular system. It has a primer pump, the heart, and the channels in the form of blood vessels.

Blood which acts as a vehicle carrying oxygen and nutrients is transported to the individual cell by contraction of the heart and movement of blood through the blood vessels.

An alternate pathway for drainage exists in the form of lymphatic system composed of lymph, lymphatic vessels, lymph nodes, thymus, and spleen. It helps in the movement of fluid and large protein molecules from the tissue spaces, the fat-related substances from the digestive system to the blood.

The internal environment of a living being is threatened by foreign substances and invading microorganisms. The individual's ability to resist infection and fight cancer and other types of diseases depends on the effective functioning of the immune and lymphatic system. **Immunology** is the study of immune responses of the body.

The metabolic waste produced by the individual cell can damage the cell or hamper its function if it accumulates at the site of production. This undesirable side effect is prevented by the transport of metabolic waste through the blood to the various organs of excretion. The solid waste is excreted through the gastrointestinal tract, excess water, and soluble waste through the renal system and the gaseous waste by the respiratory system.

An increase in the size or number of groups of cells results in growth. Growth increases the size of an individual or an organ.

During life, the aging cells loose their capacity to perform functions at the desired level, and hence, they have to be replaced at periodic intervals. New cells have to be added to the different tissues to facilitate growth. Specialized cells have to be produced to repair the damaged tissues of the body. More importantly, new individuals having the same features as the ancestors have to be produced for the propagation of generation. The formation of the new individual and new cells is the function of reproductive system.

In this book, efforts have been made to give an insight to the functional manifestation in the body, physiological control mechanisms, and integration of structures and functions.

General Physiology

Life started millions of years ago with a single cell. In the course of evolution through time, multicellular organisms with complex structures and functions have developed.

Human beings are creatures with complexities in structure and function. Each and every function of a human being is actually performed by a specific organ system of the body. Physiology is the study of the manner in which these organ systems perform their functions.

Cell

Each organ system is made up of various tissues. Each tissue is made up of millions and millions of small units, termed **cells**. Cell is the basic unit of living beings. Our body is made up of 75 trillion cells.

Components of Cell

Each cell contains

- water,
- electrolytes,
- proteins,
- lipids, and
- carbohydrates.

Water

Seventy to seventy-five percent of the cell is made up of water. It contains dissolved chemicals and suspended particles. Water helps in the transport of substances from one part of the cell to another.

Electrolytes

Major electrolytes include potassium, magnesium, sodium, phosphate, sulfate, bicarbonate, chloride, and calcium. They are dissolved in water. Electrolytes are necessary for cellular control mechanisms.

Proteins

They constitute 10–20% of the cell mass. Proteins are of two types: (i) structural proteins and (ii) globular proteins.

Structural Proteins

- Present in the form of long filaments.
- Polymers of protein molecules.
- Provide contractile mechanisms for muscles.

- Form cytoskeleton of cilia, axons, and mitotic spindles.
- Found in collagen and elastic fibers.

Globular Proteins

- Made up of individual protein molecules.
- Globular (shaped like a globe or a ball) in structure.
- Mainly enzymes.

Lipids

Lipids constitute 2% of cell mass. They are made up of phospholipids and cholesterol. They are insoluble in water.

Lipids form major constituents of cell membrane. Some cells contain triglycerides. They are present in fat cells. The fat stored is used as energy whenever needed by the body.

Carbohydrates

Carbohydrates form around 1% of cell mass. They play a major role in providing nutrition to the cell.

Carbohydrates are present in extracellular fluid (ECF) as glucose and are readily available for the cell. They are also stored as glycogen, which is used for providing energy to the body.

Structure of Cell

Cell is the structural and functional unit of all living beings (Fig. 1.1). Different cells of the body have different features. Even though the features are different, the basic component of all cells in the body remains the same.

Cell is made up of two major parts: (i) nucleus and (ii) cytoplasm. **Cytoplasm** is the fluid part of cell containing the organelles. It is covered by an envelope termed **cell membrane**.

Cell Membrane

It is a thin layer of membrane surrounding the cell (Fig. 1.2). It covers both the nucleus and the cytoplasm. It is semipermeable and is 7–10 nm thick.

The membrane is principally made up of proteins, lipids, and to a much lesser extent, carbohydrates.

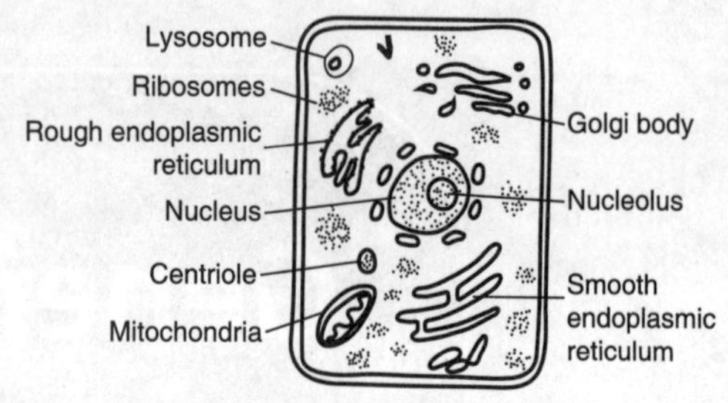

Fig. 1.1   Structure of cell.

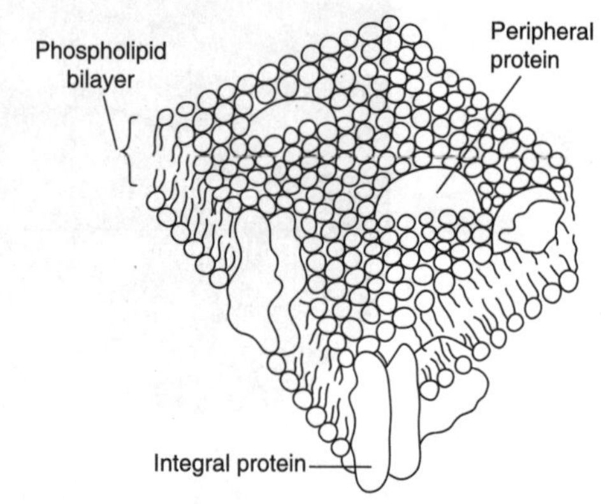

Fig. 1.2   Cell membrane.

Composition of Cell Membrane	
Proteins	55%
Phospholipids	25%
Cholesterol	13%
Other lipids	4%
Carbohydrates	3%

Various theories have been proposed to explain the cell structure. The most accepted one is the **fluid mosaic model** proposed by Singer and Nicolson.

Cell membrane is made up of two layers of lipids, which are only two molecules thick. It is mainly made up of phospholipids and cholesterol. The phosphate radical of phospholipid and hydroxyl radical of cholesterol are water soluble, i.e., hydrophilic.

The fatty acid radical of phospholipid and steroid nucleus of cholesterol are fat soluble, i.e., hydrophobic. Hydrophobic portion of both these molecules occupy the center of the membrane. Hydrophilic portion faces the surrounding water.

Lipid bilayer is impermeable to water-soluble substances such as ions and glucose, but is permeable to fat-soluble substances such as oxygen and alcohol. Lipid bilayer is fluid and solid. Therefore the fluid portion of the membrane flows from one point to another along the cell membrane.

Functions of Lipids

- Form the cell membrane.
- Selectively permeable; allow fat-soluble substances to pass through them easily.
- Provide a framework for the arrangement of protein and carbohydrate molecules on the cell membrane.

Proteins are globular masses floating in the lipid bilayer. They are mostly glycoproteins. They are of two types: (i) integral proteins and (ii) peripheral proteins.

Integral proteins pass through the entire thickness of the membrane. **Peripheral proteins** are attached only to the surface.

Functions of Proteins

- Act as structural proteins which provide framework for the cell.
- Act as pumps which help in active transport.
- Act as carriers in facilitated diffusion.
- Form ion channels.
- Act as receptors.
- Act as enzymes.

Carbohydrates are present on the outer surface of the cell. They are glycoproteins or glycolipids. Carbohydrate molecules form a thin layer throughout the surface of cell membrane called **glycocalyx**.

Functions of Carbohydrates

- Attach to glycocalyx of other cells.
- Act as receptors for binding hormones.
- Participate in immune reactions.

Nucleus

Nucleus is a spherical structure covered by a nuclear membrane (nuclear envelope). It is the control center of the cell.

It controls

- chemical reactions occurring in the cell and
- reproduction of the cell.

Nucleus contains nucleolus and chromatin material. It is mainly made up of water. Proteins account for 80% of the dry weight, 18% by DNA, and 2% by RNA. Nucleus contains a densely staining network of DNA and protein. This is called **chromatin**. Chromatin material gets organized and is readily identified as chromosomes during cell division. Each species has a fixed number of chromosomes. Human beings have 23 pairs of chromosomes.

Genes are the units of heredity. Each gene is a portion of DNA molecule. They are present on the chromosomes.

Nuclear Membrane

Nuclear membrane has two layers: (i) outer and (ii) inner. The outer layer is continuous with endoplasmic reticulum (ER). The space between the two nuclear membranes is continuous with the space inside the ER.

Nuclear membrane has several nuclear pores. These pores allow low-molecular-weight substances to pass through them.

Nucleoli

Nucleoli are lightly stained structures in the nucleus. They synthesize and store RNAs and proteins. Later, they are transported to form mature ribosomes, which play an important role in protein synthesis.

Cytoplasm

It contains a fluid portion of the cell in which organelles are present. The fluid portion is called **cytosol**. It contains dissolved proteins, glucose, and electrolytes. The contents of cytoplasm include cell organelles, inclusion bodies, and cytoskeleton.

Cytoplasm contains the following cellular organelles:

- mitochondria,
- endoplasmic reticulum,
- ribosomes,
- Golgi apparatus,

- lysosomes, and
- centrosomes.

Mitochondria

Mitochondrion is called power house of the cell. It is present in the cytoplasm. It is a sausage-shaped structure made up of an outer membrane and an inner membrane (Fig. 1.3).

The inner membrane is folded to form shelves called **cristae**. The membranes of mitochondria are similar to cell membrane. The inner portion of mitochondria is filled with matrix. Matrix contains dissolved enzymes required for the Krebs cycle. Its number varies depending on the energy requirement of the cell.

Mitochondria are self-replicative and produced in large numbers whenever extra energy is required by the cell.

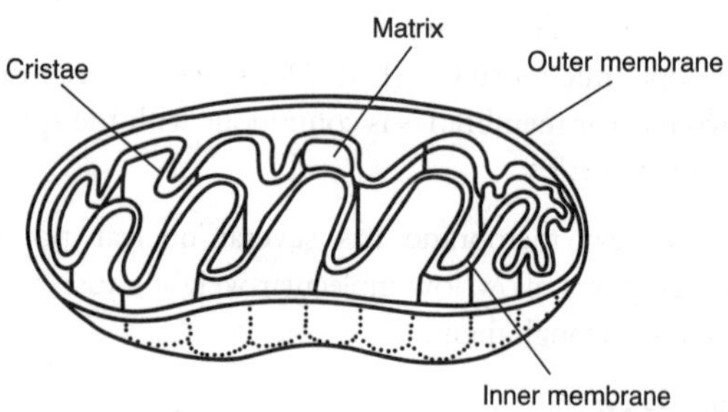

Fig. 1.3   Mitochondrion.

Functions

Mitochondria contain large quantities of enzymes that convert food products to CO_2 and water by citric acid cycle. Energy liberated during the reaction is used for the synthesis of high-energy molecules like adenosinetriphosphate (ATP). The ATP is transported out of mitochondria to the place where energy is required.

Endoplasmic Reticulum

This is a network of tubular and flat vesicular structures interconnected with each other.

The spaces between the tubules and the vesicles are filled with a watery fluid termed **endoplasmic matrix**. The surface area of ER is quite large. It is around 30–40 times the area of cell membrane.

Endoplasmic reticulum is of two types: (i) rough endoplasmic reticulum (Fig. 1.4) and (ii) smooth endoplasmic reticulum (Fig. 1.5).

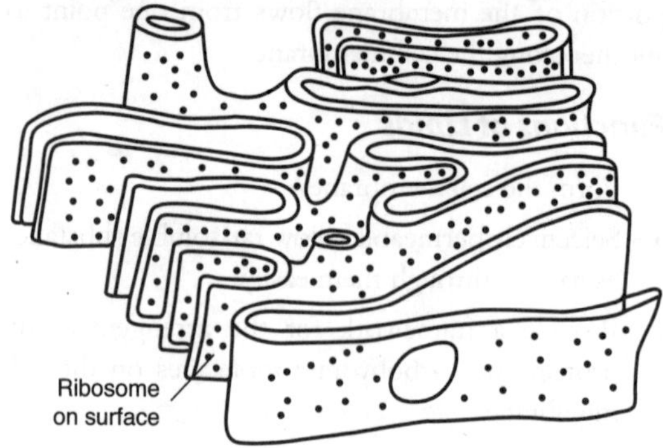

Fig. 1.4   Rough endoplasmic reticulum.

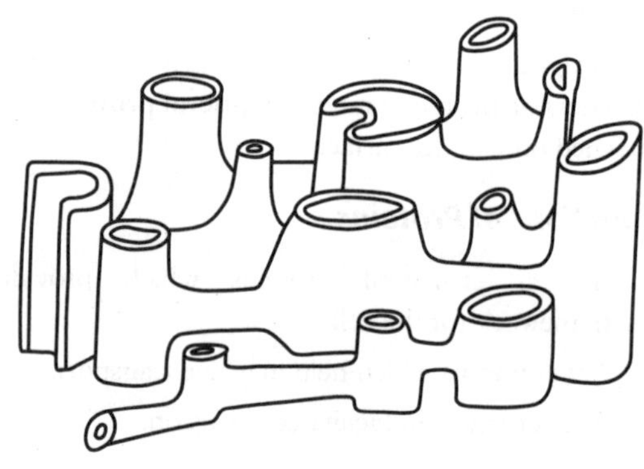

Fig. 1.5   Smooth endoplasmic reticulum.

Rough Endoplasmic Reticulum   Endoplasmic reticulum with granular structure (ribosomes) on its outer surface is called rough endoplasmic reticulum. It is well developed in cells actively involved in protein synthesis.

Nissl granules of neurons and acinar cells of pancreas have well-formed rough ER.

Function

It helps in the synthesis of proteins.

Smooth Endoplasmic Reticulum   This does not have ribosomes on its surface. It is found in abundance in Leydig cells and cells of adrenal cortex.

In skeletal and cardiac muscles, smooth ER is modified to form sarcoplasmic reticulum.

Functions

It helps in the synthesis of lipids, drug degradation, glycogen metabolism, and control of calcium ion concentration.

Ribosomes

They are spherical particles found in both free and bound forms. The bound form is present on the outer surface of ER. Ribosomes are made up of RNA and proteins.

Function

It helps in the synthesis of proteins.

Golgi Apparatus

It resembles the smooth ER. It is made of multiple layers of thin flat vesicles lying near the nucleus (Fig. 1.6).

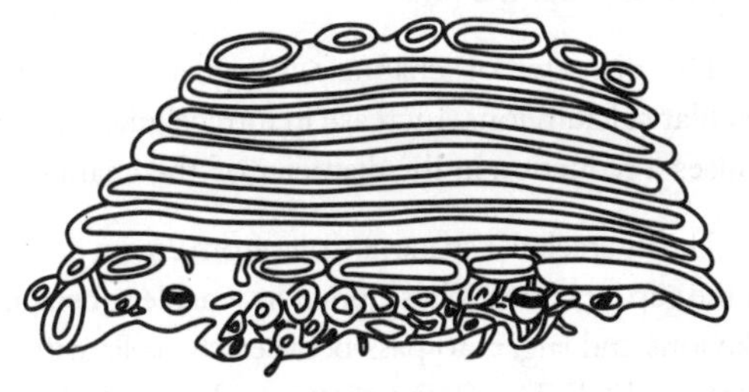

Fig. 1.6   Golgi apparatus.

Functions

It concentrates protein and polysaccharide. It helps in the synthesis of carbohydrate portion of glycoprotein. It is the site of formation of lysosomal enzymes.

Lysosomes

Lysosomes are formed by Golgi apparatus and are present throughout the cytoplasm.

They are filled with hydrolytic enzymes.

Functions

They help in the removal of unwanted, damaged substances and foreign bodies like bacteria.

They are responsible for regression of tissues, e.g., regression of uterus after pregnancy and mammary glands after lactation.

Peroxisomes

Peroxisomes are similar to lysosomes formed from smooth ER. They contain oxidases and catalyze reactions generating hydrogen peroxide.

Centrosomes

Centrosomes are structures present near the nucleus. They are made up of structures called **centrioles**. Centrioles are two short cylinders arranged at right angles to each other. They are visible only during cell division.

Microtubules in groups of three run longitudinally in the walls of each centriole.

Centrosomes divide into two during cell division and move to the opposite poles of mitotic spindle.

Function

They control the steps of cell division.

Cytoskeleton

Cytoskeleton is a system of fibers that maintains the structure of cell and permits the cell to change its shape. It helps in the movement of cell.

Cytoskeleton is made up of

- microfilaments,
- intermediate filaments, and
- microtubules.

Microfilaments   They are long solid fibers 4–6 nm in diameter. They are made of actin molecules and provide elastic support for the cell membrane. The actin molecules are G-actin. These G-actins polymerize to form F-actin. F-actin is the microfilament.

Intermediate Filaments   They are 8–14 nm in diameter. They connect nuclear membrane to the cell membrane. They are found in all types of cells.

Microtubules   They are long hollow structures with a diameter of 15 nm. They are formed by the organization of two globular protein subunits α- and β-tubulin. These subunits aggregate to form long tubes made of stacked rings.

They provide tracts for the transportation of vesicles and organelles like mitochondria from one part of cell to another. They form a spindle which moves the chromosomes during mitosis.

Microtubules assemble and disassemble as and when required. Warmth facilitates assembly and cold facilitates disassembly.

Molecular Motors

These are ATPases that move proteins, organelles, and other contents of cells from one part to the other. They bind to microtubules or microfilaments and bring about the movement of substances. They include kinesin, dynein, and myosin.

Kinesin is a double-headed molecule. One head binds to the microtubule and the other head swings forward and binds to the substance carried. Kinesins are associated with mitosis and meiosis.

Dyneins are of two types: (i) cytoplasmic dynein and (ii) axonemal dynein. The functions of cytoplasmic dynein are similar to those of kinesin. Axonemal dynein is responsible for beating of flagella and cilia. Dyneins also have two heads.

Myosin is present in multiple forms. Its functions include muscle contraction and cell migration.

Intercellular Connections

These are junctions formed between the cells. Types of intercellular connections are tight junctions and gap junctions (Fig. 1.7).

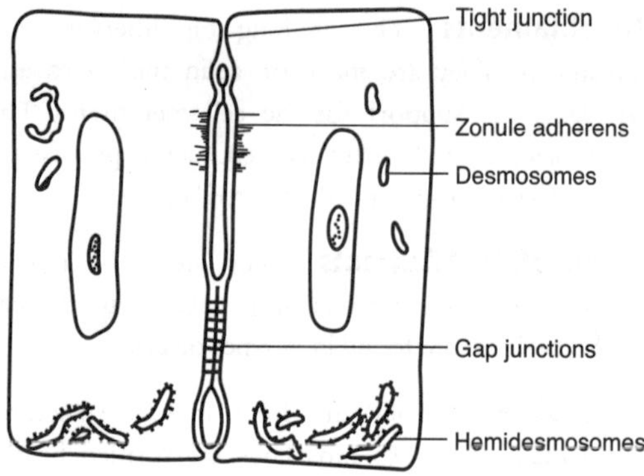

Fig. 1.7   Intercellular connections.

Tight Junctions

Tight junctions are also known as *zonula occludens*. They are present in the apical zone of the cell. They are commonly seen in cells lining the intestinal mucosa, renal tubules, and choroid plexus. They permit the passage of some ions and other solutes and prevent the movement of proteins in the plane of the membrane.

Zonule adherens is present on the basal side of zonule occludens and is the major site for attachment of actin fibers.

Desmosomes are spot-like patches present on the membranes of two adjacent cells.

Hemidesmosomes attach cells to the basal lamina.

Focal adhesions are dense plaques which also attach cells to the basal lamina.

Gap Junctions

These are channels formed by protein units called **connexons**. Each connexon is made up of six subunits surrounding a channel. The diameter of a channel is around 2 nm.

The diameter of channels is regulated by intracellular calcium ions. Increase in intracellular calcium causes a reduction in the diameter of the channel.

The intercellular space narrows from 25 nm to 3 nm at the gap junctions. These junctions enable substances like ions and sugars to pass between the cells without entering ECF. They also permit rapid propagation of electrical activity from one cell to another.

Cell Adhesion Molecules

Cell adhesion molecules (CAM) are substances which attach cells to basal lamina and also to each other. They are important in embryonic development, formation of nervous system and other tissues. They are useful in holding the cells together in adults, in inflammation and wound healing, as well as in the metastasis of tumors.

CAMs are divided into four broad groups:

1. integrins—heterodimers that bind to various receptors;
2. adhesion molecules of IgG superfamily of immunoglobulins;
3. cadherins—calcium-dependent molecules that mediate cell-to-cell adhesion by homophilic reactions;
4. selectins—they bind carbohydrates.

Cell Division

All multicellular organisms start from a single cell. Each of the human cells has 46 chromosomes (23 pairs). Out of the 23 pairs, 22 pairs are autosomes and 1 pair of sex chromosomes.

Transformation from a single cell to a multicellular organism involves the processes of cell division and cell differentiation.

Cell divides in two phases: (i) interphase and (ii) mitosis.

Interphase

It is a preparation period for mitosis. It is subdivided into G_1, S, and G_2 phase.

G₁ Phase

Decision for cell division is confirmed during this stage. The cell performs all its normal functions.

S Phase

There is duplication of DNA material. DNA double helix separates. Two strands synthesize its complement and therefore two DNA double helix are formed.

G₂ Phase

In this phase, the volume of cytoplasm increases.

Mitosis

This has four phases (Fig. 1.8):

1. prophase,
2. metaphase,
3. anaphase, and
4. telophase.

Prophase

Centrioles move apart and form poles of mitotic spindle. Chromatin material condenses into chromosomes. Each chromosome is made up of a pair of chromatids attached to the centromere. There is dissolution of nuclear membrane and nucleoli.

Metaphase

Chromosomes move to the equator of the spindle. Centromeres split and chromatids get separated.

Centrioles duplicate resulting in two centrioles at each pole of the spindle.

Anaphase

Separated chromatids move toward opposite poles with the help of spindles. A constriction appears in the middle of the cell indicating the formation of two daughter cells.

Telophase

Chromosomes are converted to chromatin network. Nucleoli reappear, new nuclei are formed, and nuclear membrane reappears. Spindle fibers disappear and finally two daughter cells are formed.

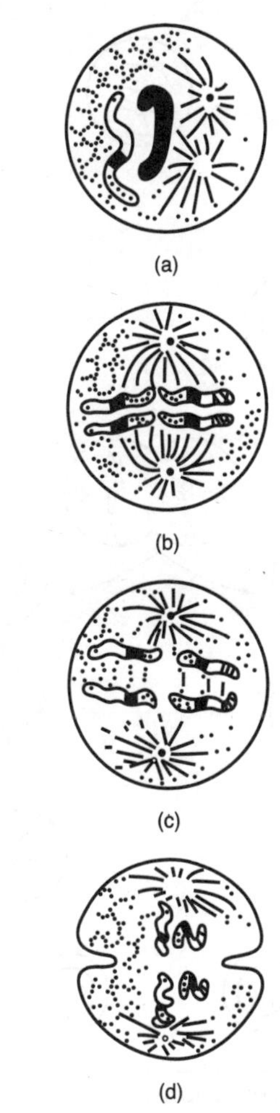

Fig. 1.8 Stages of mitosis: (a) prophase, (b) metaphase, (c) anaphase, and (d) telophase.

Meiosis

Meiosis is a process where four daughter cells with half the number of chromosomes are formed. Sex cells (gametes) are produced by this method.

Gamete formation occurs in two stages: (i) Meiosis I and (ii) Meiosis II.

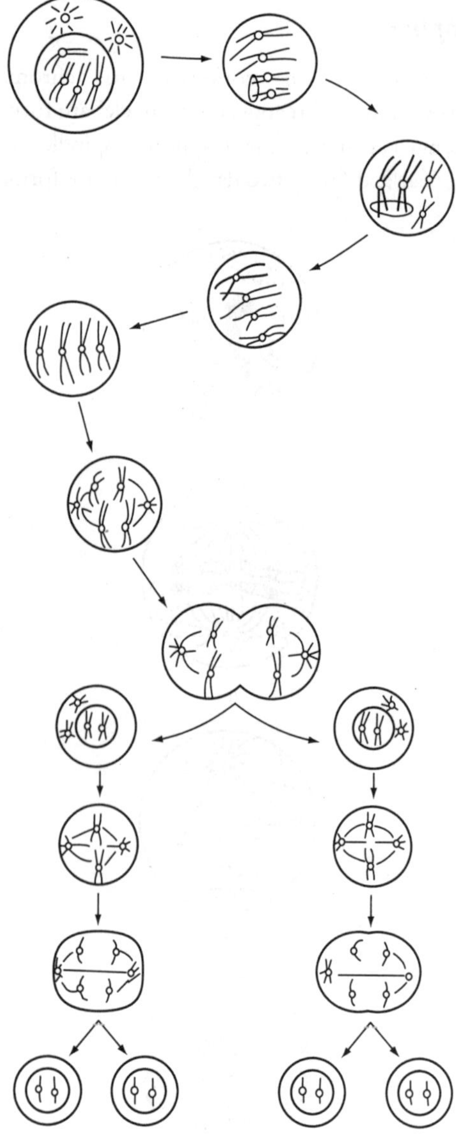

In the first division, two cells with haploid number of chromosomes are formed. In the second division, four cells are formed from these two cells without reduction in the number of chromosomes. Meiosis also occurs in four phases as seen in mitosis.

Stages (Fig. 1.9)

Prophase I   Centrioles move apart. Chromatin material condenses into chromosomes. The chromosomes separate and are attached at a few points. Exchange of genetic material occurs between the chromatids.

Metaphase I   The homologous pairs of chromosomes move toward the equator with the help of microtubules attached to centromere.

Anaphase I   One chromosome from each homologous pair moves toward the opposite pole with the help of spindles. Therefore, 23 chromosomes move to one pole, while the other 23 move to the other pole.

Telophase I   The cytoplasm divides, nuclei are formed, and two cells develop. The cell has 23 chromosomes, each chromosome with a pair of chromatids.

Prophase II   This occurs after Telophase I. There is formation of a new spindle at right angle to the earlier one.

Metaphase II   A pair of chromatids moves toward the equator with the help of microtubules attached to centromere.

Anaphase II   The two chromatids move toward the opposite poles with the body of spindles.

Telophase II   The chromatids form a network. New nuclei are formed. One cell divides into two. Finally, four daughter cells are formed from one mother cell.

Genetics

This is a branch of biology devoted to the study of genes and heredity. The science of genetics has made great advance in the recent past. The foundation for modern-day genetics was laid down by Gregor Mendel. Later, hundreds of researchers have contributed to this field and have helped in revolutionizing the study of genetics.

Chromosomes

The term *chromosome* was coined by Waldeyer in 1888. Chromosomes are thin, thread-like structures present in the nucleus of eukaryotic cells during cell division.

Chromosomes are responsible for the transmission of hereditary characters from one generation to the next.

The number of chromosomes in every cell is constant for a given species. There are 46 chromosomes (23 pairs) in all the human cells, except gametes. (Sperm and ovum contain only 23 chromosomes.)

Chromosomes are mainly composed of DNA. They also contain RNA, basic proteins called histones, complex proteins, and inorganic salts.

DNA

DNA (deoxyribonucleic acid) is a long double-stranded helical structure containing simple chemical compounds bound together in a regular pattern (Fig. 1.10).

DNA is the component of chromosomes that carries the genetic message (hereditary characteristics) from the parent to the offspring.

DNA is made of phosphoric acid, deoxyribose sugar, and four nitrogenous bases—adenine, guanine, thymine, and cytosine.

Phosphoric acid and deoxyribose sugar form the helical strands and nitrogenous bases connect the two strands. These strands are linked together by hydrogen bonds between the specific nitrogenous bases.

Adenine pairs with thymine, and guanine pairs with cytosine.

There are an estimated 30,000 genes in the human genome. The collection of genes with full expression of DNA from an organism is called **genome**.

DNAs which code for proteins are called **exons**. They make up only 3% of the human genomes. The remaining 97% of DNAs are called **introns**. Their function is not yet known. They are also referred to as **junk DNAs**.

DNA Fingerprinting

The character of DNA varies from individual to individual. A common form of variation is repetition of base pairs. This causes variation in the length of DNA chain where it is cut by restriction enzymes. This process is termed **restriction fragment length polymorphism** (RFLP). Analysis of RFLP is DNA fingerprinting. It is very accurate in differentiating two individuals since the chance of RFLP matching due to chance is one in one million to one in one lakh. DNA fingerprinting can be carried out in small quantity of specimens of semen and blood, as well as of tissues.

RNA

RNA is similar to DNA except that the sugar present is ribose. Nitrogenous base thymine is replaced by uracil. During RNA synthesis, the two strands of DNA separate and one of the strands is used as a template for RNA molecule synthesis.

There are three types of RNAs:

1. mRNA (messenger RNA),
2. tRNA (transfer RNA), and
3. rRNA (ribosomal RNA).

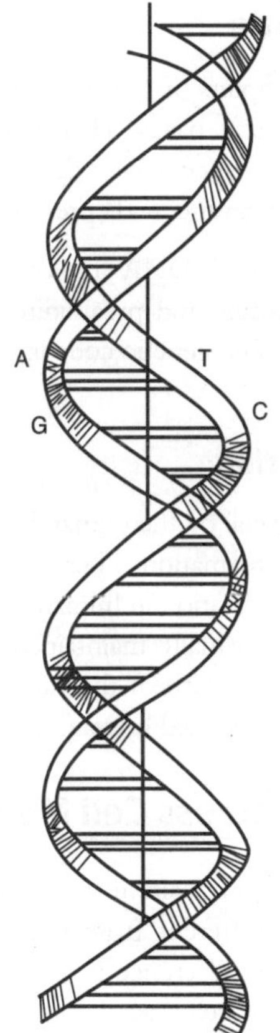

Fig. 1.10   Structure of a DNA molecule.

mRNA

This carries the genetic code from the nucleus to cytoplasm for controlling protein synthesis. It is composed of several hundred to several thousand nucleotides in a single unpaired strand. It contains codons that are complementary to triplets of DNA genes. It enters the cytoplasm and arranges itself on the ribosomes.

tRNA

tRNA contains about 80 nucleotides. It is folded to form a clover leaf. It transports amino acids to protein molecules as the protein is being synthesized.

tRNA combines with amino acids that are to be incorporated into proteins. Then it acts as a carrier to transport these amino acids to the ribosomes where protein is formed.

In the ribosomes, each specific type of tRNA recognizes a particular codon on mRNA and thereby delivers the correct amino acid for the protein molecule which is newly formed.

rRNA

This is synthesized in the nucleus. It constitutes about 60% of the ribosomes. The remainder of the ribosomes are proteins. There are 75 different types of proteins in the ribosome.

rRNA functions in association with tRNA and mRNA. tRNA transports amino acids to the ribosome for incorporation in the protein. mRNA provides the necessary information for arranging the amino acids in proper order.

Transcription

It is the process of formation of mRNA. Transcription occurs under the influence of RNA polymerase enzyme.

Steps in the Transcription Process

DNA strand contains a sequence of nucleotides called **promoter**. RNA polymerase recognizes this promoter and attaches to it. It unwinds the DNA helix and separates the two strands. As unwinding goes on, a new RNA nucleotide is added to the newly formed RNA chain. The newly formed RNA chain breaks away from the DNA template. It is released into the nucleoplasm. The DNA strand rebonds with its own complementary DNA strand.

Translation

It is the process of formation of polypeptide chain from mRNA. mRNA molecule comes in contact with the ribosomes. As it travels through the ribosomes, the protein molecule is formed. The protein molecule formation ends when the chain-terminating codon passes through the ribosome. This protein molecule is released into the cytoplasm.

Genes

Genes are the functional units of DNA. The portion of chromosome which codes a particular character is called a **gene**. The position of a gene on a chromosome is called **locus**.

Genetic Code

It consists of triplets of bases. A triplet is made up of three successive bases. This triplet is termed a **code word**. The successive triplets finally control the sequence of amino acids present in a protein.

Two strands of DNA molecules split apart, exposing the purine and pyramidine bases on each of the strands. The genetic code is formed in these exposed bases.

Gene Expression

Each and every cell of the human body contains the entire genetic information. There is a great differentiation and specialization in human cells. The genetic information is normally maintained in a repressed state and only small parts of the information are transcribed. This is mediated by transcription factors.

Transport across Cell Membrane

The chemical composition of extracellular fluid (ECF) is quite different from that of intracellular fluid (ICF). This difference is extremely important for the survival of cell.

The lipid bilayer of the cell membrane allows lipid-soluble substances to pass through it.

Lipid-insoluble substances are selectively transported by protein molecules present in the cell membrane. These proteins are called **transport proteins**.

Transport Proteins

Transport proteins are of two types: (i) channel proteins and (ii) carrier proteins.

Channel Proteins

They have watery spaces through the molecule and therefore allow free movement of certain ions and molecules.

Carrier Proteins

They bind to substances that are to be transported and undergo conformational change. This causes movement of substances from one side of the membrane to the other side.

Types of carrier-mediated transport are as follows:

- **Uniport:** There is transport of only one substance.
- **Symport:** There is transport of two substances in the same direction. Examples are sodium and glucose transport.
- **Antiport:** There is movement of two substances in opposite directions. Example is Na^+–K^+ pump.

Both the carrier and channel proteins are highly selective in allowing the passage of ions or molecules across the membrane.

Methods of Transport

Transport of ions or molecules occurs by two basic processes: (i) diffusion and (ii) active transport.

Diffusion

It is the continuous movement of molecules among one another in liquid or in gaseous states.

Diffusion is of two types:

1. simple diffusion and
2. facilitated diffusion.

Simple Diffusion (Fig. 1.11) Diffusion is the movement of molecules or ions through the cell membrane without involvement of carrier proteins. It occurs from the region of higher concentration to the region of lower concentration.

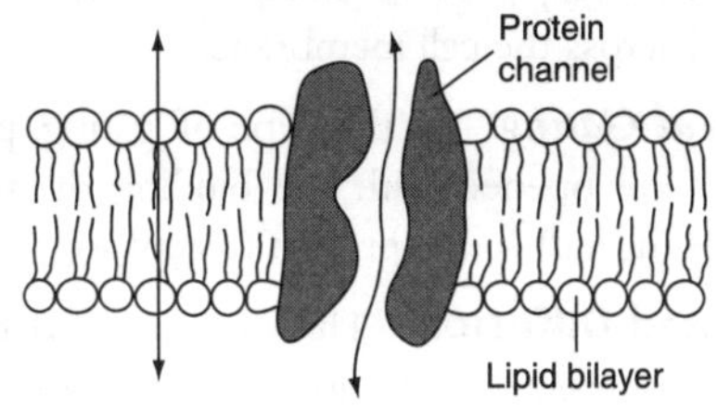

Fig. 1.11   Simple diffusion.

Diffusion depends on

- concentration of substance,
- velocity of kinetic motion, and
- number of openings in the membrane.

Simple diffusion occurs through the lipid bilayer and protein channels.

Diffusion through Lipid Layer Substances such as O_2, CO_2, alcohol, and N_2 dissolve directly in the lipid layer and diffuse through the cell membrane. The rate of diffusion of these substances is directly proportional to their lipid solubility.

Diffusion through Protein Channels Substances like water can easily pass through these protein channels. Transport of other substances depends on the character of protein channels.

Protein channels have two important characteristics:

1. They are selectively permeable to certain substances.
2. Many of the channels can be opened or closed by gates.

Selective Permeability Protein channels are highly selective for the transport of ions or molecules. It depends on the diameter, shape, and electrical charge of the channel.

Gating Gates are actually extensions of the transport protein molecule. These gates provide means for controlling the permeability of the channels. A conformational change in the shape of the protein molecule causes either opening or closing of the gate. Opening and closing of the gate are controlled by two mechanisms:

1. voltage gating and
2. chemical gating (ligand gating).

Voltage Gating   Here, the molecular conformation of the gate responds to changes in the electrical potential across the cell membrane.

Chemical Gating   In this type of gating, protein channels are opened with the binding of another molecule (ligand) to the protein (receptor).

Facilitated Diffusion   This is also called carrier-mediated diffusion. The substances are transported with the help of a specific carrier protein, e.g., glucose and amino acids (Fig. 1.12).

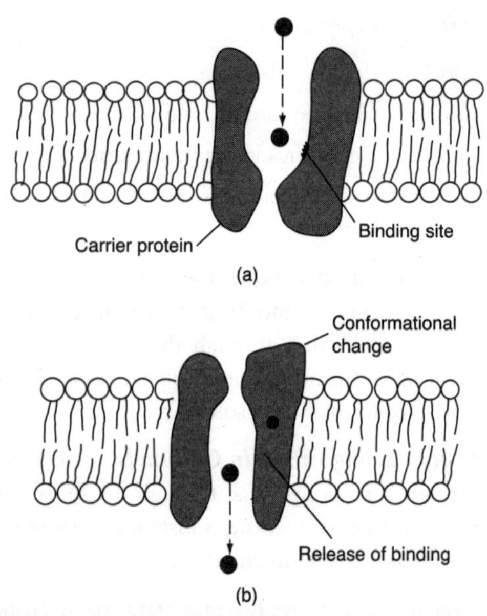

Fig. 1.12   Facilitated diffusion.

Osmosis   Osmosis is a special type of diffusion. It is the movement of water across a semipermeable membrane from a region of lower solute concentration to a region of higher solute concentration (Fig. 1.13).

The pressure required to prevent osmosis is called **osmotic pressure**. Osmotic pressure depends on the number of particles in the solution and not on the type or size of the particle.

Osmotic pressure exerted by colloidal substances in the body is called **colloidal osmotic pressure**.

Colloidal osmotic pressure due to plasma colloids is called **oncotic pressure**.

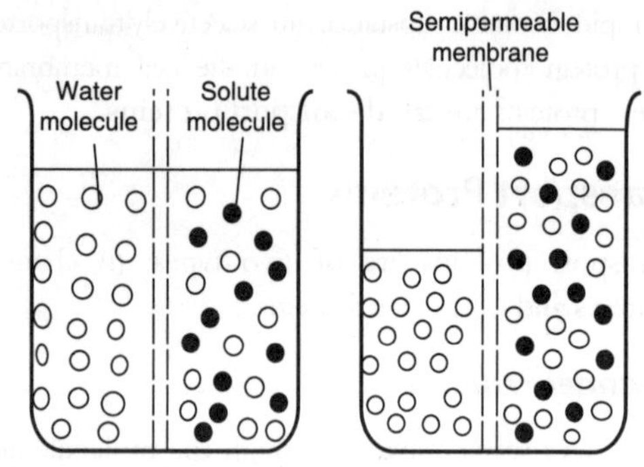

Fig. 1.13   Osmosis.

Active Transport

This is a process by which molecules or ions move uphill across the cell membrane against a concentration gradient (Fig. 1.14). Active transport needs expenditure of energy. This energy is provided by ATP.

Active transport is divided into two types: (i) primary and (ii) secondary.

Primary Active Transport   In primary active transport, energy is derived directly from the breakdown of ATP or some other high-energy phosphate compound.

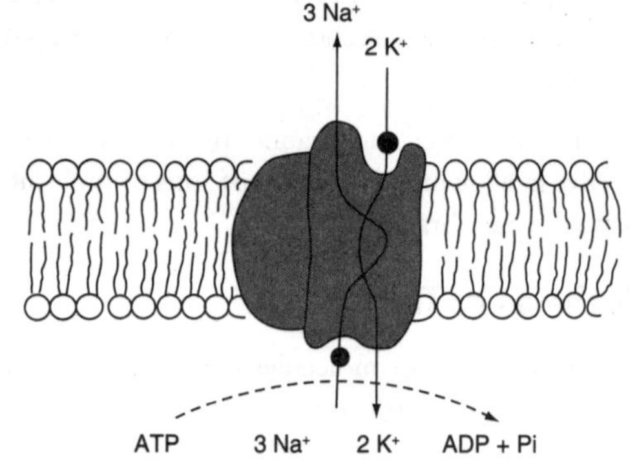

Fig. 1.14   Active transport.

Important primary active transport processes are

- sodium–potassium pump,
- potassium–hydrogen pump, and
- calcium pump.

Sodium–Potassium (Na⁺-K⁺) Pump   It is present in all the cells of the body. This pump transports sodium ions from inside the cell to the exterior. At the same time it transports potassium ions from outside to inside of the cell.

Structure $Na^+ - K^+$ pump is a carrier protein. It is made up of two globular protein subunits, α and β.

The α subunit is larger than the β subunit. The α subunit is mainly concerned with sodium–potassium transport.

This pump has

- three intracellular binding sites: one for three Na^+ ions, another for ATP, and third is the phosphorylation site;
- two extracellular sites: one for binding two K^+ ions and another for ouabain.

This pump has three receptor sites for binding sodium ions on the inside. It has two receptor sites for binding potassium ions on the outside. The inner portion near the sodium binding sites has ATPase activity.

Functions   It causes electronegativity inside the cell. It prevents accumulation of water inside the cell.

Potassium–Hydrogen (K^+–H^+) Pump   It is present in two places: at the parietal cells of gastric glands and at the renal tubules.

This pump present in the parietal cells actively transports H^+ ions out of the cells into the lumen of gastric glands and K^+ ions from the lumen into the cell.

K^+–H^+ pump present in the cells of distal tubule of nephron secretes large amounts of H^+ ions into the tubules to eliminate them from the body.

Secondary Active Transport   Energy derived from the transport of one substance helps the movement of the other substances. This transport is of two types:

1. cotransport and
2. countertransport.

Cotransport (Symport)   Two substances are simultaneously transported across the cell membrane in the same direction. Examples of this include sodium–glucose cotransport and sodium–amino acid cotransport.

Countertransport (Antiport)   A single carrier is used to transport two substances in opposite directions. Examples of this include sodium–calcium countertransport (occurs throughout the body) and sodium–hydrogen countertransport (occurs in distal convoluted tubule).

Vesicular Transport Mechanisms

They are involved in the transport of substances like protein molecules which cannot pass through the cell membrane either by diffusion or by active transport. They include

- exocytosis,
- endocytosis, and
- transcytosis.

Exocytosis

This is a process by which intracellular substances are extruded out of the cell. Granules and vesicles present inside the cell move toward the cell membrane. The membranes of granules and vesicles fuse with the cell membrane releasing the contents to the exterior. Release of hormones and enzymes by secretory cells of the body occurs by exocytosis.

Endocytosis

Endocytosis is the reverse of exocytosis. It is a process by which substances are taken into the cell.

The types of endocytosis are (i) phagocytosis and (ii) pinocytosis.

Phagocytosis (Fig. 1.15)   This is a process in which bacteria, dead tissue, etc., are engulfed by the cells.

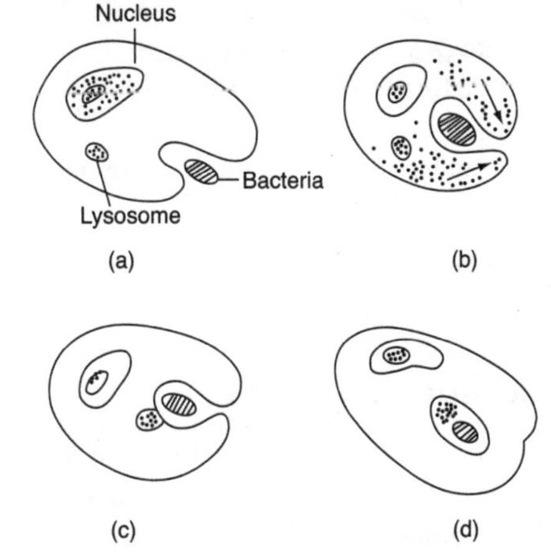

Fig. 1.15   Phagocytosis.

When the bacteria come in contact with the cell membrane, there is invagination of the cell membrane. Later, this invagination is pinched off from the cell membrane, making it a membrane-enclosed vacuole.

Pinocytosis   Pinocytosis is similar to phagocytosis, but the substances ingested are in fluid form. It is, therefore, called **cell drinking**.

Transcytosis

This is vesicular transport within the cell. It is also called **cytopempsis**. Transcytosis makes use of caveolin-coated vesicles.

Body Fluids

Water is an essential component of our body. The major portion of our body is composed of water. Total body water (TBW) is around 60% of the body weight, i.e., 42 L in a 70-kg adult male. The total body water is about 10% less in a normal adult female as compared to a male. This is due to relatively greater amounts of fat tissue in females. TBW decreases with age.

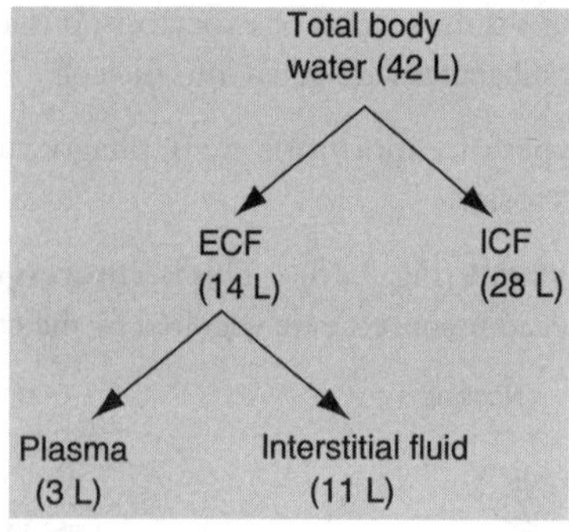

Body fluids are divided into two compartments, namely,

- intracellular fluid and
- extracellular fluid.

Intracellular Fluid (ICF)

This is the total amount of fluid present inside the 75 trillion cells of our body. Although the fluid is distributed among the 75 trillion cells of our body, it is considered as one single unit because the composition of fluid in all these cells is similar. ICF compartment comprises about 40% of the body weight.

Normal volume of ICF is 28 L.

Constituents

Intracellular fluid contains large amounts of potassium, phosphate, magnesium, and sulfate ions. It contains small quantities of sodium and chloride ions and almost no calcium ions. It also contains large amounts of protein.

Extracellular Fluid (ECF)

This is the fluid present outside the cells. It constitutes about 20% of the body weight. Normal volume of ECF is 14 L.

It has two parts: (i) interstitial fluid (11 L) and (ii) plasma (3 L).

Interstitial fluid surrounds the cells. **Plasma** is the noncellular part of blood. Plasma communicates continuously with interstitial fluid through the pores of capillaries. Therefore plasma and interstitial fluid have almost similar composition.

Constituents

ECF contains large amounts of sodium and chloride ions, and moderate amounts of bicarbonate ions. Potassium, calcium, magnesium, and phosphate ions are present in very minute quantities.

Transcellular Fluid

This is a special type of ECF. It includes synovial, peritoneal, pericardial, intraocular, and cerebrospinal fluid.

Transcellular fluid totally constitutes 1–2 L.

Composition of Body Fluids		
	ECF (mOsm/L H_2O)	ICF (mOsm/L H_2O)
Na	142	14
K	4.2	140
Ca	1.3	0
Mg	0.8	20
Cl	108	4
Protein	1.2	4

Measurement of Body Fluids

Total Body Water

Total body water (TBW) is measured by using radioactive water, heavy water, and antipyrine. These substances mix well with body water within few hours after injection. Total body water is calculated by estimating the degree of dilution of these substances:

$$TBW = \frac{\text{Amount of substance injected}}{\text{Concentration of the substance after dilution}}.$$

Extracellular Fluid

It is measured by using substances that disperse in ECF and plasma but do not enter the cell. Substances used are radioactive sodium, sucrose, thiosulfate ion, and inulin.

Plasma Volume

Substances that remain in the vascular system but do not readily penetrate the capillary membranes are used to measure the plasma volume—e.g., serum albumin labeled with radioactive iodine and Evans blue (a dye) by dilution technique.

Intracellular Fluid

It is the fluid present within the cells. It cannot be measured directly. It is calculated from

$$ICF = TBW - ECF.$$

CHAPTER 2

Blood

Blood is a fluid connective tissue present in the circulatory system. It is red in color due to the presence of hemoglobin.

Blood is made up of

- **Fluid component:** Plasma
- **Formed elements:** Erythrocytes (RBCs), leukocytes (WBCs), and thrombocytes (platelets)

Plasma constitutes 55% of blood and formed elements constitute 45%.

The pH of blood is 7.4. Its specific gravity is 1055–1060.

Functions of Blood

- **Transport of oxygen and carbon dioxide:** Blood helps in the transport of oxygen from the lungs to the tissues and carbon dioxide from the tissues to the lungs.
- **Supply of nutrition to various tissues:** Blood supplies absorbed food materials from the gastrointestinal tract to the tissues.
- **Transport of waste products:** Metabolic waste products like urea, uric acid, and creatinine are transported by blood to the kidneys and other excretory organs.
- **Transport of hormones, vitamins, drugs, and chemicals:** Blood is the vehicle through which various substances like hormones and drugs are transported from one part of the body to the other.
- **Maintenance of acid–base balance:** Blood has various buffers which maintain the acid–base balance.
- **Regulation of body temperature:** Blood distributes the heat generated at a particular organ to all parts of the body.
- **Protection against infection:** Leukocytes present in the blood help in protecting the body against invading microorganisms.
- **Helps in blood clotting:** It forms a clot during injury, preventing blood loss.

Blood Volume

It is the total amount of blood present in the body.

Total volume of blood is around 5 L in an average adult male (70 mL/kg body weight).

Females have a lower blood volume than males.

Variations

Blood volume increases during pregnancy and after meals. It decreases on prolonged standing.

Pathological Variation

Blood volume increases in polycythemia and congestive cardiac failure. It decreases after hemorrhage, burns, vomiting, and diarrhea.

Determination

Blood volume is determined by measuring the plasma volume and cell volume separately. It can also be determined by measuring the plasma volume and calculating the volume of formed elements.

Determination of Cell Volume

The RBCs from O^- individuals can be tagged with radioactive compounds like radioactive iron and radioactive phosphorus. A known amount of these tagged RBCs is injected into the individuals whose blood volume is to be measured. The RBC with radioactive substance is diluted in the blood of the individual, and from this dilution, the RBC volume can be calculated.

Determination of Plasma Volume

Plasma volume can be determined by dye dilution technique. In this method, a known amount of nontoxic dye is injected into the individual. Time is allowed for the distribution of the dye. After a reasonable time, plasma sample is collected and the concentration of the dye in plasma is measured. The plasma volume is measured by the following formula:

$$\text{Plasma volume} = \frac{\text{Amount of dye injected}}{\text{Concentration of dye in plasma}}.$$

Plasma

Plasma is the fluid portion of blood. Its normal volume is 3500 mL. It is mainly composed of water (91%).

Other substances present in plasma are as follows:

- **Inorganic substances:** Na^+, K^+, Ca^{++} ions, iron, and copper

- **Organic substances:** Proteins, lipids, glucose, urea, and creatinine

Serum is plasma without clotting factors. It is obtained by allowing the blood to clot and later removing the clot. The remaining fluid is called serum.

Plasma Proteins

They are the proteins present in plasma.

Formation

Most of the plasma proteins are synthesized in the liver. Albumin, prothrombin, and fibrinogen are synthesized in the liver. Globulin is formed by the reticuloendothelial cells, plasma cells and lymphocytes.

Types

Important plasma proteins are **albumin**, **globulin**, **fibrinogen**, and **prothrombin**.

Albumin   It has a molecular weight of 66,000. It is produced in the liver. The plasma half-life of albumin is 19 days. Albumin is mainly responsible for the maintenance of colloidal osmotic pressure. It also helps in the transport of bilirubin, hormones, and drugs.

Globulin   It has a molecular weight ranging from 90,000 to 1,56,000. Globulins include transport proteins, lipoproteins, and immunoglobulins. There are three fractions:

1. α-globulin,

2. β-globulin, and

3. γ-globulin.

Fibrinogen   It has a molecular weight of 3,40,000. It plays an important role in blood coagulation. It is mainly responsible for the viscosity of blood due to its asymmetrical shape.

Prothrombin   Prothrombin is the inactive precursor of thrombin. It is a plasma protein with molecular weight of 68,700. The normal concentration in plasma is 15 mg/dL. It is formed in the liver with the help of vitamin K.

Total proteins	6.0–8.0 g/dL
Albumin	4.5–5.5 g/dL
Globulin	1.3–2.5 g/dL
Fibrinogen	0.2–0.4 g/dL
Prothrombin	0.1 g/dL
Albumin/globulin ratio	1.7:1

Functions

1. **Maintenance of colloidal osmotic pressure:** The normal colloidal osmotic pressure of plasma is 25 mm Hg. Plasma proteins are responsible for this pressure. The capillary wall is impermeable to plasma proteins. Therefore, water is drawn into the blood.

2. **Maintenance of viscosity of blood:** Blood is four to five times more viscous than water. The viscosity of blood depends on the shape and size of the protein molecules in plasma.

3. **Buffering action:** Plasma proteins act as buffers. They maintain pH at 7.4 by accepting or donating H^+ ions. They are responsible for 15% of buffering capacity of the blood.

4. **Protein reserve:** Plasma proteins present in the blood act as reservoir of the proteins. They are especially helpful during starvation.

5. **Immunity:** γ-Globulins are antibodies that protect the body against the invading micro-organism.

6. **Blood clotting:** Fibrinogen and prothrombin are responsible for blood coagulation.

7. **Transport:** Plasma proteins transport hormones, drugs, and metabolites by forming a loose bond with them.

Separation

The separation of plasma proteins is done to study them and also to diagnose diseases.

The different methods for separation of plasma proteins are

- salt separation,

- paper electrophoresis,

- Cohn's fractional precipitation,

- immunoelectrophoresis, and

- ultracentrifugation technique.

Applied Physiology

Plasma protein levels decrease in prolonged starvation and malabsorption. They also decrease in liver and kidney diseases.

In liver diseases, plasma protein levels decrease due to the reduced synthesis.

The normal albumin/globulin ratio is reversed in liver diseases.

In renal diseases, more amount of proteins is lost in the urine.

Edema develops in these patients due to a decrease in the plasma oncotic pressure.

Afibrinogenemia is a disease due to congenital deficiency of fibrinogen. It is characterized by defective blood clotting. The symptoms include bruising, bleeding in joints and nose, and excessive bleeding after injury.

Plasmapheresis

This was an experiment performed in dogs by Whipple to determine the role of plasma proteins in diet. In this experiment, the whole blood is withdrawn and the cellular elements are injected back into the body. The process is repeated till plasma protein levels fall to 4 g/100 mL. Thereafter, different diets are given and their effect on protein synthesis is studied.

Erythrocytes

The erythrocytes or RBCs are the most abundant cells present in blood.

The mean red cell diameter is 7. 2 μ. Thickness is 2.2 μ at the periphery and 1 μ at the center. Its surface area is 135 μ^2. The normal volume is 80–94 μ^3. The normal life span of an RBC is 120 days.

RBC surface has a negative charge. RBCs do not have nucleus, mitochondria, or ribosomes. Therefore, a mature RBC cannot divide. RBCs contain the pigment hemoglobin in jelly form.

RBCs can easily pass through narrow capillaries because of their biconcave shape and flexibility.

Normal Erythrocyte Count	
Males	5–5.5 million cells/mm³
Females	4.5–5 million cells/mm³
Infants	6–7 million cells/mm³

Structure

RBCs contain 61% water, 28% Hb, 7% lipids, 3% carbohydrates, electrolytes, and metabolites.

RBC membrane is made up of lipids and proteins.

- **Lipids:** Cholesterol, phospholipid, and glycolipids
- **Proteins:** Spectrin, actin, ankyrin, and band 3 and 4 proteins

The glycolipids constitute the ABO blood group substances (agglutinogens).

Metabolism

The metabolic need of RBCs is very less. It is met by the glucose metabolism through the anaerobic Embden–Meyerhof (EMF) pathway (90%) and the pentose phosphate shunt (10%).

Functions

The functions of RBCs are due to the presence of Hb.

They include

- transport of oxygen from lungs to tissues,
- transport of CO_2 from tissues to lungs, and
- regulation of acid–base balance.

Erythropoiesis

Erythropoiesis is the process of formation of RBCs.

Sites

Erythropoiesis starts in the third week of intrauterine life in the mesoderm of the yolk sac.

From the third month of intrauterine life erythropoiesis takes place in the liver and spleen.

After the fifth month of intrauterine life, the fetal bone marrow starts producing RBCs.

By birth, the bone marrow becomes the only place of erythrocyte production.

Bone marrow is of two types:

1. red bone marrow and
2. yellow bone marrow.

Red bone marrow produces RBCs. At birth, it is present in all the bones. In adults, it is present in flat bones (membranous bones) like cranial bones, vertebrae, pelvic bones, ribs, sternum, and upper ends of long bones like femur and humerus.

Yellow bone marrow is mainly made up of adipose (fat) tissue.

Stages (Fig. 2.1)

All blood cells are produced from stem cells. They have the capacity to form different types of blood cells and are termed pluripotent hemopoietic stem cells.

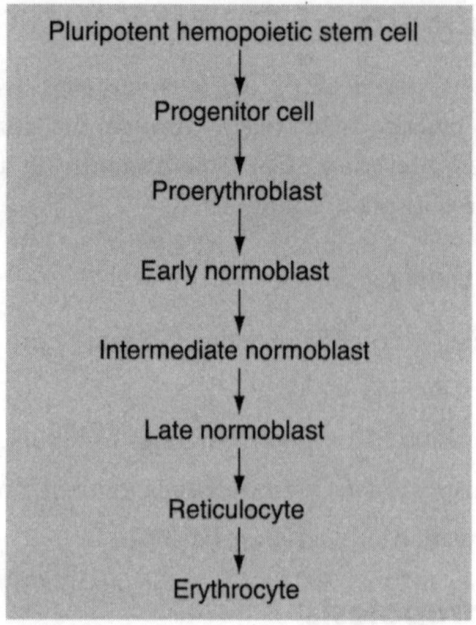

Pluripotent Stem Cells   The pluripotent stem cell differentiates to form the committed stem cell. The committed stem cell of the myeloid series gives rise to all blood cells except the lymphocytes.

The committed stem cells for the erythrocyte give rise to the progenitor cells.

Progenitor Cells   The progenitor cells are of two types:

1.   BFU–E (burst-forming units) and

2.   CFU–E (colony-forming units).

BFU–E   They form large multilobulated colonies from progenitor cells. The development of colonies requires the presence of factors called burst-promoting activity (BPA).

The cells are immature blast cells oval in shape with moderately basophilic cytoplasm, occasional pseudopods, fine chromatin, and nucleoli. BFU–E is the progenitor of CFU–E.

CFU–E   They form small colonies. They do not require BPA but require other factors like erythropoietin. BFU–E give rise to CFU–E. CFU–E cells give rise to blast cells.

CFU–E cells are more mature than BFU–E cells. Morphologically, they are similar to BFU–E cells.

Proerythroblast   These cells develop from CFU–E. They are large cells, 15–20 μ in diameter. The nucleus is large containing basophilic nucleoli. It occupies 80% of the cells. The cytoplasm is scanty and basophilic. These cells actively divide by mitosis. They do not have hemoglobin.

Early Normoblast   These cells are 10–16 μ in diameter. They also show active mitosis. The nucleus is large, the cytoplasm is basophilic, and hemoglobin begins to appear. The nucleoli disappear and condensation of chromatin begins in this stage.

Intermediate Normoblast   These cells are 10–14 μ in diameter. The nucleus becomes small. Mitosis stops

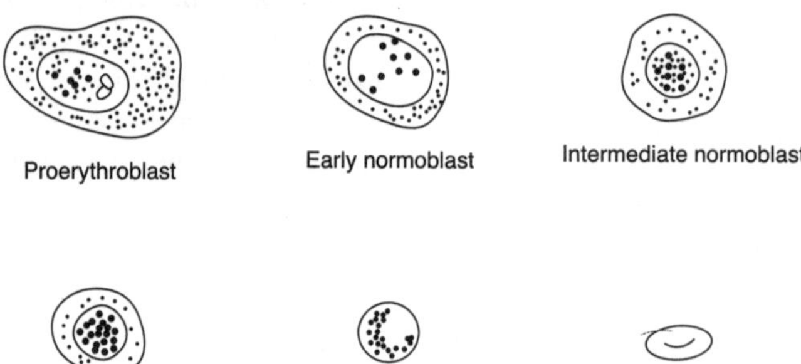

Fig. 2.1   Stages of erythropoiesis.

at this stage. Hemoglobin concentration increases and cells become acidophilic due to Hb. The condensation of nuclear chromatin increases in this stage.

Late Normoblast These cells are 8–10 μ in diameter. The cytoplasm is acidophilic. The nucleus is very small, becomes pyknotic (small), and is lost by extrusion.

Reticulocyte This is a flat, disk-shaped, non-nucleated cell, slightly bigger than the mature RBC. It is slightly basophilic. Hb content increases to reach the level of the mature cell. The remaining chromatin is organized in the form of a network (reticulum); hence, it is called a reticulocyte. RBC attains maturity in 1–2 days after the loss of the basophilic material.

Erythrocyte This is a mature cell, 7.2 μ in diameter, eosinophilic, non-nucleated; it resembles a biconcave disk.

The process of erythropoiesis takes 7 days.

Factors Influencing Erythropoiesis

Erythropoietin This is a glycoprotein hormone that stimulates erythropoiesis. It increases RBC production, enhances synthesis of Hb, and hastens maturation of RBC.

Androgens They stimulate erythropoiesis. Therefore, men have a higher RBC count compared to women. Androgens stimulate the production of erythropoietin. In addition, they directly stimulate erythropoiesis.

Estrogens They have inhibitory effect on the erythropoiesis by suppression of erythropoietin production.

Hormones Thyroxine, cortisol, and growth hormone are necessary for RBC production. Interleukin 1, 5, and 3, granulocyte macrophage colony-stimulating factor (GM-CSF), and BPA all act as local hormones and help in the conversion of stem cells to progenitor cells.

Dietary Factors Iron is necessary for Hb synthesis. The deficiency of iron leads to hypochromia and decrease in the size of RBC.

Vitamin B_{12} and folic acid are necessary for maturation of RBC.

Vitamin B_6, vitamin C, copper, and cobalt act as cofactors.

Intrinsic Factor This is produced from the parietal cells of the gastric mucosa. It helps in the absorption of vitamin B_{12}.

Erythropoietin

It is a glycoprotein hormone having a molecular weight of 46,000. It is made up of 74% protein and 26% carbohydrate.

Formation

It is mainly formed in the kidney and partly in the liver. In the kidney it is produced by the endothelial cells of the peritubular capillaries.

Functions

- Increases RBC production.
- Enhances synthesis of Hb.
- Hastens maturation of RBC.

Factors Influencing Erythropoietin Production

The basic stimulus for erythropoietin production is hypoxia.

- Androgens increase erythropoietin production.
- Estrogens depress erythropoietin production.
- Products of RBC destruction increase erythropoietin production.
- Vasoconstrictors produce renal hypoxia. They cause formation of erythropoietin.
- Erythropoietin is inactivated in the liver and is excreted through the kidneys.

Fate of RBC

The old and fragile RBC is phagocytosed by the reticuloendothelial system. In the reticuloendothelial cells, they are broken down and Hb is released. Subsequently, Hb is broken down into heme and globin. Globin is added to the amino acid pool. Iron liberated from heme is used again for the synthesis of new Hb. The remaining portion of heme is called biliverdin. It is reduced to bilirubin in the liver and secreted through the bile.

Hemoglobin

Hemoglobin (Hb) is a conjugate protein present in the RBC. It forms 95% of dry weight of RBC.

The molecular weight of Hb is 64,450.

Hemoglobin is a globular molecule made up of four subunits. Each subunit contains a heme moiety conjugated to a polypeptide. Four polypeptides form the globin portion of Hb molecule.

There are two pairs of polypeptides in each Hb molecule. In normal adult Hb (HbA), two types of polypeptide chains are α chains and β chains. Therefore, HbA is $\alpha_2\beta_2$.

About 2.5% of Hb is HbA_2, which has α_2 and δ_2 polypeptide chains.

Human fetus has HbF. It has α_2 and γ_2 polypeptide chains.

Fetal hemoglobin is replaced by adult Hb soon after birth. O_2 binding capacity of fetal Hb is greater than adult Hb. This helps in the movement of O_2 from the maternal to fetal circulation.

Normal Value	
Males	14–18 g/dL
Females	12–16 g/dL
Infants	Up to 20 g/dL

Functions

- It carries oxygen from lungs to the tissues. (1 g of hemoglobin carries 1.34 mL of oxygen.)
- It is also involved in the transport of CO_2.
- It acts as a buffer.

Synthesis

The substances required for the synthesis of heme are succinyl-CoA and glycine. It is synthesized in the normoblastic stage of the developing RBC.

Two molecules of succinyl-CoA and two molecules of glycine combine to form a pyrrole ring. Four pyrroles combine together to form protoporphyrin IX. Protoporphyrin IX combines with iron and polypeptide chain to form hemoglobin chain. Four such hemoglobin chains make up hemoglobin molecule.

Heme is located in the periphery of Hb molecule which helps in its easy binding to O_2.

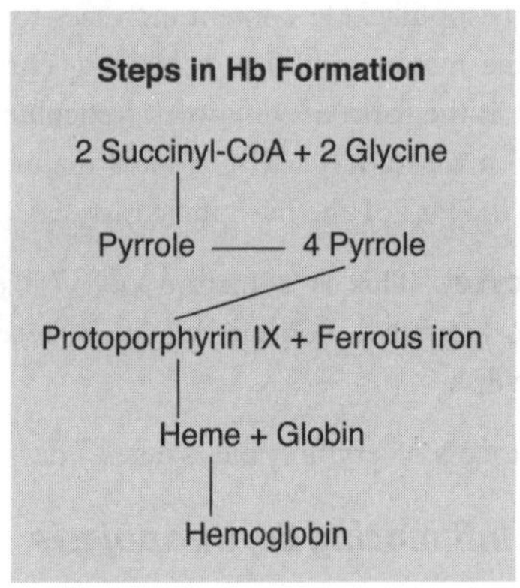

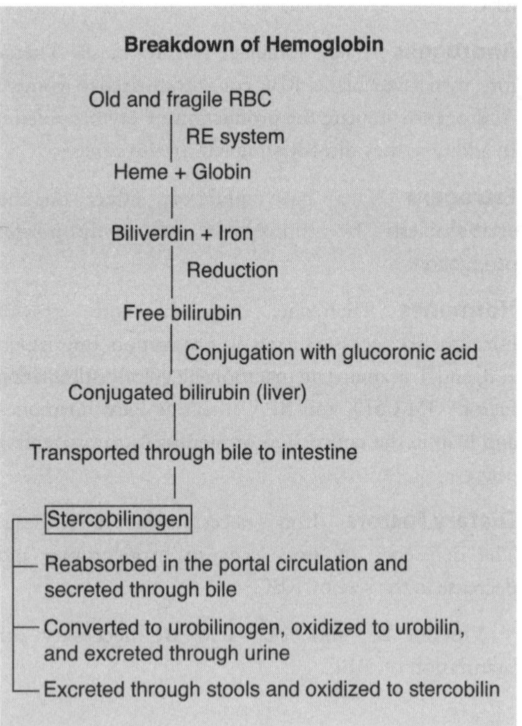

Compounds

Oxyhemoglobin Hemoglobin combines with oxygen readily and reversibly to form oxyhemoglobin.

The affinity of Hb to O_2 depends on various factors like temperature, pH, and 2,3-diphosphoglyceric acid (DPG) (2,3-DGP).

Methemoglobin Iron in Hb is converted from ferrous to ferric state to form methemoglobin. It occurs normally within the body to some extent.

The ferric form is converted back to ferrous form by methemoglobin reductase. Deficiency of this enzyme results in methemoglobinemia.

Carboxyhemoglobin The combination of Hb with carbon monoxide forms carboxyhemoglobin. The affinity of Hb to CO is much greater than its affinity for O_2. Therefore, CO displaces O_2 from Hb causing reduced O_2 carrying capacity of blood.

Carbaminohemoglobin CO_2 combines with globin part of Hb to form carbaminohemoglobin.

Acid Hematin The combination of acid with Hb forms acid hematin. This forms the basis for estimation of Hb by Sahli's method.

Abnormal Hemoglobin

They are produced due to the defective synthesis of either heme or globin portions. The defect in the heme part is usually rare. The defect in the globin chain is more frequent.

There are two major types of inherited disorders of hemoglobin synthesis: hemoglobinopathies and thalassemias.

Hemoglobinopathies The defects are due to the abnormalities in the polypeptide chain. The abnormal hemoglobins produced are HbS, HbC, and HbE.

HbS In this type of hemoglobin, valine replaces glutamic acid at the sixth position in the β chain. When HbS is exposed to hypoxia, it becomes insoluble leading to a change in the shape of RBC. The sickle-shaped deformity developed in RBC results in its excessive destruction.

They are less flexible than normal RBCs. This leads to the blocking of capillaries. The homozygous individuals suffer from this condition leading to sickle cell anemia. The heterozygous individuals have sickle cell trait. They do not suffer severely with this problem. HbS individuals are resistant to one form of malaria.

Thalassemia In this condition, α and β chains of globin are normal, but they are produced in lesser number or absent.

The decrease in α chain synthesis is called α-thalassemia.

α-Thalassemia is of two types: (i) α-thalassemia major and (ii) α-thalassemia minor.

α-Thalassemia major is usually incompatible with life. In α-thalassemia minor, the persons have less number of α chains than normal and are usually symptom free.

β-Thalassemia is caused due to reduced synthesis of β chains.

It is of two types: (i) β-thalassemia major and (ii) β-thalassemia minor.

In β-thalassemia major, the patients suffer from anemia due to rapid destruction of RBCs. They need frequent blood transfusion. They accumulate iron. There is increased bone marrow activity, leading to frontal bossing, splenomegaly, repeated fever, and failure to thrive.

Iron

The normal iron content of an adult is 3–5 g. It is more in males than females.

About 60–70% of the total body iron is in hemoglobin.

Iron is derived from the breakdown of RBCs. It is carried by iron-binding protein transferrin and reutilized for hemoglobin synthesis.

Biological Forms

Tissue Iron It is nonavailable iron present in myoglobin and enzymes such as cytochrome, catalase, and peroxidase.

Storage Iron The storage iron (available iron) can be utilized for Hb synthesis. The storage iron is 1–2 g.

It is stored as

- ferritin and

- hemosiderin.

Ferritin is normally predominant. Iron is stored in reticuloendothelial cells, hepatic parenchymal cells, and skeletal muscles.

Plasma Iron Three to four milligrams of iron present in the plasma is bound to a transport protein called transferrin.

Absorption

Only 10% of iron in the diet is absorbed. A major portion of iron is reused in the body. Iron absorption occurs in the duodenum and proximal jejunum.

The liver produces a substance called **apotransferrin**. This flows through the bile into the duodenum. In the intestine, apotransferrin binds with iron to form transferrin. Transferrin is absorbed into the epithelial cells and later released into the blood capillaries in the form of plasma transferrin.

Applied Physiology

Anemia

This is a clinical condition wherein RBC count or Hb% or both are decreased. In anemia, O_2 carrying capacity of blood is reduced.

Classification

Depending on the cause of anemia, they are classified as

1. anemia due to decreased RBC formation,
2. anemia due to increased RBC destruction, and
3. anemia due to blood loss.

Anemia due to Decreased RBC Formation

(a) **Iron-deficiency anemia:** Iron is required for the formation of hemoglobin. Nutritional deficiency of iron causes anemia. This is the commonest type of anemia occurring in India. RBCs are microcytic and hypochromic.

(b) **Vitamin B_{12} and folic acid deficiency:** Vitamin B_{12} and folic acid are required for the development and maturation of RBCs. Deficiency of these vitamins causes megaloblastic anemia. RBCs are macrocytic and normochromic.

(c) **Pernicious anemia:** Vitamin B_{12} requires intrinsic factor for its absorption. The deficiency of intrinsic factor leads to pernicious anemia.

(d) **Aplastic anemia:** This is caused due to suppression of bone marrow by drugs, toxins, and exposure to X-rays.

Anemia due to Increased RBC Destruction   Also termed hemolytic anemia.

(a) **Thalassemia:** There is a defect in the synthesis of globin chain of Hb. This causes premature destruction of red cell due to membrane damage.

(b) **Sickle cell anemia:** RBCs contain abnormal hemoglobin termed HbS. This leads to a sickle-shaped deformity on exposure to hypoxia, resulting in early rupture and destruction of the cell.

(c) **Hereditary spherocytosis:** In this condition, RBCs become excessively permeable to Na^+. They assume a biconvex shape and are prone to hemolysis.

(d) **Glucose-6-phosphate dehydrogenase (G6PD) deficiency:** The deficiency of this enzyme causes damage to RBC membrane leading to hemolysis. G6PD is required for the formation of NADPH which maintains glutathione in reduced state. The decreased concentration of reduced glutathione causes damage of RBC membrane.

Anemia due to Blood Loss

(a) **Acute blood loss:** Hemorrhage occurs due to accidents or during surgery. Sudden blood loss results in RBCs being normocytic and normochromic. However, anemia is due to reduction in its number.

(b) **Chronic blood loss:** It is seen in peptic ulcer, hemorrhoids, hookworm infestation, and menstrual irregularities. The RBCs are microcytic and hypochromic.

Morphological Classification

(a) **Microcytic hypochromic anemia**: In this type of anemia, RBCs are smaller in size. Hb content of the cell is also reduced and RBCs look pale. Mean corpuscular volume (MCV), mean corpuscular hemoglobin (MCH), and mean corpuscular hemoglobin concentration (MCHC) are reduced, e.g., iron-deficiency anemia.

(b) **Normocytic normochromic anemia:** In this type of anemia, RBCs are normal in size, Hb content is also normal, but the number of cells is reduced. MCV, MCH, and MCHC are within normal range, e.g., anemia due to hemorrhage.

(c) **Macrocytic anemia:** RBCs are larger in size. The Hb content of these cells is normal or reduced. MCV is above normal, e.g., vitamin B_{12} deficiency anemia.

Clinical Manifestations

The clinical signs and symptoms are not found in mild anemia. They are manifested only in moderate and severe anemia.

Patients have

- pallor, dyspnea, palpitations, and heart murmurs;
- headache, vertigo, restlessness, and muscle weakness;
- glossitis and atrophy of papillae of tongue, mouth ulcers, and dysphagia.

Polycythemia

This is a condition where RBC count is increased above 8 million cells/mm^3.

There are two types of polycythemia:

1. polycythemia vera and
2. secondary polycythemia.

Polycythemia Vera

Polycythemia vera is produced due to genetic abnormality. The blast cells start producing too many cells. This increases the hematocrit value, total blood volume, and viscosity of blood.

It is a chronic, progressive, and ultimately fatal disease.

Secondary Polycythemia

Physiological polycythemia occurs at high altitude due to hypoxia. This is seen in people who live at altitudes of 17,000–18,000 ft.

Pathological polycythemia occurs in pulmonary disease, hydronephrosis of kidney, and tumors of the liver and kidneys.

Functions

Iron is required for the synthesis of hemoglobin, myoglobin, and heme enzymes like cytochrome C and catalase.

Iron Balance

The total body content of iron remains within a narrow range of variation. The loss of iron from the body is matched by the absorption of it from the gastrointestinal tract (GIT). Iron is not excreted from the body. It is lost during the removal of epithelial cells of GIT.

Daily Requirement

The human beings require around 1 mg of iron every day. Females in the reproductive age require little more iron compared to males due to its loss during menstruation.

Certain foods like phytates, which are present in grains, inhibit iron absorption. Calcium, zinc, and cadmium also interfere with the absorption of iron.

Hematological Investigation

Erythrocyte Sedimentation Rate

Erythrocyte sedimentation rate (ESR) is the rate at which red blood cells settle down. It is the measure of supernatant plasma separated out at the end of 1 h when a column of blood (mixed with an anticoagulant) is kept undisturbed.

> **Normal Value**
>
> 0–5 mm at the end of 1 h in males
> 0–8 mm at the end of 1 h in females

The sedimentation rate is influenced by rouleaux formation, viscosity, fibrinogen, and globulin content of blood.

ESR is increased in pregnancy and during menstruation.

It is increased in infections like tuberculosis, rheumatoid arthritis, malignancy, and anemia.

ESR decreases in polycythemia and sickle cell anemia.

Significance ESR is of prognostic importance than of diagnostic value. It helps to assess the effect of treatment and progress of the disease. It has limited value in detecting a disease.

Determination ESR can be determined by two methods:

1. **Westergren's method:** Westergren's tube is 300 mm long, open at both ends. Blood mixed with anticoagulant is filled in Westergren's tube and placed vertically in a stand and left undisturbed. The height of the column of plasma separated is read directly from the tube at the end of 1 h.
2. **Wintrobe's method:** Wintrobe's tube is a short tube open at one end and closed at the other. Blood mixed with anticoagulant is filled in the tube and placed vertically in a stand for 1 h. The value is read directly at the end of 1 h.

Packed Cell Volume

Packed cell volume (PCV) is the percentage of red cells present in the blood. It is also called hematocrit value.

> **Normal Value**
>
> | Males | 42–48% |
> |---|---|
> | Females | 38–42% |

PCV is increased in polycythemia, diarrhea, and excessive vomiting.

It is decreased in anemia and pregnancy.

Determination

- **Wintrobe's method:** Wintrobe's tube is filled with blood mixed with anticoagulant. Tube is then centrifuged at 3000 RPM for 20 min. The red cells settle at the bottom and the clear plasma is separated at the top. A buffy coat is present between the packed cells and the supernatant plasma containing WBCs and platelets. The mark up to which red cells are packed indicates the PCV.

Blood Indices

Blood indices indicate the health status of an individual. They also help in the diagnosis of various types of anemia.

They include MCV, MCH, MCHC, and CI.

Mean Corpuscular Volume   It is the average volume of a single red cell. It ranges from 87 to 93 μ^3.

MCV is reduced in microcytic anemia. It is increased in megaloblastic anemia.

$$\text{MCV} = \frac{\text{PCV per 100 mL of blood}}{\text{RBC in millions/mm}^3 \text{ of blood}} \times 10.$$

Mean Corpuscular Hemoglobin   This is the average Hb present in a single red cell. Normal value ranges from 28 to 32 pg. It is reduced in microcytic anemia.

$$\text{MCH} = \frac{\text{Hb in g per 100 mL of blood}}{\text{RBC in millions/mm}^3 \text{ of blood}} \times 10.$$

Mean Corpuscular Hemoglobin Concentration   It is the relative percentage of Hb in a single red cell. Normal value is 33%.

It is decreased in megaloblastic anemia.

$$\text{MCHC} = \frac{\text{Hb in g per 100 mL of blood}}{\text{PCV per 100 mL of blood}} \times 100.$$

Color Index (CI)   This is the ratio between Hb% and RBC%.

It is reduced in hypochromic anemia.

$$\text{CI} = \frac{\text{Hb\%}}{\text{RBC\%}}.$$

Normal range is 0.85–1.15.

$$\text{Hb\%} = \frac{\text{Hb measured}}{\text{Normal Hb (15 g\%)}}.$$

$$\text{RBC\%} = \frac{\text{RBC counted}}{\text{Normal RBC count (5 million/mm}^3)}.$$

Microcyte	RBC with reduced volume
Macrocyte	RBC with increased volume
Hypochromia	Hb less than normal

Leukocytes (WBCs)

We are exposed to a variety of harmful pathogens such as bacteria, viruses, fungi, and parasites which can cause diseases. To combat these pathogens, we have a specific defense system in the body. Leukocytes or white blood cells form a major part of this defense mechanism.

Classification

Based on their staining properties, leukocytes are classified as

- granulocytes and
- agranulocytes.

Granulocytes

Neutrophils	60–65%
Eosinophils	1–4%
Basophils	0–1%

Agranulocytes

Lymphocytes	25–30%
Monocytes	2–8%

Functions

- Neutrophils and monocytes are phagocytic.
- Eosinophils are antiallergic and antiparasitic.
- Basophils liberate heparin and histamine.
- Lymphocytes are involved in immunity.

Leukopoiesis (Fig. 2.2)

Leukocytes develop from the pluripotent stem cells of the myeloid series. These cells give rise to committed stem cells also called progenitor cells. These committed stem cells differentiate into various types of leukocytes.

Two different lineages of leukocytes are formed:

1. myelocytic lineage and
2. lymphocytic lineage.

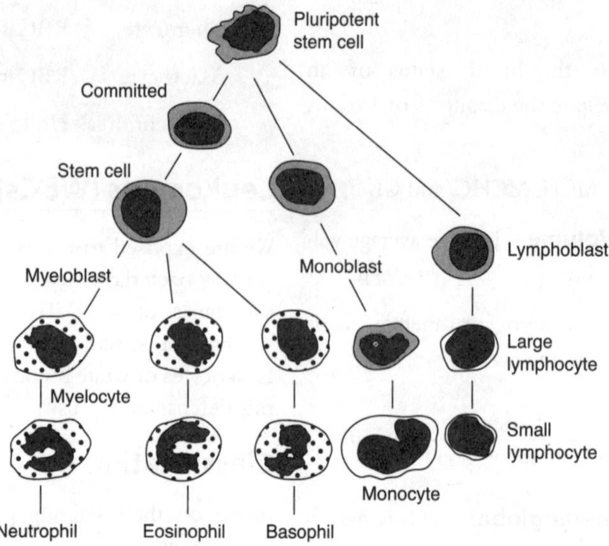

Fig. 2.2   Leukopoiesis.

The neutrophils, eosinophils, basophils, and monocytes are formed from the myelocytic lineage. Lymphocytes are formed from the lymphocytic lineage.

Myelocytic Lineage

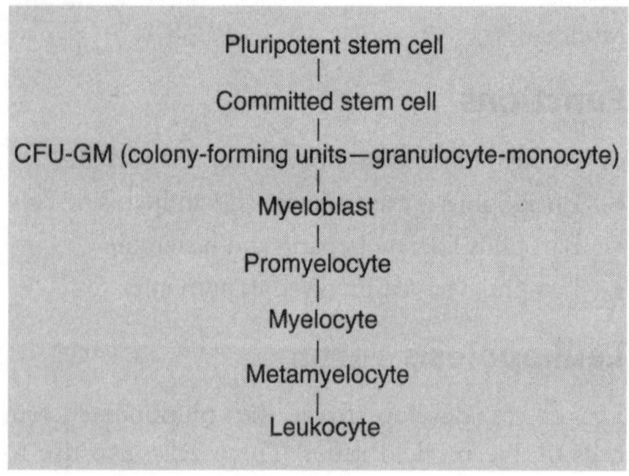

Myeloblasts   Myeloblasts are large cells 12–18 μ in diameter. They have a round nucleus, they are nonmotile, and they do not contain granules.

Myelocytes   The cells multiply, the cytoplasm becomes less basophilic, and the granules appear in the cytoplasm. The size of the nucleus decreases.

Metamyelocytes   The nucleus develop lobes, and cells stop multiplying and start maturing. They become fully mature and functional to form a leukocyte.

The formation of granulocyte from myeloblast takes around 10 days.

Monocytes are also formed from the myelocytic lineage.

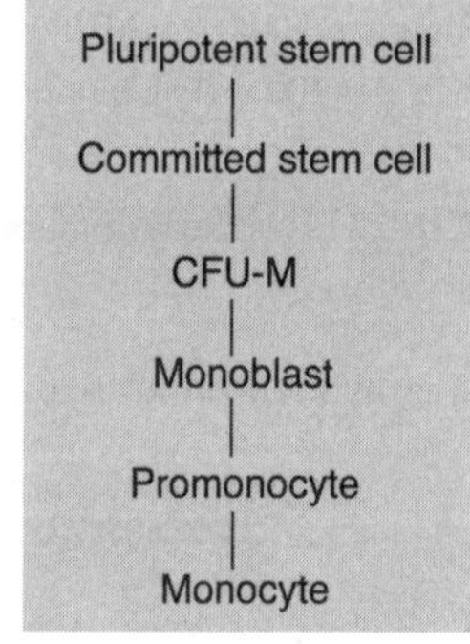

Monocytes require 6 days for their formation.

Lymphocytic Lineage

Lymphocytes are produced in the bone marrow and processed in the thymus. They are finally lodged in the peripheral lymphoid organs like the lymph node, spleen, tonsils, and the lymphoid tissues of the intestine.

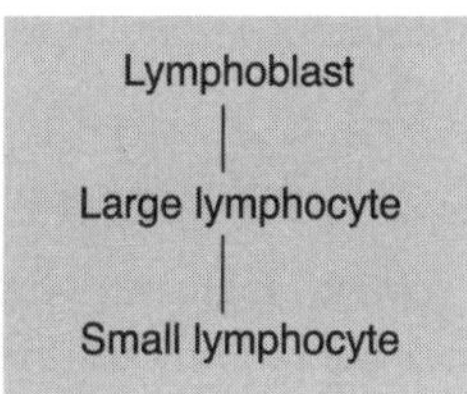

Lymphoblasts They are large cells, 12–20 μ in diameter with round nucleus. These cells undergo division to form large lymphocytes.

Large Lymphocytes They stop dividing and only mature. They appear in circulation.

Small Lymphocytes They are formed by further maturation of large lymphocytes.

Regulation of Leukopoiesis

- Protein formed by **scl gene** (stem cell leukemia) is responsible for the production of pluripotent stem cell.

- Colony-stimulating factor is a protein produced by the T-lymphocytes, fibroblasts, macrophages, and endothelial cells.

  They are of three types:

  (a) **CSF-GM** stimulates the production of neutrophils, monocytes, eosinophils, erythrocytes, and megakaryocytes.
  (b) **CSF-G** stimulates the production of neutrophil.
  (c) **CSF-M** stimulates the production of monocytes.
- **Interleukins** are hormone-like substances regulating immune responses. Interleukin-1, -3, and -6 convert pluripotent uncommitted stem cells to committed stem cells.
- Prostaglandins, cortisol, and adrenocorticotropic hormone (ACTH) play an important role in control of leukopoiesis.

Morphology of Leukocytes

Neutrophils (Fig. 2.3)

Neutrophils are about 10–12 μ in diameter. They form about 60–65% of the total leukocytes. Nucleus is multilobed. The number of lobes vary from 2 to 7.

Cytoplasm contains fine granules.

The granules are of two types:

1. **Primary azurophilic granules**: They contain various proteolytic substances, myeloperoxidase enzymes, and lysosomal enzymes.
2. **Secondary granules**: They contain lactoferrin, alkaline phosphate, and vitamin B_{12} binding protein.

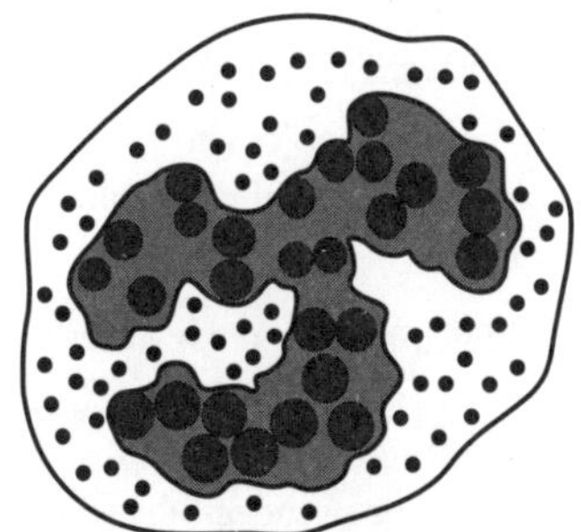

Fig. 2.3   Neutrophil.

Life span of neutrophil is about 6–7 h in the blood and 1–4 days in the tissues.

Functions The main function of a neutrophil is destruction of microorganisms by phagocytosis. These cells are considered the first line of defense against infection.

The substances called **selectins** attract the neutrophils toward the vascular endothelium.

Attachment of the neutrophils to the endothelium is **margination**.

Later, the neutrophils squeeze through the pores of blood vessels by the process of **diapedesis**.

The neutrophils are attracted to the site of inflammation by a process called **chemotaxis**.

The invading bacteria are coated with certain plasma factors which make it suitable for phagocytosis. This process is called **opsonization**.

Neutrophils project pseudopodia in all directions around the bacteria and it is engulfed. This process is termed **phagocytosis**.

Phagocytosis

It is a process of ingestion and destruction of microorganisms by the cells.

Phagocytosis is the most important function of neutrophils and macrophages.

The phagocytes first recognize the microorganism to be phagocytosed. The immune system of the body develops antibody to the microorganism. The antibodies adhere to the membrane of the microorganism. It also combines with C3 product of complement system. These C3 molecules attach to the membrane of the microorganism.

Neutrophils approach these antibody-coated microorganisms and attach to them. They project pseudopodia in all directions around the microorganism. The pseudopodia fuse to form a closed cavity inside the cytoplasm of neutrophil. This is called a **phagocytic vesicle**.

A neutrophil can phagocytose 3–20 bacteria before it dies.

Macrophages are more powerful phagocytes than neutrophils. They engulf as many as 100 bacteria. They phagocytose red cells and malarial parasites.

Digestion of Ingested Particle

Once ingestion has occurred, the proteolytic enzymes present in the neutrophils and macrophages come in contact with phagocytic vesicle and empty the digestive enzymes into it. This causes digestion of foreign particle. Phagocytic vesicle is converted into a digestive vesicle.

Eosinophils (Fig. 2.4)

They are around 10–14 μ in diameter. They form 1–4% of total leukocytes. The nucleus has two (spectacle-shaped) lobes. The cytoplasm contains coarse granules, oval or round in shape, which take up acid stain and appear orange colored with eosin.

The eosinophilic granules contain major basic protein, eosinophilic peroxidase, eosinophilic cationic protein, arylsulfatase B, and lysophospholipase.

They stay in blood for 6–8 hours and in the tissues for 4–5 days.

Functions   They are antiallergic in function.

Eosinophil count increases during parasitic infestations. They migrate toward the larvae of the parasite, bind to it and destroy them by releasing hydrolytic enzymes and major basic proteins and by forming superoxides.

Eosinophils are attracted toward the site of inflammation by various chemotactic factors. These eosinophils cause detoxification of inflammation inducing substances released by the mast cells and basophils.

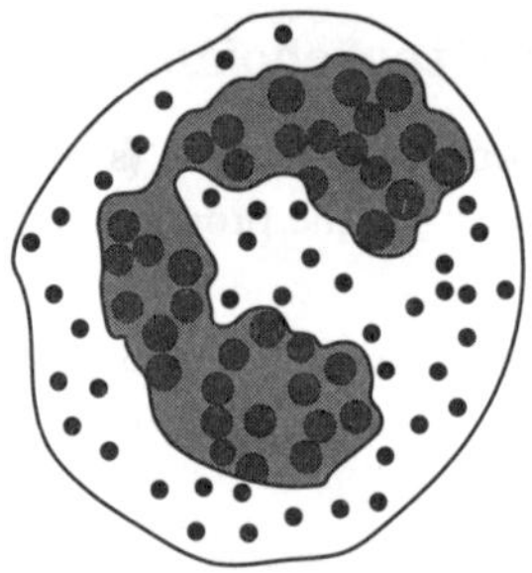

Fig. 2.4   Eosinophil.

Basophils (Fig. 2.5)

Basophils are the least numerous of leukocytes forming less than 1% of the total leukocytes. They are around 8–10 μ in diameter. The nucleus is irregular or S-shaped; the cytoplasm contains coarse granules which take up the basophilic stain.

Basophils remain in blood for short duration and later migrate to the tissues.

Granules of basophils contain histamine, heparin, acid peptides, and protease.

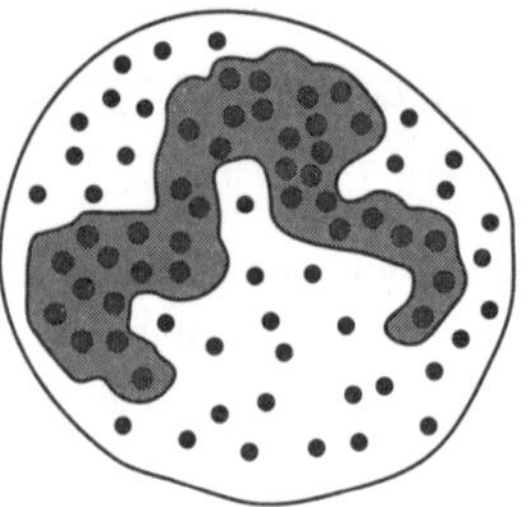

Fig. 2.5   Basophil.

Functions   Basophils liberate heparin, which is an anticoagulant substance.

They liberate histamine, which produce allergic reactions.

They also liberate small quantities of bradykinin and serotonin, which participate in the inflammatory process.

Monocytes (Fig. 2.6)

These are very large cells, around 12–18 μ in diameter. They form 2–8% of total leukocytes. The nucleus is indented (kidney-shaped or horseshoe-shaped) and does not have lobes. The cytoplasm is pale blue on staining and does not contain granules.

The life span of monocytes in blood is around 10–20 h and later they migrate to the tissues. In the tissues they become large in size to form the **tissue macrophages**. They remain in the tissues for months to years.

Functions   They form the second line of defense. Monocytes are also phagocytic. They are immature cells in the blood and do not have the full ability to fight against infection. But once they enter the tissues, they are converted to tissue macrophages which enlarge to attain a size of about 80 μ. A single macrophage can digest around 100 bacteria. After digestion, the digested particles are extruded out. Thus, macrophages can survive for months.

The dead neutrophils, macrophages, necrotic tissue, and dead bacteria all combine together to form the **pus**.

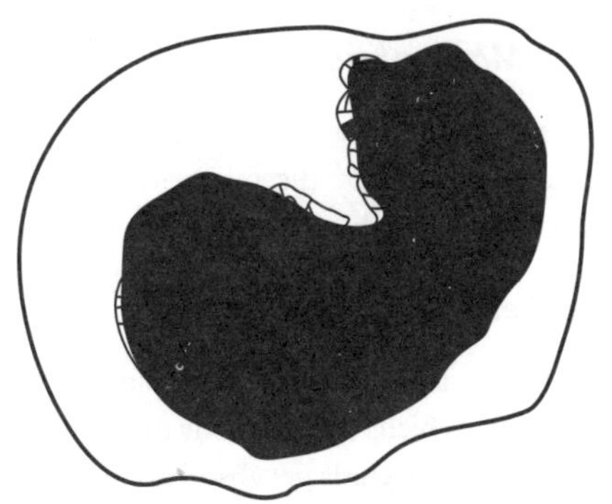

Fig. 2.6   Monocyte.

Lymphocytes (Fig. 2.7)

They form around 25–30% of total leukocytes. Morphologically, they are of two types, large and small lymphocytes.

Large lymphocytes are about 10–12 μ in diameter. The quantity of cytoplasm is more compared to that of small lymphocytes. There are no granules in the cytoplasm.

Small lymphocytes are about 7 μ in diameter. They have a large nucleus occupying the major part of the cell with a thin rim of pale basophilic cytoplasm.

Functions   They are involved in immunity. Functionally, lymphocytes are of two types:

1. **T-lymphocytes:** Processed in the thymus.
2. **B-lymphocytes:** Processed in bursa of Fabricius in lower animals. They are also processed in fetal liver and bone marrow in humans. These are equivalent to bursa of Fabricius.

T-lymphocytes are concerned with cell-mediated immunity. They are of four types:

1. cytotoxic T cells,
2. helper T cells,
3. memory T cells, and
4. suppressor T cells.

B-lymphocytes get transformed into **plasma cells**. They form immunoglobulins and are responsible for humoral immunity.

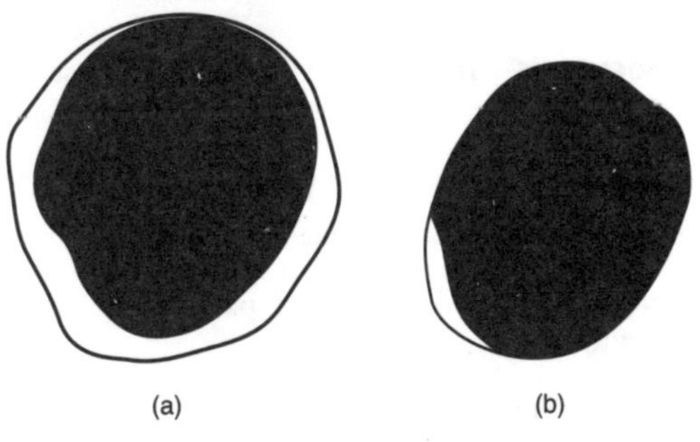

Fig. 2.7   Lymphocyte: (a) large and (b) small.

Leukocyte Count and Its Variations

The normal WBC count is 4,000–11,000 cells/mm^3 of blood.

Physiological Variations

The count is increased in

- emotion and exercise;
- menstruation, pregnancy, and labor;
- newborns and infants.

  It is decreased in

- starvation and severe cold;
- diurnal variation.

  Lowest in the morning and increased during evening.

Pathological Variations

Leukocytosis   It is an increase in the leukocyte count above 11,000 cells/mm³.

The causes of leukocytosis include acute bacterial infections, hemorrhage, burns, and malignancy.

Neutrophilia   Increased neutrophil count is observed in acute bacterial infections, myocardial infarction, and tissue injury.

Eosinophilia   It is seen in parasitic infestations, allergic conditions like asthma, hay fever, and some skin diseases.

Basophilia   It is seen in viral infections like influenza and chicken pox.

Lymphocytosis   It is seen in tuberculosis, measles, and mumps.

Monocytosis   It is seen in Hodgkin's disease and Crohn's disease.

Leukopenia   Decrease in WBC count below 4000 cells/mm³ is termed leukopenia.

- **Neutropenia:** Typhoid and paratyphoid fevers, and bone marrow depression
- **Eosinopenia:** Seen after injection of ACTH
- **Lymphopenia:** AIDS

Leukemia   Abnormal, uncontrolled increase in leukocytes is termed leukemia. It is a malignant condition associated with increased number of premature cells in the blood.

Reticuloendothelial System (Monocyte Macrophage System)

Reticuloendothelial (RE) system consists of monocytes, wandering macrophages, tissue macrophages, and specialized endothelial cells in the bone marrow, spleens, and lymph nodes.

Monocytes wandering in the blood enter the tissues and become larger cells called **macrophages**. These macrophages get attached to the tissues and phagocytose bacteria, viruses, and necrotic tissue.

Macrophages remain in the tissues for months and years. Some of the macrophages can break away from their attachments and again become mobile.

Macrophages are present as tissue macrophages in the lymph nodes, alveolar macrophages in the lungs, Kupffer cells in the liver, macrophages in the spleen, histiocytes in the skin, and glial cells in the CNS.

Type of Macrophages

Tissue Histiocytes

When the skin is broken and gets infected, local tissue macrophages attack and destroy the infective agents.

Macrophages in Lymph Nodes

The microorganisms which are not destroyed at the tissues enter the lymphatic stream. These microorganisms are trapped in the lymph nodes. Macrophages present in the lymph nodes kill these microorganisms.

Alveolar Macrophages

They are present in the alveolar walls of lungs. These cells invade and destroy the microorganisms which enter the body through lungs.

Kupffer Cells

These cells are present in the liver sinusoids. They destroy bacteria which enter the body through the GIT. Large numbers of bacteria get absorbed in the mucosa of the gastrointestinal wall and enter the portal blood. They are destroyed by the Kupffer cells.

Macrophages in Spleen and Bone Marrow

If the microorganism succeeds in entering the general circulation, macrophages present in the spleen and bone marrow trap and destroy them.

Glial Cells

These cells are present in the CNS. They destroy the microorganisms which gain entry into the CNS.

Functions of Macrophages

Phagocytosis

Macrophages play an important role in the defense mechanism of the body. They engulf microorganisms like bacteria and viruses and destroy them.

Destruction of RBC

RE cells in the spleen cause destruction of the old and fragile RBC.

Secretion of Interleukins

Macrophages secrete various interleukins which regulate immune response. They play an important role in inflammation. They form colony-stimulating factor resulting in increased production of blood cells. They ingest and process the antigen which later stimulates the formation of antibody.

Immunity

Immunity is the ability of the body to resist invasion by the microorganism and influence of the toxins that cause tissue damage.

Factors Influencing Immunity

- **Age:** Newborn and old people have low levels of immunity. The immune mechanisms in newborn are not fully developed. In old age there is a gradual decrease in immune response.
- **Hormones:** Change in hormonal levels leading to various endocrine disorders increases the susceptibility to infections due to reduced immunity.
- **Nutrition:** Immunity is reduced in malnutrition.

Types

There are two types: (i) innate immunity (nonspecific) and, (ii) acquired immunity (specific).

Innate Immunity

This is present since birth. It is effective against all invading organisms and is not specific to a particular type of organism. It does not depend on previous contact with microorganism.

This type of immunity includes

- phagocytosis of bacteria by neutrophils and macrophages,
- skin and mucus membrane act as barrier against infections;
- acid secretion of stomach which destroys the swallowed pathogenic organisms;
- lysosomes present in blood;
- complement system of the body;
- natural killer cells which recognize and destroy tumor cells and infected cells.

Acquired Immunity

This is ability of the body to develop specific immunity against invading agents like bacteria, viruses, and foreign substances.

It is of two types:

1. **Humoral immunity:** Humoral immunity is mediated by immunoglobulins. These immunoglobulins are produced by B-lymphocytes. B-lymphocytes specific for the antigen enlarge to form lymphoblast in response to challenge by an antigen. Lymphoblast differentiates into plasma blast and plasma blast produces *plasma cells.*

   The mature plasma cells produce *immunoglobulins,* or antibodies.

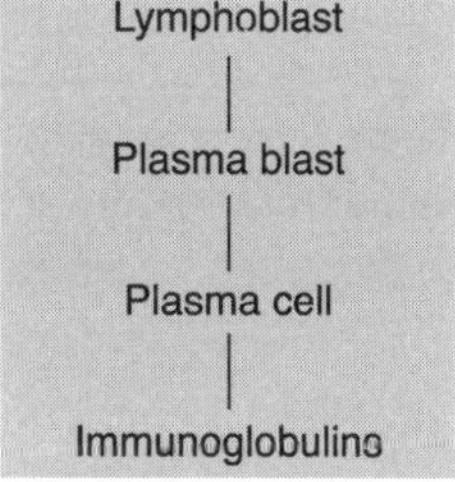

Immunoglobulins are of five types: IgG, IgA, IgM, IgD, and IgE.

Immunoglobulins, in general, contain four polypeptide chains. Two long chains are called *heavy chains* and the two short chains are called *light chains*. In different types of immunoglobulins, there is variation in heavy chains.

- *IgG:* This consists of γ (gamma) heavy chains. It is present in plasma and ECF. It is the most abundant immunoglobulin. IgG passes through the placenta. It is involved in complement activation and phagocytosis.

- *IgA:* It contains α (alpha) heavy chains. It is called the secretory antibody. It is present in body secretions (milk, tears, saliva, and gastrointestinal secretions).

- *IgM:* This contains μ (mue) heavy chains. It is responsible for complement activation. It also forms ABO antibodies.

- *IgE:* It contains ε (epsilon) heavy chain. It causes the release of histamine from basophils and mast cells. It is increased in atopic allergy and parasitic infestations.

- *IgD:* This contains δ (delta) heavy chain. It is involved in the antigen recognition by B cells.

These immunoglobulins act by

(a) directly attacking the invading organism by agglutination, precipitation, and neutralization reactions;

(b) activation of the complement.

Complement System

This is a system of enzymes present in the serum that are activated by the antigen–antibody interaction. These factors mediate a number of biologically significant consequences.

The enzymes present in the complement are named C1 to C9.

Complement is present in the body in an inactive form. Antigen–antibody reaction induces the activity of complement.

Activation of complement occurs through two pathways:

1. classic pathway and

2. alternate pathway.

Classic Pathway

It is a chain of events in which components of complement react in a specific sequence ending in immune cytolysis. Activation of C3 by C3 convertase is the major step in this pathway.

Alternate Pathway

In this pathway, activation of C3 occurs without C3 convertase. Properdin pathway is an example for this pathway.

Biological Effects of Complement

- Mediates immunological membrane damage causing bacteriolysis or cytolysis.

- Amplifies the inflammatory response.

- Participates in the pathogenesis of certain hypersensitivity reactions.

- Exhibits antiviral activity.

- Promotes phagocytosis.

2. Cell-mediated immunity: This is produced by T-lymphocytes. They are of four types:

(a) *Helper T cells:* These cells constitute about 75% of T-lymphocytes. They form a series of protein mediators called **lymphokines.** These lymphokines cause

- stimulation and growth of cytotoxic and suppressor T cells;

- stimulation and growth of B cells with the formation of antibodies;
- activation of macrophage system;
- feedback stimulation of other helper T cells.

(b) *Cytotoxic T cells:* These cells directly attack and kill the microorganisms. The cells get attached to the microorganism. They create holes in cell membrane of the microorganism and release cytotoxic substances causing death of the microorganism.

(c) *Suppressor T cells:* They are capable of suppressing the functions of both the cytotoxic and helper T cells. They prevent excessive immune reactions that might cause damage to the body. Thus, they act as regulatory cells.

(d) *Memory T cells:* After the exposure to an antigen, a small number of T cells (and also B cells) persist as memory cells. Whenever the same antigen enters the body, these cells are activated to produce a rapid antibody response.

Applied Physiology

AIDS (Acquired Immune Deficiency Syndrome)

This disease is caused due to infection by a retrovirus called human immunodeficiency virus (HIV).

Infection occurs when the virus enters the body of the person and comes in contact with a suitable host cell–like T_4 lymphocyte. It causes destruction of helper T cells and reduces their number. Loss of T helper cells results in decreased activity of B cells and cytotoxic T cells.

Clinical Features

The infected person after an acute illness with low-grade fever, headache, etc., is asymptomatic for months to years. Later, the patient develops unexplained fever, diarrhea, weight loss, and generalized lymphadenopathy. The patient is more prone to opportunistic infections and malignancies.

Autoimmune Diseases

In this condition, the body produces antibodies against its own proteins. There is widespread destruction of antigenic substance by antigen–antibody reaction.

Autoimmune diseases include Type I diabetes mellitus, myasthenia gravis, Grave's disease, and rheumatoid arthritis.

Allergy and Hypersensitivity

Antigenic substances present in chemicals, drugs, and cosmetics can cause allergy by activation of T cells. This is characterized by skin rashes due to the release of histamine.

Urticaria, hay fever, and asthma are examples of hypersensitivity.

Anaphylaxis

This is a widespread allergic reaction affecting the vascular system and related tissues. It is caused by IgE antibodies reacting with the antigens.

Antigen

It is a substance which stimulates the production of an antibody with which it reacts specifically in the body. Antigens are normally proteins or heptans.

Antibody

It is the substance produced in the body in response to an antigenic stimulation.

Natural Killer Cells

They are the third type of lymphocytes present in the body apart from T- and B-lymphocytes.

They are large lymphocytes that make up for 10–15% of the circulating lymphocytes.

Functions

They destroy malignant cells in the body, thereby preventing cancerous growth. They attack viruses and help in destroying them.

Antigen–Antibody Reaction

It is the reaction between antigen and antibody specifically in an observable manner.

Cytokines

These are hormone-like substances produced from lymphocytes and macrophages. Cytokines with known amino acid sequences are called **interleukins**.

Earlier, substances secreted by lymphocytes were called **lymphokines**. Since these substances are also secreted from other cells, they are now called **cytokines**.

Effects of Interleukins

- B-cell proliferation and immunoglobulin production
- Activation of phagocytes
- Inflammation and febrile response
- Eosinophil growth and function

Cytokines like tumor necrosis factor α and β cause necrosis of tumor and blood vessels.

Vaccination (Immunization)

Vaccination is used to produce acquired immunity against specific diseases.

Vaccines

They are prepared from live or killed microorganisms or their products. They are used for immunization.

Live Vaccines   Live vaccines (e.g., BCG, measles, and oral polio) cause an infection without producing disease. Immunity lasts for years. They can be given orally (polio vaccine) or parenterally (measles).

Killed Vaccines   These vaccines (e.g., tetanus toxoid and diphtheria toxoid) are less immunogenic than live vaccines and protection lasts only for a short period. Therefore, they have to be administered repeatedly. At least two doses are required. First dose is called primary dose. Subsequent doses are called booster doses. Killed vaccines are usually administered through injections.

Lymphatic System

Lymphatic system is an accessory route through which fluid flows from the interstitial spaces into the blood.

Almost all tissues of the body have lymphatics, exceptions being the skin, brain, and bones.

Lymph

It is a modified tissue fluid derived from interstitial fluid. It flows in the lymphatic channels.

Composition

It contains proteins, fats, clotting factors, ions like Na^+, K^+, Cl^-, Ca^{++}, lymphocytes, few RBCs, and platelets.

Functions

- Absorbs nutrients from the GIT
- Maintains the normal interstitial fluid pressure
- Transports proteins
- Transports foreign particles to lymph nodes
- Helps in immunity

Lymph from lower parts of the body and left upper parts of the body pass through lymphatic channels and empty into the venous system via the thoracic duct.

Lymph from the right upper part of the body enters the right lymphatic duct which later empties into the venous system at the junction of right subclavian and internal jugular veins.

Formation

Lymph is formed from the interstitial fluid. Therefore, the composition of lymph initially is similar to interstitial fluid.

Most of the fluid filtered from the blood capillaries flows around the cells and is reabsorbed back at venous end of the capillaries. About 10% of the fluid flows through the lymphatic capillaries and forms lymph. This fluid returning through the lymphatics contains high-molecular-weight substances like proteins that cannot be absorbed into the blood directly.

Normal lymphatic flow is 2–4 L/day.

Lymphatic flow is determined by two factors:

1. **Interstitial fluid pressure:** Increase in the interstitial fluid pressure increases lymph flow. Increased capillary pressure and decreased interstitial fluid colloid osmotic pressure increase the interstitial fluid pressure causing an increase in lymph flow.
2. **Activity of lymphatic pump:** Lymphatic channels have valves. These valves prevent backflow of lymph. The portion of lymphatic channels between two valves forms a segment. Stretch of these segments by lymph causes contraction of the smooth muscles causing pumping of lymph into the next segment. This continues in the subsequent segments until the fluid is emptied into the veins.

The lymphatic pump can generate pressures up to 100 mm Hg.

Thrombocytes (Platelets)

These are small, colorless, round, or oval disks, 2–4 μ in size. They do not have a nucleus (Fig. 2.8).

Normal count is 1.5–4 lakh cells/mm^3.

Their life span is 9–12 days.

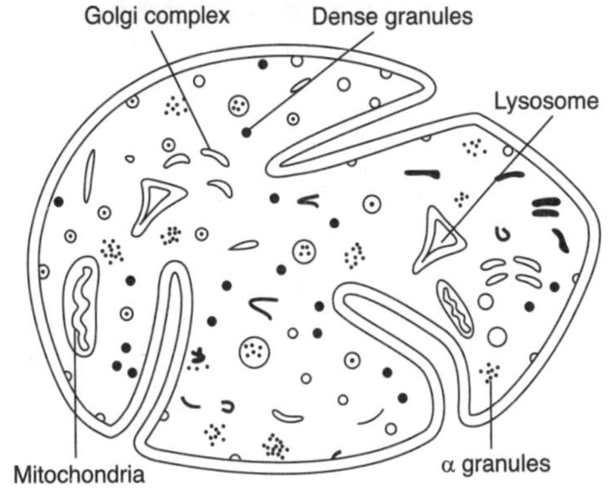

Fig. 2.8   Thrombocyte (platelet).

Formation

They are formed in the bone marrow from megakaryocyte, which is a large multinucleated cell. Megakaryocytes develop pseudopod-like extensions that break into fragments to form platelets. One megakaryocyte forms around 2000–4000 platelets.

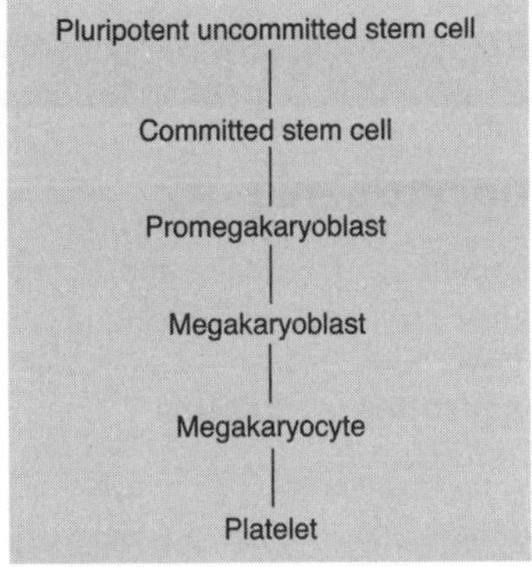

Applied Physiology

Edema

It is accumulation of abnormally large quantities of fluid in the interstitial space. Reduced lymphatic drainage causes edema. This is due to the leakage of protein into the interstitial space that raises the interstitial fluid colloid osmotic pressure.

Structure and Contents

The cell membrane of platelet has a coating of glycoprotein that prevents adhesion to the normal endothelium. It also contains large amounts of phospholipids. Platelet membrane contains receptors, which attach them to the von Willebrand factor, collagen, and fibrinogen. Platelets contain mitochondria and various enzymes that form ATP and ADP. They contain contractile proteins: actin, myosin, and thrombosthenin.

Platelets contain three types of granules: α granules, dense granules, and lysosomal granules. The α granules have platelet-derived growth factor, von Willebrand factor, and thrombospondin. Dense granules contain nonprotein substances like serotonin, ADP, ATP, and Ca^{++}.

Functions

- Help in hemostasis by forming a platelet plug
- Cause vasoconstriction by releasing serotonin, and thromboxane A_2
- Accelerate the process of clotting
- Involved in phagocytosis of antigen–antibody complexes and viruses
- Help in the repair of damaged endothelium

- Store and transport 5-hydroxytryptamine and histamine
- Play a role in inflammation

Platelet Reaction

Injury to blood vessel exposes its endothelium. Platelets adhere to the vessel wall. These adherent platelets become activated. They change their shape, become motile, and release their granular contents. Platelets become stickier and promote adhesion of greater number of platelets to the vessel wall. They ultimately form a platelet plug. This plug helps in the arrest of bleeding in small blood vessels. If the damage is large, bleeding is arrested by the formation of a clot.

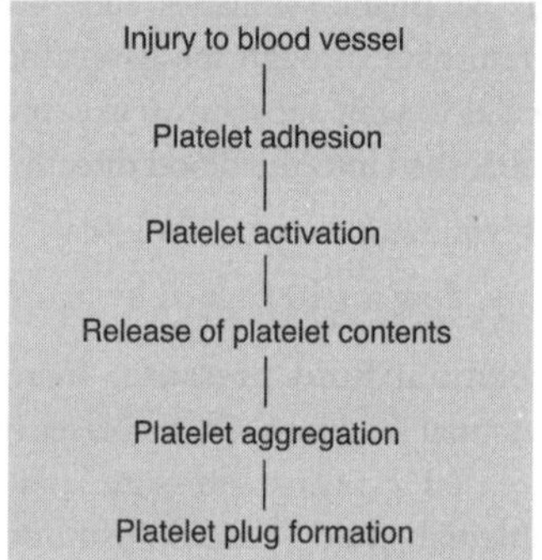

Applied Physiology

Thrombocytopenia

This is a condition of reduced number of platelets in circulation. The individuals with thrombocytopenia have a tendency to bleed. This bleeding is from small capillaries.

Thrombocytopenic Purpura

The disease is characterized by the formation of purplish spots beneath the skin due to spontaneous bleeding. In this condition, clot retraction is delayed and there is poor constriction of ruptured vessels.

In this condition, bleeding time is prolonged but clotting time is normal. Manifestation of disease is seen when the platelet count is less than 50,000 cells/mm^3.

Thrombasthenic Purpura

This is a condition with normal platelet count but the circulating platelets are abnormal.

Treatment   Infusion of fresh blood or infusion of platelet concentrate.

In nonresponding cases, splenectomy (removal of spleen) is advised.

Hemostasis and Blood Coagulation

An injury causes rupture of the vessel resulting in hemorrhage. The body mechanisms try to arrest the bleeding. This is termed **hemostasis**.

Hemostasis is achieved by several mechanisms:

- vascular spasm or vasoconstriction;
- formation of a platelet plug;
- formation of a blood clot as a result of blood coagulation;
- deposition of fibrous tissue in the clot and permanent closure of defect in blood vessel.

Vascular Constriction

Whenever a blood vessel is ruptured or cut, the vessel automatically constricts. This causes reduction of blood flow through that vessel. Vasoconstriction is produced by nervous reflexes, local myogenic reflexes, humoral factors released from traumatized tissues, and blood platelets.

Formation of Platelet Plug

If the damage in the blood vessel is small, it is sealed by means of a platelet plug.

Formation of Blood Clot

This is a powerful mechanism for hemostasis. In severe trauma, there is rupture of blood vessel and blood gets exposed to exterior. Blood, when it is shed, forms a semisolid jelly-like substance in about 15–20 s. Within 3–6 min, the opening in the vessel is filled with clot. After 20 min to an hour, clot retracts and completely seals the defect in the blood vessel.

Formation of Fibrous Tissue in the Clot

After the blood clot is formed, either it is invaded by fibroblasts or it dissolves.

Fibroblasts are formed within few hours following clot formation. Later in 1–2 weeks, clot is completely organized into the fibrous tissue.

The clot dissolves by the action of special enzymes. This occurs in places where the clot is not required and patency of the vessel has to be maintained.

Mechanism of Blood Coagulation

About 50 different substances that affect blood coagulation have been identified. The substances that promote coagulation are called **procoagulants**. The substances inhibiting coagulation are called **anticoagulants**. In normal state, the anticoagulants predominate over procoagulants and therefore blood does not clot. But whenever the vessel ruptures, procoagulants in that area become activated and override the effect of anticoagulants producing the clot.

Clotting or coagulation occurs in three basic stages:

1. The rupture of blood vessel results in a cascade of chemical reactions in blood involving 12 coagulation factors. They finally form a complex of activating substances called the **prothrombin activator**.
2. Prothrombin activator catalyzes the conversion of the **prothrombin** to **thrombin**.
3. Thrombin acts as an enzyme to convert **fibrinogen** to **fibrin**.

Fibrin forms a mesh in which the blood cells, platelets, get entangled and form a clot.

Clotting Factors

The formation of prothrombin activator requires 12 different coagulation factors. They are as under:

- **Factor I—fibrinogen:** Fibrinogen is a soluble plasma protein having a molecular weight of 3,30,000. Plasma contains about 100–700 mg/dL.

  It is acted upon by thrombin to form insoluble fibrin clot. Absence of factor I is termed **afibrinogenemia**.

- **Factor II—prothrombin:** Prothrombin is the inactive precursor of thrombin. It is a plasma protein with molecular weight of 68,700. The normal concentration in plasma is 15 mg/dL. It is formed in the liver with the help of vitamin K.

- **Factor III—thromboplastin:** This converts prothrombin to thrombin in the presence of factors V, VII, X, Ca^{++}, and phospholipids.

- **Factor IV—calcium:** Ionic calcium is required for clotting. This is required for the formation of prothrombin activator, for the conversion of prothrombin to thrombin, and for the formation of insoluble fibrin clot.

- **Factor V—labile factor (proaccelerin):** This is required for the conversion of prothrombin to thrombin by tissue extract and plasma factors.
- **Factor VI:** Absent.
- **Factor VII—stable factor (proconvertin):** This is required for the formation of prothrombin activator from tissue extracts.
- **Factor VIII—antihemophilic factor A:** This is required for the formation of prothrombin activator by tissue extract. Absence of this factor leads to disease termed *hemophilia*.
- **Factor IX—Christmas factor (antihemophilic factor B):** This is needed for the formation of prothrombin activator from blood constituents. Lack of factor IX results in Christmas disease.
- **Factor X—Stuart–Prower factor:** This is also required for the formation of prothrombin activator. Absence of this factor leads to hemorrhage.
- **Factor XI—plasma thromboplastin antecedent (antihemophilic factor C):** This is required for the formation of prothrombin activator from blood constituents. Absence of this factor leads to hemorrhage.
- **Factor XII—Hageman factor:** Deficiency of this factor leads to delayed clotting. This factor is activated by glass and water-wettable surfaces. It also takes part in the formation of prothrombin activator.
- **Factor XIII—fibrin-stabilizing factor:** This is a plasma protein which causes polymerization of soluble fibrin to produce insoluble fibrin.

Clotting Mechanisms

Clotting occurs by two pathways:

1. extrinsic pathway, and
2. intrinsic pathway.

Clotting factors are necessary for the formation of prothrombin activator. Prothrombin activator is formed by two pathways.

Extrinsic Pathway

Trauma to the tissue releases complex tissue factors composed of phospholipids and lipoprotein. Tissue factor and factor VII in the presence of Ca^{++} ions act on factor X to form activated factor X. Activated factor X combines with tissue phospholipids, platelet phospholipids, and factor V to form the complex called **prothrombin activator**.

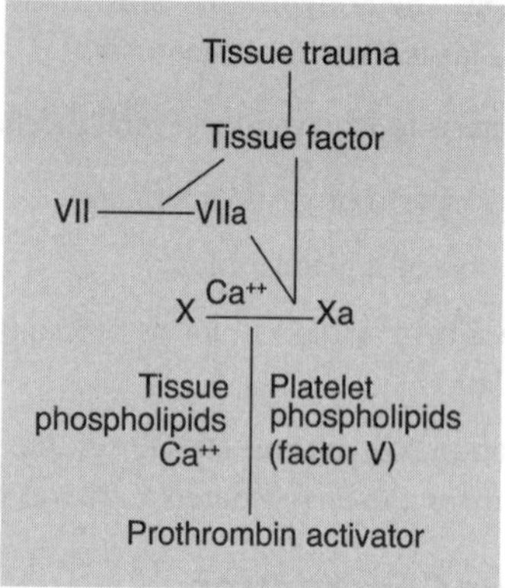

Intrinsic Pathway

This begins with damage to blood cells or exposure of blood to collagen in traumatized vessel wall. It results in activation of factor XII to activated factor XII (XIIa). It also causes damage to platelets and this releases platelet phospholipids. Activated factor XII acts on factor XI and activates it. Activated factor XI causes activation of factor IX. Activated factor IX along with activated factor VIII and traumatized platelets cause activation of factor X. Activated factor X combines with factor V and platelet or tissue phospholipids to form the complex called **prothrombin activator**.

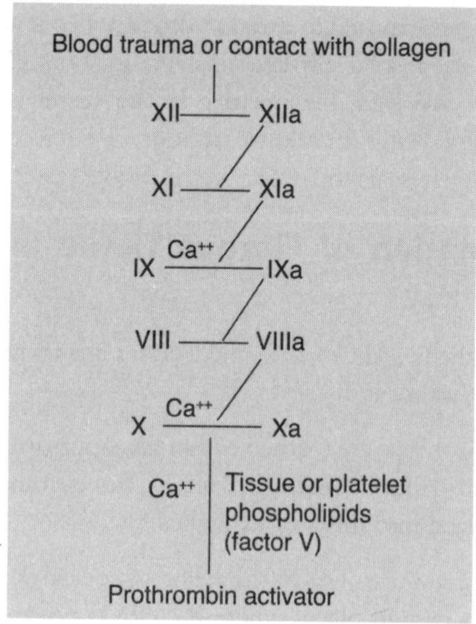

After formation of prothrombin activator, the second step in clotting is the conversion of prothrombin to thrombin:

$$\text{Prothrombin} \xrightarrow[\text{Ca}^{++}]{\text{Prothrombin activator}} \text{Thrombin}.$$

The third step in clotting mechanism is conversion of fibrinogen to fibrin:

$$\text{Fibrinogen} \xrightarrow{\text{Thrombin}} \text{Fibrin}.$$

Thrombin acts on fibrinogen and converts it to fibrin monomer by removing four low-molecular-weight peptides from each molecule of fibrinogen. Many fibrin monomers polymerize within seconds to form long fibrin fiber.

These fibers ultimately form a meshwork in which platelets, blood cells, and plasma get entangled. This is known as a **clot**. The fibers are strengthened by a substance known as fibrin-stabilizing factor.

Clot formation by extrinsic pathway is rapid. Intrinsic pathway is much slower, requiring 1–6 min to produce clotting. Ca^{++} ions are absolutely necessary for both the pathways. Therefore in the absence of Ca^{++} ions clotting does not occur.

Once a blood clot is formed, it follows one of the two courses:

1. It can be invaded by fibroblasts and form fibrous tissue within about 1–2 weeks.
2. It can be dissolved by substances such as plasmin or fibrinolysin.

Applied Physiology

Bleeding Disorders

1. Hemophilia
2. Vitamin K deficiency
3. Afibrinogenemia
4. Thrombocytopenia

Hemophilia

Hemophilia major is due to deficiency of factor VIII. It is a sex-linked hereditary disease which occurs exclusively in males. Females are the carriers. This disease is genetically transmitted recessive disorder. Persons suffering from this disease have bleeding tendencies after a minor trauma. The clotting time is prolonged and bleeding time is normal in hemophilia. Treatment is by injection of the purified factor VIII.

Absence of factor IX is termed **hemophilia minor** or **Christmas disease**.

Vitamin K Deficiency

Vitamin K is necessary for the formation of five clotting factors—prothrombin, factor VII, factor IX, factor X, and protein C—in the liver. Absence or deficiency of vitamin K leads to deficiency of these factors and defective clotting. Diseases of the liver like hepatitis and cirrhosis can also cause impaired absorption of vitamin K leading to decreased production of clotting factors.

Afibrinogenemia

There is deficiency of fibrinogen. This can occur due to genetic defect, liver diseases, and prostatic cancer. Treatment is supplementation of fibrinogen through injections or fresh blood transfusion.

Thrombocytopenia

It has been discussed earlier.

Plasmin is formed from a substance called plasminogen under the influence of tissue plasminogen activator. Plasmin is a proteolytic enzyme which digests fibrin as well as other clotting substances in blood.

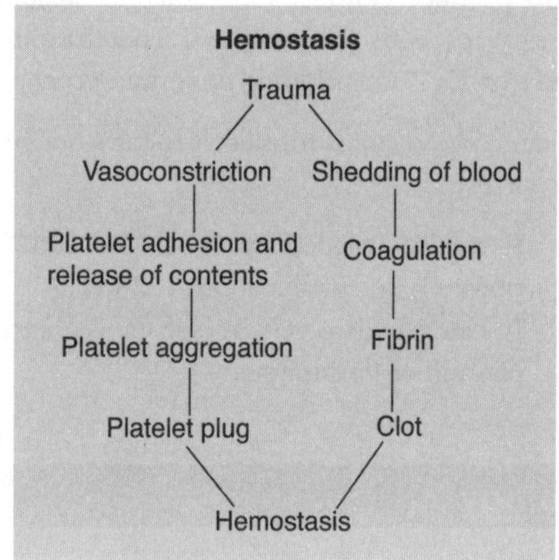

Tests for Coagulation

Bleeding Time

It is the time interval from the onset of bleeding to its spontaneous arrest.

The normal bleeding time is 2–4 min. It is prolonged in thrombocytopenic purpura.

Clotting Time

It is the time lag from the onset of bleeding to the appearance of first fibrin thread. Normal duration is 2–8 min. It is prolonged in hemophilia.

Prothrombin Time

Normal prothrombin time is 11–16 s. It varies with alteration in prothrombin level in the blood. Prothrombin time gives an indication about the total amount of prothrombin present in the blood. Increased prothrombin time delays coagulation. It is increased in liver diseases and vitamin K deficiency.

Anticoagulation

This is a process of limiting blood clotting within the body to optimum levels. This is brought about by the following:

1. **Prostacyclin:** It is formed at the site of injury in the initial layer. This prevents extension of the clot.
2. **Antithrombin III:** It is a protease inhibitor present in plasma. It prevents activity of factor IXa, Xa, XIa, and XIIa.
3. **Thrombomodulin:** It is a protein present on the endothelial cells which bind to thrombin. Thrombin–thrombomodulin complex activates protein C. This inactivates factor V and VIII, thereby preventing coagulation.

Fluid State of Blood/Blood in Circulation

Blood is kept in fluid state mainly due to continuous motion.

Other factors helping this are

- smoothness of endothelium,
- negative charge of endothelium,
- natural anticoagulants like heparin, and
- anticlotting mechanisms.

Fibrinolytic System

This system dissolves clot and keeps the lumen of blood vessel patent. Lysis (break down) of fibrin is brought about by plasmin.

Streptokinase and urokinase are used in lysis of clots in conditions of intravascular clotting, e.g., management of early stages of myocardial infarction.

Anticoagulants

Anticoagulants prevent coagulation of blood.

Heparin

This is a naturally occurring anticoagulant found in basophils and mast cells. It is used both in vivo (inside the body) and in vitro (outside the body). It acts by neutralizing the action of thrombin.

Vitamin K Antagonists

They include warfarin, sodium, and dicumarol. They inhibit the formation of vitamin K–dependent clotting factors.

Calcium-Chelating Agents

They include EDTA (ethylene diamine tetracetate), citrates, and oxalates of sodium and potassium. These substances form insoluble salts with calcium and precipitate them. Thus calcium is not available for the process of clotting.

Blood Groups

Blood is categorized into different groups based on their antigenic properties. Antigenic and immunologic properties of blood have clinical, genetic, and medicolegal importance.

Karl Landsteiner discovered blood groups. There are around 23 blood group systems containing more than 400 antigens. Of these 400 antigens only about 30 occur commonly and most of them are weak antigens.

Blood group systems include ABO system, Rh system, M and N system, Lewis system, P system, Kell system, and Duffy system. Most important are the ABO and Rh systems.

Uses of Blood Grouping and Rh Typing

- Proper blood transfusion
- Medicolegal importance—paternity testing and crime detection
- Genetic studies
- Study the influence of blood group in evaluation of diseases

ABO System

Human blood is categorized into four major groups depending on the presence or absence of antigens. Antigens are present on the surface of RBC. They are called **agglutinogens**.

There are two agglutinogens in ABO system: A and B.

Further, A agglutinogen is of two types:

1. A_1: Contains A and A_1 agglutinogens
2. A_2: Contains only A agglutinogens

Group	Agglutinogen	Agglutinin
A	A	Anti-B (β)
B	B	Anti-A (α)
AB	Both A and B	Nil
O	Nil	Anti-A and Anti-B

Blood contains antibodies in plasma. These are called **agglutinins**. They are IgM and IgG immunoglobulins. They are absent at birth and develop within 2–8 months after birth, reaching a maximum by 8–10 years and gradually decline thereafter.

Landsteiner's Law

If an agglutinogen is present on RBCs of an individual, the corresponding agglutinin must be absent in plasma.

If the agglutinogen is absent on the RBC, corresponding agglutinen must be present in the plasma.

Thus, group A individuals have A agglutinogen and β agglutinin.

Group B individuals have B agglutinogen and α agglutinin.

Group AB individuals have A and B agglutinogens and no agglutinin.

Group O individuals have no agglutinogen and α and β agglutinins.

ABO Incompatibility

When mismatched blood is transfused to a person, serious reactions can occur resulting in death of the person.

The affected person develops hemolysis resulting in shock and renal failure.

Rh System

It is also an important system of blood grouping. The term Rh is derived from Rhesus factor since the original discovery was made in Rhesus monkeys. There are six agglutinogens in Rh system. They are C, D, E, c, d, e. Out of the six agglutinogens only D agglutinogen is potent and therefore Rh group is described only in relation to D agglutinogen. Individuals having D agglutinogen are said to be Rh+ (positive) and individuals not having D agglutinogen are said to be Rh– (negative). About 85% of the population is Rh+ and 15% of the population is Rh–.

Applied Physiology

Rh Incompatibility

An Rh– individual transfused with Rh+ blood develops anti-Rh agglutinins slowly. If this person is later exposed to Rh+ blood, severe transfusion reactions occur.

Erythroblastosis Fetalis

This is a disease of neonates with Rh incompatibility. There is agglutination and destruction of fetal red cells. In this condition, mother is Rh– and fetus is Rh+. There is no complication in first pregnancy but problem occurs in subsequent pregnancies. If Rh+ baby is born to an Rh– mother, some fetal erythrocytes pass to the mother during childbirth. This produces anti-D antibodies in the mother. In the next pregnancy, if the fetus is Rh+, these antibodies from the mother destroy fetal erythrocytes leading to hemolytic disease of the newborn.

Clinical Features

The fetus is jaundiced, anemic; liver and spleen are enlarged. Increased concentration of bilirubin in the brain tissue can damage the nerve cells leading to kernicterus. In severe form it presents as hydrops fetalis.

Prevention

Administration of anti-D antibodies to the mother soon after delivery of the first child. This causes destruction of Rh+ fetal cells in maternal blood.

Treatment

Replacement of blood of the newborn with Rh– blood repeatedly during the first few weeks. About 400 mL of Rh– blood is infused and at the same time equal amount of Rh+ neonatal blood is removed.

Blood Transfusion

It is a procedure in which blood collected from the donor is transfused to the recipient.

Indications:

- Sudden blood loss due to accidents
- During major surgeries
- Patients with bleeding disorders
- Patients with severe burns
- Patients with severe anemia, thalassemia, and leukemia
- Hemolytic disease of newborn

Collection and Storage of Blood

Blood is collected from a healthy donor free of all infectious diseases like HIV, hepatitis, malaria, and syphilis.

It is collected under strict aseptic precautions and mixed with anticoagulant (acid citrate dextrose).

One unit of blood (420 mL) can be collected from a donor at a time. This is stored at 2–4°C in blood bank. The stored blood has to be used within 3 weeks from the time of its collection.

Leukocytes and platelets are absent after 24 h of storing blood. Therefore patients requiring leukocytes or platelets should be transfused fresh blood.

Precautions during Blood Transfusion

- Temperature of the blood to be transfused must be brought to room temperature.
- Transfusion should be done under strict aseptic precautions.
- Transfusion must be very slow since rapid infusion can lead to excessive load on the heart resulting in cardiac failure.

Blood Grouping and Cross-matching

Blood grouping and cross-matching has to be done to prevent complications of blood transfusion.

Blood Grouping

Saline suspension of RBC is mixed with anti-A, anti-B, and anti-D sera. Presence or absence of agglutination helps to identify the blood group.

Cross-matching

Erythrocyte of the donor is matched with serum of recipient in **major cross-matching**.

In **minor cross-matching**, erythrocyte of recipient is matched with serum of the donor.

Hazards of Blood Transfusion: Hazards of Mismatched Blood Transfusion

Immediate   This includes hemolysis leading to shock and renal failure due to precipitation of Hb in the nephrons.

Delayed   Jaundice

Hemolysis   Mismatched blood transfusion results in antigen–antibody reaction inside the recipient's body causing massive destruction of red blood cells.

Shock   This is caused due to loss of circulating RBCs and also production of toxic substances from the hemolysed cells. The arterial pressure falls leading to decreased renal blood flow.

Renal Failure   This occurs within few minutes to few hours of blood transfusion.

Renal failure is due to

(a)   constriction of renal blood vessels by toxins released,
(b)   reduced blood flow secondary to circulatory shock, and
(c)   precipitation of Hb in the nephrons.

Jaundice   It occurs due to release of hemoglobin from hemolysed RBCs. Hemoglobin released is converted to bilirubin. Bilirubin concentration in the body fluids increases resulting in jaundice.

Other Hazards of Blood Transfusion

Immediate   Pyrogen reactions, shock, circulatory overload, hyperkalemia, and hypocalcemia.

Delayed   Transmission of diseases, and iron overload.

Pyrogen Reactions   Fever with chills and rigors can develop during transfusion.

Circulatory Overload   Rapid transfusion of blood can lead to hypervolemia resulting in circulatory overload.

Hyperkalemia   This occurs due to loss of K^+ ions from red cells into plasma in stored blood.

Hypocalcemia   Addition of citrate to blood results in lack of ionized calcium resulting in hypocalcemia.

Transmission of Diseases   Malaria, syphilis, and HIV can be transmitted through blood.

Iron overload   This occurs in patients receiving repeated blood transfusion.

Autologous Blood Transfusion

This refers to transfusion of an individual's own blood which has been drawn earlier and stored. This can be done in the case of elective surgeries.

Nerve–Muscle Physiology

The muscles and nerves are the excitable tissues. There are about 100 billion neurons in the human central nervous system (CNS). The neurons are the building blocks of the nervous system. They respond to various types of stimuli. The generation and transmission of impulse is the specialized function of a neuron. The neurons develop from the primitive neuroeffector cells.

The muscle cells in addition to the property of excitability have the capacity to contract. The contractile mechanism of the muscle is activated by an action potential. Actin and myosin are the contractile proteins present in the muscle, which bring about contraction.

This chapter deals with the excitation, the integration, and the activity of the excitable tissues of the body.

Neuron

Neuron is the structural and functional unit of the nervous system (Fig. 3.1).

Structure

A neuron has the following structures:

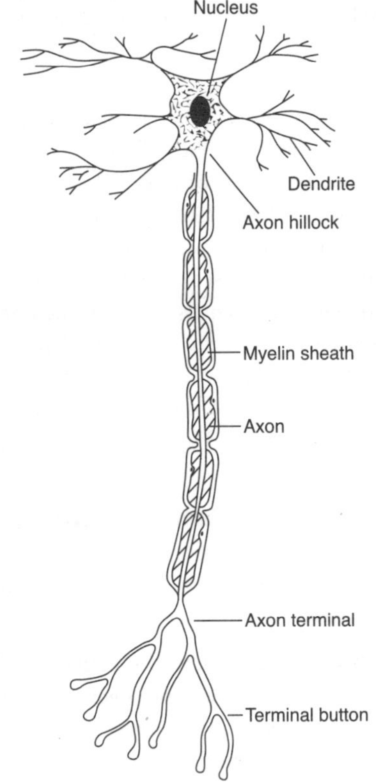

Fig. 3.1 Neuron.

Cell Body (Soma)

The cell body contains the nucleus, endoplasmic reticulum, ribosome, and Golgi apparatus having similar structure and function as in other cells. It has genetic information and system required for protein synthesis. In addition, it has Nissl granules.

Nissl Granules   These are also called tigroid bodies. They are present all over the cell except the axon hillock. They resemble ribosomes and help in the synthesis of proteins needed for the transmission of impulses from one neuron to another. The proteins produced by them are useful in the maintenance and regeneration of the nerve fibers. They disappear when the nerve is injured. This process is called *chromatolysis*. They reappear during the regeneration of neuron.

Dendrites

These are five to seven short branching processes. They carry information toward the cell body. Dendrites in the cerebral and cerebellar cortex have small projections, termed the **dendritic spines**. The branching dendrites increase the cell's receptive area and thereby increase its capacity to receive signals.

Axon

It is the long process of a neuron. It carries information away from the cell body. It arises from the prominent portion of the cell body called the **axon hillock**. The portion of the axon close to cell body (near the site of origin) is termed the **initial segment**. The initial segment is the trigger zone where the electrical signals are generated and then propagated away from the cell body. The axons are also called nerve fibers. The axons vary in length and diameter. Length of the axon varies from a few millimeters to a meter. The diameter ranges from 1 to 20 micron.

Axon Telodendria (Terminal Buttons)   These are the terminal portions of the axon which divides into branches. They contain vesicles filled with neurotransmitter.

Neurofibrils and Neurofilaments   These are bun-dles of microtubules and microfilament. They form the cytoskeleton and provide structural support to the neuron. The neurofibrils form a pathway for the rapid transport of molecules from the far end of the neuron.

The nerve fibers are covered by a connective tissue layer called the **endoneurium**. Several such fibers form a bundle and are enclosed in a sheath called the **perineurium**. These bundles are termed **fascicles**. Several bundles are enclosed by the outermost layer called the **epineurium**.

Myelination of Axon   The axons of many neurons are covered by a myelin sheath. They are called **myelinated nerve fibers**. The cells of Schwann form the myelin sheath in the peripheral nervous system. The myelin sheath is a protein–lipid complex that wraps around the neuron. The myelin sheath is formed when the cells of Schwann wrap its membrane about 100 times around the axon. Later, the layers of the membrane are compacted to form the myelin sheath. The process of formation of myelin sheath is termed **myelinogenesis** (Fig. 3.2). The myelin sheath acts as an insulator around the axon. It is interrupted at periodic intervals at the nodes of Ranvier. The cells of Schwann form the myelin sheath for a single neuron.

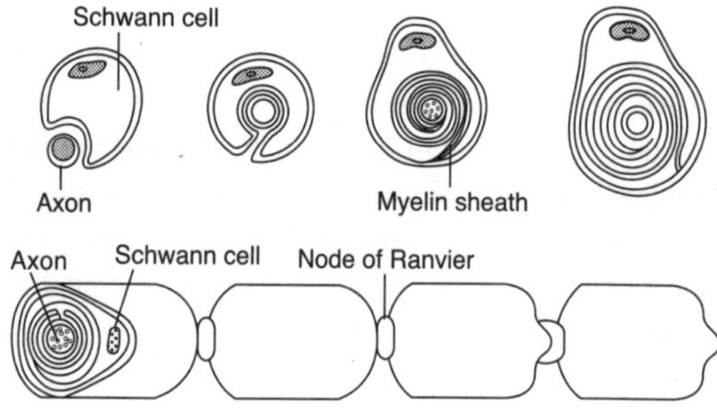

Fig. 3.2   Myelin sheath formation.

The oligodendrocytes form the myelin sheath for the neurons of the CNS. A single oligodendrocyte forms myelin sheath for multiple neurons. The majority of the mammalian neurons are myelinated. The neurons in invertebrates are unmyelinated.

Loss of the myelin sheath is associated with a delay or block in the conduction of impulses. This is the characteristic feature of an autoimmune disease, termed **multiple sclerosis**. In this disease, there is patch destruction of the myelin sheath in the CNS.

In the peripheral neuron, the *neurilemma* covers the nerve fiber. It is the basement membrane of the cells of Schwann. During nerve injury, if the neurilemmal tube is intact, the nerve can regenerate.

The neurilemma is absent in the neurons of the CNS. Hence, regeneration of the nerve is not possible in the CNS.

Transport in the Axon   The axon does not have the ability to synthesize proteins. Hence, the proteins formed in the cell body are transported through the axon by the *axoplasmic flow*. If the movement is from the cell body to the axon terminal, it is called the **orthograde transport**. The substances and organelles to be moved are connected to the microtubules present in the cell body and the axon with the help of proteins. The microtubules serve as the pathway through which the substances are transported. The linking proteins act as motors to move the substance and ATPase enzymes provide the energy.

The flow of substances in the opposite direction is called the **retrograde transport**. Growth factors and harmful substances, such as tetanus toxin and herpes and polio viruses, reach the CNS by the retrograde transport.

Classification

1. Based on the number of processes
   (a) **Unipolar neuron:** The neuron has a single pole. The processes arise from this pole. The unipolar neurons originate in the embryo as bipolar neurons. Later, the processes fuse into one for a short distance beyond the cell body. Then, they separate into the axon and the dendrite. The sensory neurons are unipolar.
   (b) **Bipolar neuron:** The neuron has two poles. The axon and dendrite arise from these poles. The bipolar neurons are present in the retina of the eye.
   (c) **Multipolar neuron:** The neuron has multiple poles. The neuronal processes arise from these poles.

2. Based on myelination
   (a) **Myelinated nerve fiber:** The nerve fiber is covered by the myelin sheath.
   (b) **Nonmyelinated nerve fiber:** The nerve fiber lacks the covering of the myelin sheath.

3. Based on functions
   (a) **Sensory or afferent neurons:** They carry information from the periphery to the CNS.
   (b) **Motor or efferent neurons:** They carry motor impulses from the CNS to the effector organs.
   (c) **Interneurons:** They connect neurons within the CNS.

4. Depending on the neurotransmitter secreted
   (a) **Adrenergic neurons:** These neurons secrete adrenaline at the nerve terminal.
   (b) **Cholinergic neurons:** These neurons secrete acetylcholine at the nerve terminal.

5. Based on diameter and conduction velocity

Erlanger and Gasser's Classification			
Type	**Function**	**Diameter (μm)**	**Conduction Velocity (m/s)**
Aα	Proprioception	12–20	70–120
Aβ	Touch, pressure	5–12	30–70
Aγ	Motor to muscle spindle	3–6	15–30
Aδ	Pain, temperature	2–5	12–30
B	Preganglionic autonomic	<3	3–15
C	Dorsal root: Pain, temperature	0.4–1.2	0.5–2.0
	Sympathetic postganglionic	0.3–1.3	0.7–2.3

Electrical Properties of Nerve

Principles

The body fluid is distributed in the intracellular and extracellular compartments. The extracellular fluid (ECF) has greater concentration of sodium and chloride ions. The intracellular fluid has greater concentration of potassium ions and nondiffusible protein molecules. The distribution of these charged particles on either side of the cell membrane plays a major role in the cell integration and communication.

The movement of electric charges is called the **electrical current**. The electrical forces between the charges make them flow producing a current. The current depends on the difference in potential between the charged areas and nature of the membrane through which they pass.

The difficulty experienced by the electrical charge for its movement is known as **resistance**. The materials having high resistance are termed **insulators** and those with low resistance are called **conductors**. Water containing dissolved ions is a good conductor of electricity. Lipids contain few charged particles. Hence, they cannot carry current. The lipid layers of the plasma membrane have a high electrical resistance.

Resting Membrane Potential

It is the potential difference existing across the cell membrane at rest. It keeps the cell in an excitable state. Interior of the cell is negatively charged in relation to the exterior. Sodium and potassium ions play an important role in the generation of resting membrane potential (RMP).

In a motor nerve, the RMP is about −70 mV. It means that the intracellular fluid has an excess of negative charge.

The potential difference across the membrane has a magnitude of 70 mV. In the muscle RMP ranges from −80 to −90 mV.

Molecular Basis for RMP

- The concentration of sodium ions is greater outside the cell (150 mmol/L outside and 15 mmol/L inside the cell). The concentration of potassium ions is greater inside the cell (150 mmol/L inside and 5.5 mmol/L outside the cell). There is a natural concentration gradient for sodium ions directed inward and for potassium ions outward.

- In the resting state, permeability of membrane is greater for potassium ions. (Plasma membrane has 50–75 times greater number of potassium channels as compared to sodium channels.) Hence, potassium ions move out of the cell. This takes away the positive charges from within the cell.

- Sodium–potassium ATPase pump. It pumps three sodium ions to the exterior in exchange for two potassium ions pumped in. This differential pumping makes inside of the cell more negative. A pump that moves net charges across the

membrane and helps in the genesis of membrane potential is called the **electrogenic pump**.

- Large, nondiffusible, negatively charged protein molecules present within the cell add negativity to the inside of the cell.

Graded Potential

A sudden change in the environment around the excitable tissue alters the permeability of the membrane to different ions. This changes membrane potential over a small area of the membrane. The response dies down exponentially at the site of stimulation. The magnitude of response depends on the intensity of stimulation. This type of local potential without the period of latency is termed the **graded potential**.

The graded potentials in different regions are named as the receptor potential, pacemaker potential, and synaptic potential. The graded potential and action potential are the important ways by which the nerve cells process and transmit the information. The graded potentials transmit the signals for a short distance, whereas the action potentials transmit them over long distances.

Action Potential

It is an electrochemical change occurring in the excitable tissue in response to the threshold stimulus (Fig. 3.3). It has the phases of depolarization and repolarization.

The action potentials are large, rapid alterations in the membrane potential showing a fluctuation of about 100 mV (from −70 mV to +30 mV).

The nerve, muscle, endocrine, immune, and reproductive cells have the plasma membrane capable of producing the action potential.

Ionic Basis for Action Potential

- Stimulation of the motor nerve with minimal stimulus increases permeability of the membrane to the sodium ions.

- The sodium ions start entering into the cell.

- Inside of the cell tends to move toward the positive side. (A slight decrease in RMP potential leads to increased potassium efflux and chloride influx restoring RMP.)

- At around −55 mV (firing level), permeability of the membrane increases to sodium ions significantly resulting in its explosive entry.

- Sudden influx of sodium makes inside of the cell relatively positive. There is reversal of polarity. This phase is termed **depolarization**.

- During depolarization, the potential difference across the membrane becomes zero. This is termed the **isoelectric potential**. Subsequently, it becomes positive inside.

- On reaching a maximum potential of +35 mV (spike potential), the sodium channels are inactivated and the potassium channels open.

- The potassium ions move out of the cell.

- There is restoration of potential. This phase is termed **repolarization**.

- The potassium ions continue to move out of the cell in spite of reaching the resting level. Inside of the cell becomes relatively more negative. This phase is termed **hyperpolarization**. Hyperpolarization reduces excitability of the cell.

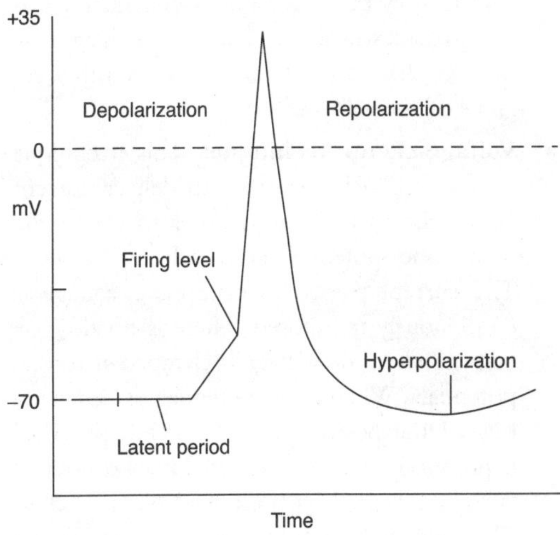

Fig. 3.3   Action potential in a neuron.

Influence of Ions on RMP and Action Potential

Sodium Ions   Decrease in the sodium ion concentration outside the cell reduces the size of the action potential. However, there is little influence on the RMP.

Potassium Ions   Increase in the potassium ion concentration outside the cell decreases the RMP.

Calcium Ions   Reduction in the extracellular calcium ion concentration increases excitability of the cell. This action is brought about by reducing depolarization necessary to alter the sodium and potassium conductance.

An increase in the calcium ion concentration decreases the excitability and stabilizes the membrane of the cell.

Local Response

When a subminimal stimulus is given to an excitable tissue, there is a depolarizing change. However, the number of ions entering the cell is unable to depolarize the cell up to the firing level. Hence, the response dies down exponentially at the site of stimulation. This is a **local response**.

The local response recorded at the anode is termed the **anelectrotonic potential**. The response recorded at the cathode is termed the **catelectrotonic potential**.

Graded Potential	Action Potential
Amplitude of response varies with strength of stimulus	Response shows all-or-none pattern
It does not have a threshold	It has a threshold (15 mV less than resting level)
The response can be summated	The response cannot be summated
There is no latent and refractory period	It has a latent and refractory period
It is a nonpropagated response	It is a propagated response
It can be depolarization or hyperpolarization	It is normally depolarization
Duration depends on the character of stimulus	Duration is fixed for a particular cell type
It depends on ligand-gated channels	It depends on voltage-gated channels

Types of Action Potential

Types of action potential are as follows:

(a) **Monophasic action potential:** The action potential is recorded by placing one electrode within and the other electrode outside the cell. The recording is in one direction. This is called the monophasic action potential.

(b) **Biphasic action potential:** The biphasic action potential is recorded when both the recording electrodes are placed over the surface of the cell (Fig. 3.4).

When the nerve is stimulated, the electrode nearest to the point of stimulation becomes positive. An upward deflection is recorded. The impulse gets propagated and reaches a point in between the two recording electrodes. At this point, no potential is recorded by both the electrodes. Hence, the recording returns to zero potential, or *isoelectric potential.* Later, impulse moves toward the second electrode. The first electrode becomes positive with respect to the second electrode. The recording shows a negative deflection. Thus, a biphasic action potential shows an upward deflection followed by an isoelectric line and then a downward deflection. Duration of the isoelectric potential depends on the speed of conduction.

The ionic basis for monophasic and biphasic action potentials are the same.

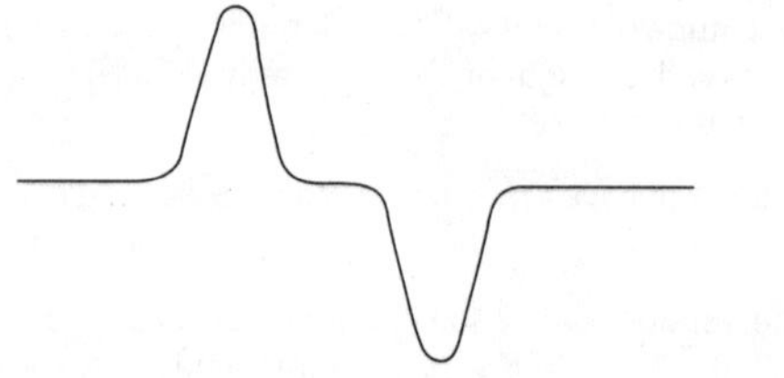

Fig. 3.4 Biphasic ation potential.

(c) **Compound action potential:** The action potential recorded from a group of nerve fibers results in compound action potential (Fig. 3.5). The mixed nerve is made up of groups of fibers with different conduction velocities. When all the fibers are stimulated simultaneously, impulses reach the recording electrode at different times. Hence, the recording shows multiple peaks. The number and size of peaks vary with the type of fiber stimulated in the nerve. The separation of peaks depends upon the conduction velocity and the distance of recording electrode from the point of stimulation. Greater the distance, greater is the separation of peaks.

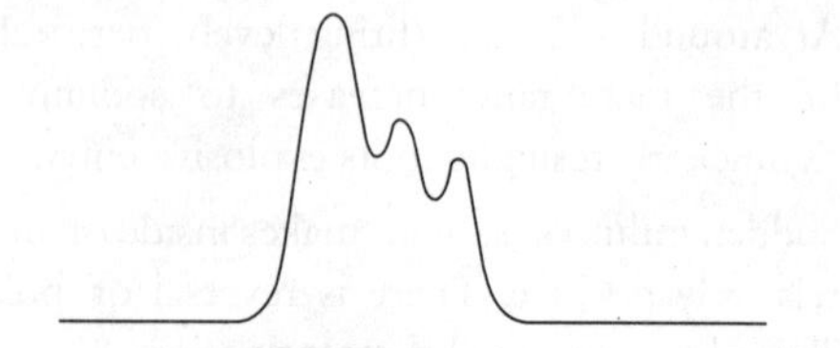

Fig. 3.5 Compound action potential.

The movement of ions across the membrane during electrical activity is determined by patch-clamp and voltage-clamp techniques.

- **Patch-clamp technique:** This technique allows determination of the activity of a single membrane channel. A specially designed micropipette is placed over the membrane and a tight seal of the membrane is obtained. A small patch of the membrane covering the tip of the pipette is isolated. This patch of the membrane contains one to several ion channels. The membrane is later perfused with fluids with different ionic concentrations on the outer or inner surface. This technique allows recording of the current flow through an individual channel. It also provides facility to study the behavior of the ion channels not influenced by other regions of the cell.

- **Voltage-clamp technique:** This technique uses a feedback apparatus to deliver current across the membrane in order to clamp the membrane potential at a selected voltage. The current passed to clamp the voltage is continuously monitored. There is no flow of current when the voltage is clamped at resting potential. When the potential is changed toward the positive side, an action potential is produced. There is an initial inward flow of current followed by prolonged outward flow. The voltage-clamp technique helps to study the changes in the ionic conductance underlying an action potential.

Nerve Impulse

The action potential is generated at the site of stimulation. It travels along the nerve fiber (Fig. 3.6). The traveling action potential constitutes an impulse. Thus, an impulse is defined as self-propagating physicochemical change.

Transmission

- Stimulation of the motor nerve results in the depolarization at the site of stimulation.
- Inside of the cell becomes positive in relation to the exterior.
- Positive charges move forward to the segment ahead within the cell.
- Positive charges are drawn backward from the segment ahead outside the cell.
- There is a drop in the positive charges outside the cell. It is termed the **current sink**.
- This results in depolarization of the next segment or the next node of Ranvier.
- Thus, the spread of depolarization wave results in transmission of impulse.

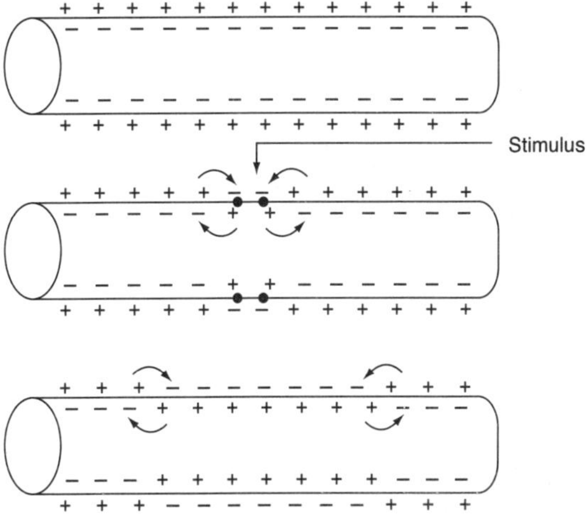

Fig. 3.6 Propagation of action potential.

Saltatory Conduction

In a myelinated nerve fiber, the myelin sheath is interrupted at periodic intervals called the nodes of Ranvier. During the impulse transmission, depolarization jumps from one node to the next node. This type of conduction is called saltatory conduction (from the Latin word *saltare*, meaning to hop or jump; Fig. 3.7).

Orthodromic Transmission

It is the conduction of impulse in normal direction (from the cell body toward the nerve terminal).

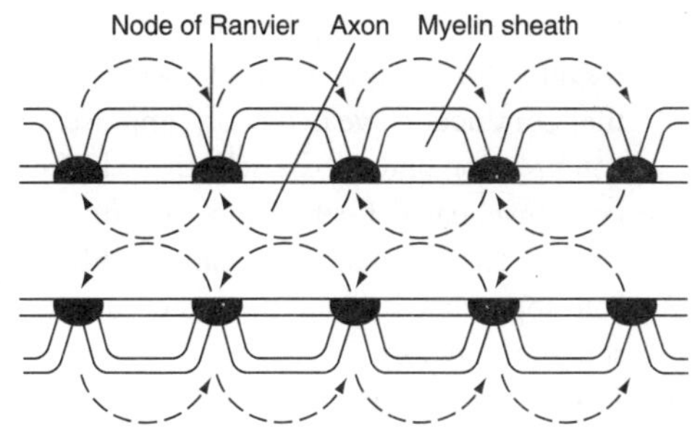

Fig. 3.7 Saltatory conduction.

Antidromic Transmission

Transmission of impulse in opposite direction is antidromic transmission.

Velocity

The factors influencing conduction velocity are as follows:

1. **Diameter of the nerve fiber:** An increase in the diameter increases the velocity of conduction. An increase in the diameter decreases the resistance to the flow of ions. The larger fibers have more ions to carry the current. The extracellular resistance does not influence the ionic movement because of a large volume of the ECF.

2. **Myelination:** The velocity of conduction in the myelinated fibers is 50 times greater than that in the unmyelinated fibers. Myelination restricts the generation of action potential to the nodes of Ranvier.

   The benefits of myelination are

   (a) higher conduction velocity for rapid transmission of impulse,
   (b) smaller diameter of nerve fiber to conserve space, and
   (c) higher metabolic efficiency because of reduced movement of ions and expenditure of energy.

3. **Temperature:** Increased temperature increases the conduction velocity. The conduction velocity decreases by about 3% for a fall of 1°C. The conduction block occurs at 7°C in large myelinated nerve fibers and at 3°C in unmyelinated fibers.

4. **Pressure:** The application of pressure resulting in compression of nerve reduces the conduction velocity of impulse. The compression and anoxia selectively block the large myelinated fibers. Thus, painful stimuli transmitted by small unmyelinated fibers are still appreciated when the other modes of sensation are lost.

5. **Local anesthetics:** The local anesthetics reduce the rate of conduction of nerve impulse or may even block its transmission. They prevent the generation of action potential by inhibiting the voltage-dependent opening of sodium channels.

6. **pH:** The decrease of pH decreases the velocity of the nerve impulse. A change in the conduction velocity can occur as a result of a disease or accident. The neural degeneration followed by regeneration leads to the formation of thinner fiber with a lower conduction velocity. The diseases like multiple sclerosis can reduce the thickness of the nerve fiber and localized loss of the myelin sheath. During the process of remyelination, the distance between the nodes of Ranvier is reduced. This reduces the conduction velocity.

Properties of a Nerve Fiber

1. **Resting membrane potential:** The nerve fiber shows a potential difference across its membrane at rest. This is resting membrane potential. In a motor nerve it is about −70 mV.

2. **Action potential:** It is an electrochemical change occurring in the excitable tissue in response to an adequate (threshold) stimulus. When a threshold stimulus is given, the membrane potential reaches the firing level, resulting in an action potential. However, a subthreshold stimulus fails to take membrane potential up to the firing level. This results in a local response. In a given nerve, the size (amplitude) of the action potential remains constant in spite of a variation in the intensity of stimulus. The difference in the intensity of stimulus is appreciated by a varying number of action potentials transmitted per unit time and not by its magnitude.

3. **Latent period:** It is the time interval between the application of a stimulus and the beginning of a response. It is the time required for the occurrence of electrochemical changes in the nerve to form an action potential (in response to a stimulus).

4. **Excitability:** It is the responding property of the tissue to a stimulus. It is also termed irritability. A threshold stimulus can excite the tissue. It causes a drop in the membrane potential to take it to the critical level and produces an action potential. A subthreshold stimulus produces a local response. The nerve fibers with larger diameter are more excitable and fibers with smaller diameter are less excitable.

5. **Conductivity:** The action potential generated at the point of stimulation is conducted along the nerve fiber. The conduction velocity in a nerve fiber depends on its myelination and diameter. In a myelinated fiber, the impulse is transmitted by the saltatory conduction. Hence, the conduction velocity is greater in a myelinated nerve fiber. The conductivity of nerve impulse is influenced by anoxia, pressure, and local anesthetics.

6. **All-or-none law:** When a nerve is stimulated with a threshold stimulus (or above the threshold strength), it responds to its maximum by producing an action potential. However, if the stimulus is subthreshold, there is no recordable response. Hence, action potential fails to occur.

7. **Refractory period:** It is of two types:

   (a) *Absolute refractory period:* It is the period during which a second stimulus of any magnitude fails to produce a response. The cell is refractory because a large number of sodium channels are voltage inactivated. Hence, these channels cannot be reopened until the membrane is repolarized.

   (b) *Relative refractory period:* It is the phase during which a second stimulus of greater intensity produces a response. During this phase, some of the sodium channels remain in an inactive state. Hence, a stronger stimulus is required to open a critical number of sodium channels to produce a response.

In a motor nerve, the entire phase of depolarization and first one-third of repolarization are absolutely refractory. The last two-thirds of repolarization is relatively refractory.

8. **Accomodation:** When a low-intensity stimulus is given to an excitable tissue, it responds initially. As the stimulus is continued for a prolonged duration, the magnitude of response gradually declines and may finally stop. This is termed accommodation. Accommodation is due to slower opening and delayed closing of the potassium channels. If the process of depolarization is rapid, opening of the sodium channel overrides the repolarizing forces and an action potential is produced. However, when the depolarization is produced slowly, opening of the potassium channels balances gradual opening of the sodium channels. Hence, the action potential is not produced.

9. **Infatigability:** The metabolic activity is very low in a nerve fiber during the conduction of an impulse. Hence, the nerve is resistant to being fatigued.

Nerve Injury

The neurons are liable to injury due to its cutting or crushing. The damage to the neurons is variable and it depends on the type and extent of injury. The neurons do not multiply during life. Fortunately, an injury to a peripheral nerve fiber (axon) does not destroy the neuron. The damaged neuron can undergo repair and become functional.

Types (Fig. 3.8)

Neuropraxia (First-Degree Injury)

In this type of injury, there is only pressure on the axon causing local anoxia. Recovery is possible within a few hours to a few days. The functions are lost temporarily. However, the structures remain intact.

Axonotmesis (Second-Degree Injury)

In this injury, the axon is divided but the endoneural sheath is continuous. This is due to prolonged and severe pressure on a part of the neuron. It is caused due to a crushing injury. Regeneration is possible in this type of injury. Recovery from the injury is complete.

Neurotmesis (Third-, Fourth-, and Fifth-Degree Injury)

In this injury, the axon and endoneural tube are divided. Regeneration is more complex. It depends on the alignment of the endoneural tube. If the alignment is restored, regeneration is possible.

Effect of Injury to the Neuron

The manifestation of injury depends on the site of injury. The injury close to the cell body results in destruction of the neuron. If the injury occurs to the axon away from the cell body, it results in degeneration followed by regeneration.

Wallerian Degeneration

When a nerve fiber is injured, a part of the nerve fiber distal to the site of injury undergoes changes. This process is known as the Wallerian degeneration. It is named after a person Waller, who first described the following changes:

(a) **Changes in nerve fiber distal to injury**
   - The peripheral part remains alive, conducting impulses up to 3 days from the day of injury.
   - The axis cylinder swells and breaks down into small rodlets.
   - The myelin sheath begins to disintegrate and is replaced by fatty droplets. This can be noted by about 8th day after injury and completed by 32nd day.
   - The phagocytes invade the peripheral part and engulf the broken-down processes of the axis cylinder and fat droplets. The hollow tube of the neurilemma with phagocytes is known as the **ghost tube**. If the neurilemma remains intact, the cells of Schwann multiply rapidly. These cells can bridge a gap of about 3 mm. If the gap at the site of injury is greater than 3 mm, repair occurs by the formation of scar tissue.

(b) **Changes proximal to injury**
   - The part of axon between the site of injury and the cell body constitutes the proximal part.

- Similar degenerative changes are seen in the proximal stump up to the nearest node of Ranvier. The changes are called **retrograde degeneration**.
- The cell body undergoes swelling with degeneration of Nissl granules. The neurofibrils disappear associated with a reduction in the number of Golgi apparatus. The nucleus is pushed to the periphery. This is called **chromatolysis**.

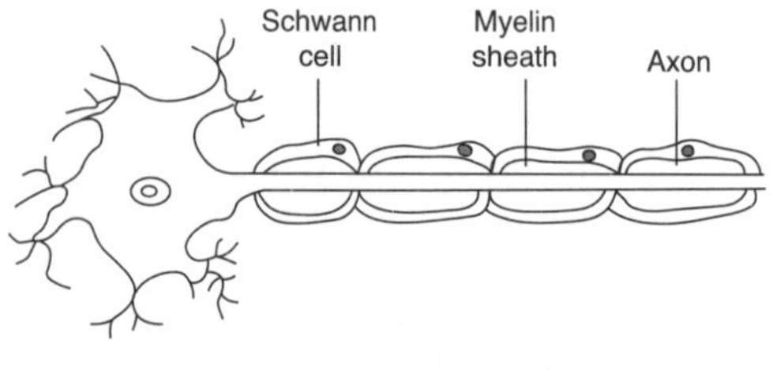

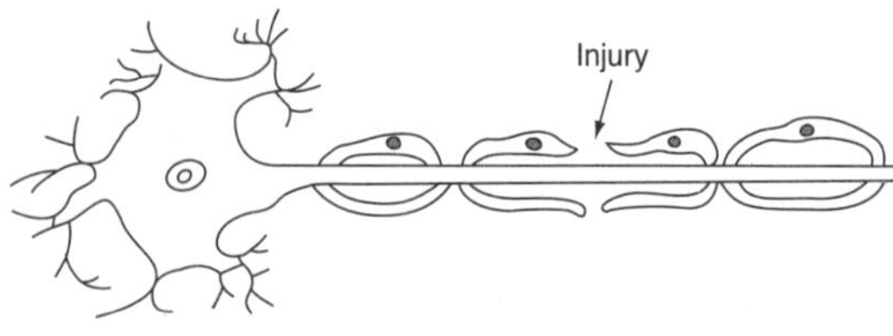

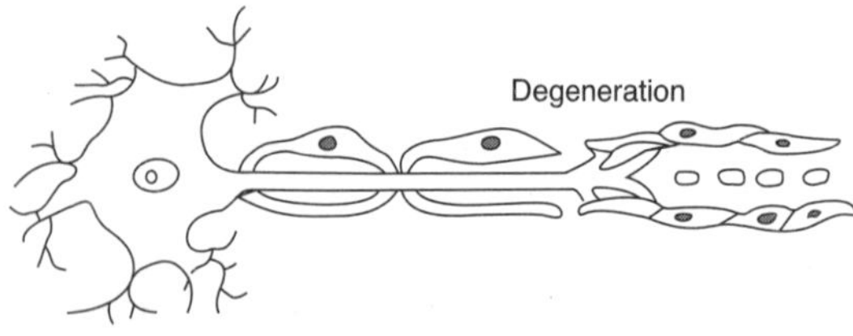

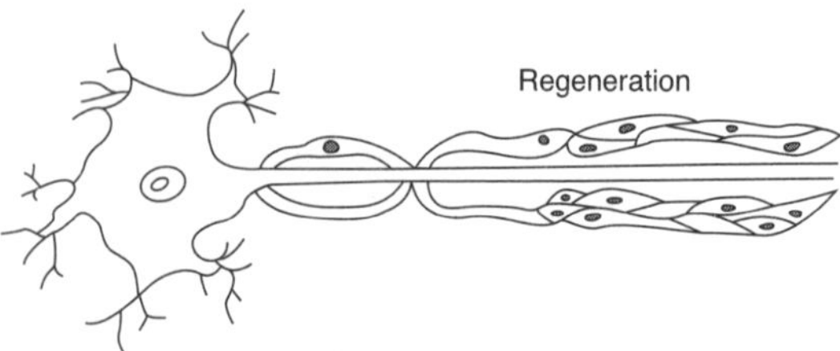

Fig. 3.8   Changes after nerve injury.

Regeneration of Damaged Nerve Fiber

If the cut end of the neurilemma is brought close to each other (less than 3 mm), the axis cylinder grows into the neurilemmal tube. Alignment of the neurilemmal tube is a critical factor for regeneration of the neuron.

The cut end of the axis cylinder gives out fine branches called **regenerative sprouting**. One of these branches reaches the cut end of the original tube and starts growing rapidly. The other branches disappear. The newly formed fibers are thin and unmyelinated. Later, the cells of Schwann and the myelin sheath are formed. The regeneration and growth of the nerve fiber through the site of injury is a very slow process. The presence of a scar tissue retards the growth of fibers. It results in the formation of a **neuroma**, which is the swollen central portion of the nerve fiber.

During the process of regeneration, the cell regains normal size. The Nissl granules reappear.

In reconstruction surgery (surgery done to repair the cut limb or fingers during an accident) care is taken to bring the cut ends of the neurilemmal tube as close as possible and to establish a good alignment.

Degeneration in CNS

The damage to neurons in the CNS results in its degeneration similar to that in the peripheral nervous system. However, regeneration does not occur due to the absence of neurilemma. The site of injury is covered by neuroglia with the formation of the glial scar.

Nerve Growth Factor

The nerve growth factor (NGF) is a protein necessary for the growth and maintenance of the sympathetic neurons. NGFs are picked up by neurons and transported to the cell body in a retrograde manner. The NGF present in the brain is responsible for the growth and maintenance of the cholinergic fibers. Other factors affecting the neuronal growth are

- ciliary neurotrophic factor,
- glial cell line–derived neurotrophic factor,
- leukemia inhibitory factor,
- insulin-like growth factor I,
- transforming growth factor,
- fibroblast growth factor, and
- platelet-derived growth factor.

Neuroglia (Fig. 3.9)

These are supporting cells present in the CNS. Their number is about 10–50 times that of neurons.

Types

The types of glial cells are as under.

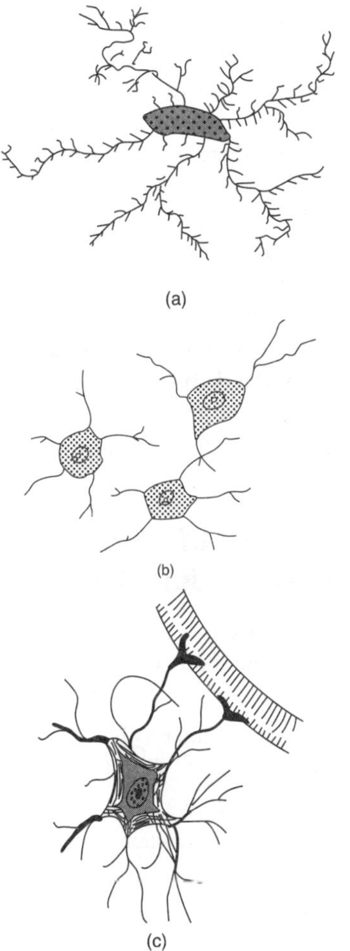

Fig. 3.9   Neuroglia: (a) microglia, (b) oligodendrocyte, and (c) astrocyte.

Microglia

The microglia resembles tissue macrophages. It consists of small cells with branching protoplasmic processes. The cytoplasm is scanty. The nucleus is oval and deeply stained. These microglia cells are derived from the mesoderm. They come from the bone marrow and enter the CNS through blood vessels.

The microglia cells acts as scavenger cells. They remove debris and dead bacteria from the CNS by the process of phagocytosis.

The microglia cells exhibit amoeboid movement and assemble in the region of damage from a considerable distance.

The microglia cells are usually found in the gray matter of the CNS close to the surface and ventricles of brain.

Oligodendroglia

The oligodendrocytes are present in both the gray and white matter, but more in the the white matter. The cells have a darkly stained spherical nucleus. The cytoplasm is dense with rough endoplasmic reticulum. The dendrites are fewer in number.

Their RMP depends on the extracellular potassium ion concentration.

The oligodendrocytes perform the following functions:

- They are helpful in the formation of myelin sheath around the axons. Each oligodendroglia cell forms myelin sheath for multiple neurons. Its function is similar to cells of Schwann of the peripheral nervous system.

- They insulate the axon and limit the flow of current around it.

Astrocytes

They are of two types:

(a) fibrous astrocytes and

(b) protoplasmic astrocytes.

The fibrous astrocytes are found in the white matter. They contain intermediate filaments.

The protoplasmic astrocytes are present in the gray matter. They have the granular cytoplasm.

- They are responsible for the formation of blood–brain barrier.

- Both the types of astrocytes send processes to blood vessels to form tight junction.

- The processes also envelop synapses and the surface of nerve cells.

- Resting membrane potential of the cell depends on extracellular K^+ concentration.

- They do not produce propagated action potential.
- They maintain a constant level of K^+ ion concentration in the CNS.
- They are helpful in the resynthesis of neurotransmitter glutamate.
- They produce substances that are trophic to the neuron.

Ependymal Cells

These cells line the ventricles of the brain and the central canal of the spinal cord. Their processes fuse with the processes of the astrocytes to form brain–CSF and blood–CSF barriers.

Neuromuscular Junction

The neuromuscular junction is a specialized area where a motor nerve ends on the skeletal muscle fiber (Fig. 3.10). Thus, it is a junction between a motor nerve and the muscle fiber.

The junction between the autonomic neurons with smooth and cardiac muscle is not well formed. Therefore, the transmission of impulse across these junctions is diffuse.

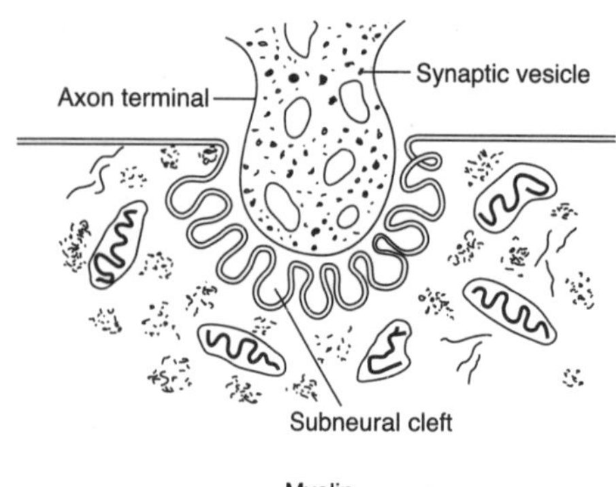

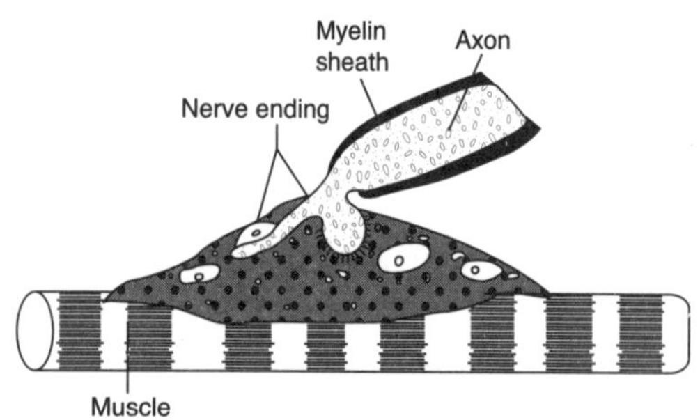

Fig. 3.10   Neuromuscular junction.

Neuromuscular junction consists of

1. **Prejunctional membrane:** This is the terminal part of the motor nerve with vesicles containing acetylcholine. The motor nerve supplying the muscle breaks into several branches called the axon telodendria. These terminals supply muscle fibers. The swollen part of nerve terminal (terminal button) fits into depression on the muscle membrane.
2. **Synaptic cleft or gutter:** It is a potential space between the nerve terminal and the muscle. This cleft produces structural discontinuity. However, there is functional continuity due to the presence of the neurotransmitter, acetylcholine.
3. **Motor end plate:** This is the muscle membrane containing the acetylcholine receptors. It forms the postjunctional membrane. The membrane is thrown into a number of folds termed the **subneural cleft**. The folding of membrane increases the surface area to accommodate more number of acetylcholine receptors.

Transmission of Impulse across Neuromuscular Junction

- Impulses arrive at the nerve terminal and increase the permeability of the membrane to calcium ions.
- Calcium ions enter the nerve terminal from ECF.
- Calcium binds to the anchoring proteins and releases the vesicles containing acetylcholine.
- Vesicles move to the nerve terminal and release neurotransmitter by either rupture or exocytosis.
- Neurotransmitter crosses the cleft and binds to the receptors present on postjunctional membrane.
- This increases the permeability of the membrane to sodium ions.
- Entry of **sodium** ions result in **end-plate potential** (EPP).
- EPP on reaching the firing level produces an action potential.
- Generated action potential travels over sarcolemma and passes through to sarcoplasmic reticulum

to activate contractile process in the muscle.

- Acetylcholine is destroyed by cholinesterase after completion of its function.

End-Plate Potential

It is a potential generated at the motor end plate during transmission of impulse across the neuromuscular junction. It is a graded, nonpropagated response without a period of latency. The EPP is due to increase in permeability of motor end plate to Na^+ ions.

When the EPP reaches the firing level, it forms an action potential.

Miniature End-Plate Potential

During rest, small quantity of acetylcholine is released from the presynaptic terminal. This alters permeability of the motor end plate to produce depolarizing change. This is called the miniature end plate potential (MEPP). It is incapable of producing an action potential.

Neuromuscular Blocking Agents

1. **Succinylcholine:** It binds to the acetylcholine receptors in the motor end plate. This produces prolonged depolarization as succinylcholine is destroyed slowly by the cholinesterase.
2. **Botulinum toxin:** It is a bacterial toxin produced by the organism clostridium botulinum. It prevents the release of acetylcholine from the presynaptic terminal.
3. **D-tubocurare:** It blocks the acetylcholine receptors in the motor end plate by competitive binding and prevents action of acetylcholine.
4. **Physostigmine and neostigmine:** They destroy the enzyme cholinesterase and prolong the action of acetylcholine. There is sustained depolarization at the motor end plate.
5. **Organophosphorus compounds (insecticides):** The mechanisms of action of these compounds are similar to the actions of physostigmine. Their effect is produced by sustained depolarization of motor end plate.

Applied Physiology

Myasthenia Gravis

It is an autoimmune disease caused by the destruction of acetylcholine receptors on the postjunctional membrane. This destruction is due to the formation of circulating antibodies to the nicotinic acetylcholine receptors. The disease is characterized by a failure in the neuromuscular transmission with repetitive nerve stimulation. The symptoms are weakness and fatigue of extraocular muscles, difficulty in speech, and in advanced stages, respiratory failure. In a patient of myasthenia gravis, intercostal muscles show a reduction in the amplitude of EPP and MEPP. In this condition, the release of acetylcholine is normal, but the receptors are reduced in numbers. The disease is associated with hyperplasia of thymus gland.

The patient has severe weakness in eyelid and respiratory muscles.

This condition can be managed by using anticholinesterase or cholinesterase inhibitors like physostigmine or neostigmine.

The cholinesterase inhibitors delay the destruction of acetylcholine. The neurotransmitter remains in contact with the receptor for a longer time, resulting in the depolarization of the motor end plate. The removal of thymus gland has beneficial effect in some patients.

Lambert–Eaton Syndrome

It is also a condition affecting the neuromuscular junction. The antibodies damage the calcium channels at the nerve terminal. The release of the neurotransmitter is defective and is associated with muscle weakness. However, the strength of the muscle increases with prolonged contraction due to greater release of the calcium ions.

Muscle Physiology

The muscles are excitable tissues similar to nerves. They are capable of contracting in response to a stimulus. They are classified as follows:

1. **Skeletal muscle:** It is a voluntary muscle, attached to the skeletal system. The muscle fibers show alternate dark and light bands called striations. They are supplied by the somatic nerves.

2. **Smooth muscle:** These are the involuntary muscles and do not have striation. They are supplied by the autonomic nervous system. The smooth muscles are present in the wall of GIT and the hollow internal organs. Hence, they are also called visceral muscles.

3. **Cardiac muscle:** They are striated muscles, but involuntary. They are regulated by input from the autonomic nervous system. These are muscles of the heart.

   The contraction of all types of muscles results in movement. The skeletal muscle contraction moves the joints, the smooth muscle contraction moves the contents of the hollow viscera, and the contraction of cardiac muscle causes the movement of blood. Hence, the muscles are termed *biological motors*.

4. **Other classifications:**
   (a) Histological appearance (based on striations)
       - striated muscle and
       - nonstriated muscle
   (b) Depending on the control
       - voluntary and
       - involuntary.

Structure of Muscle (Fig. 3.11)

A typical skeletal muscle consists of the tendon at either end. The muscle belly is enclosed in a connective tissue covering called the **epimysium.**

The muscle belly is made up of a number of muscle bundles called the **fascicles**. A layer called the perimysium covers each fascicle.

Each muscle fascicle is made of a large number of muscle fibers arranged parallel to each other. A single bundle of muscle fibers is covered by the **endomysium.**

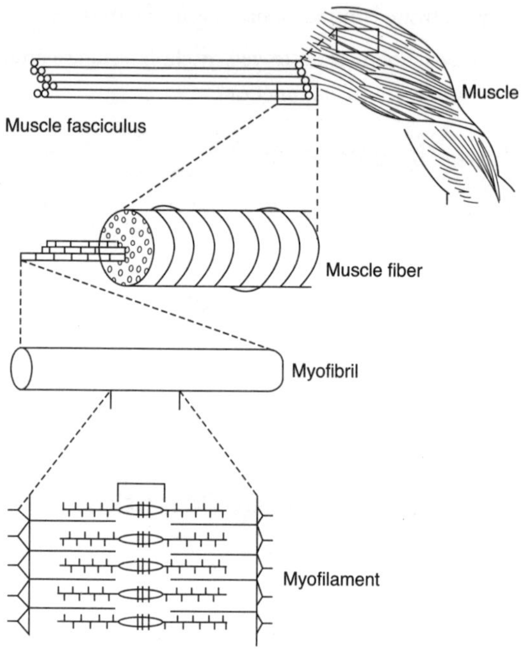

Fig. 3.11   Structure of muscle.

Each muscle fiber is a single-cell, cylindrical, and multinucleated, and is surrounded by a cell membrane called **sarcolemma.**

The muscle fiber contains several thousand myofibrils.

Each myofibril is in turn made up of around 1500 myosin and 3000 actin filaments. These are large protein molecules which cause muscle contraction.

The cytoplasm of the muscle cell is called the **sarcoplasm.**

The endoplasmic reticulum is called the **sarcoplasmic reticulum.**

Sarcomere

It is the structural and functional unit of the muscle bounded by two Z-lines (Fig. 3.12). The muscle fiber shows alternate light and dark bands.

The A (anisotropic) band is formed by myosin filaments. The I (isotropic) band is formed by thin filaments made of troponin, tropomyosin, and actin. The Z-line bisects the I-band. The center of A-band where the thin filaments do not overlap the thick filament forms the H-zone. The center of H-zone has a globular prominence and it forms the M-line.

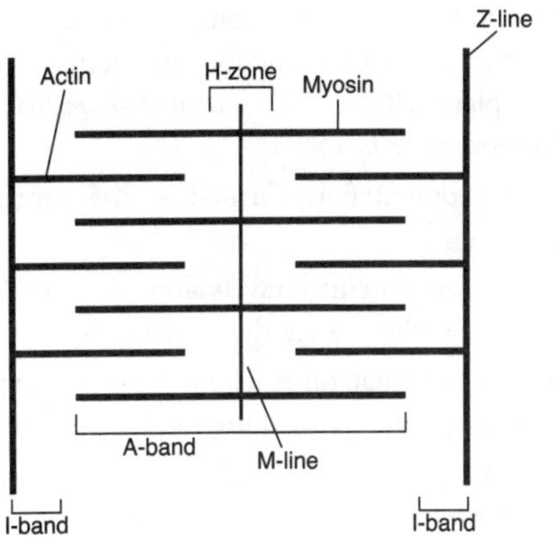

Fig. 3.12   Sarcomere.

Muscle Proteins

The various types of muscle proteins are

- myosin,
- actin,
- troponin, and
- tropomyosin (Figs. 3.13a–3.13c).

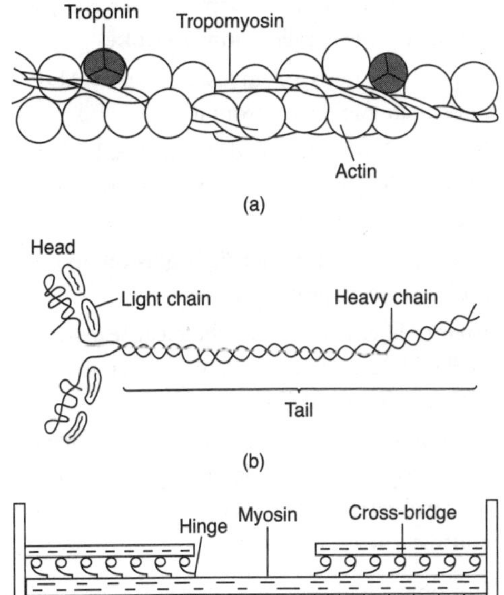

Fig. 3.13   (a) Actin, (b) myosin, and (c) arrangement of actin and myosin.

Myosin (Thick Filament)

It is composed of six polypeptide chains, two heavy chains and four light chains.

The two heavy chains wrap around each other to form a double helix. One end of each chain is folded into a globular head. The other portion forms the tail. The light chains are present near the myosin head.

The tails of the myosin molecules join together to form the body of the myosin filament. The head of myosin protrudes beyond the body. The portion of myosin connecting the head and body forms the arm. The head and arm together form the cross-bridges.

Thin Filament

The muscle proteins actin, troponin, and tropomyosin are present in the thin filament.

Actin   Each actin filament contains a double helix made of F-actin molecules. The F-actin molecules contain polymerized G-actin molecules. The ADP (adenosinediphosphate) molecules are present on the actin filaments. The actin filament has active binding sites. These are the sites where the cross-bridges of myosin interact to cause the muscle contraction.

Tropomyosin   It is a double helix structure. It lies in the groove between the two strands of F-actin filaments. In the resting state, tropomyosin covers the active binding sites on the actin molecule.

Troponin   This is a protein associated with thin filaments. Troponin is a globular protein with three subunits, namely, troponin I, troponin T, and troponin C.

Troponin I has affinity for actin.

Troponin T has affinity for tropomyosin.

Troponin C has affinity for calcium ions.

Sarcotubular System

It is the system of communication between the outer sarcolemma (cell membrane of the muscle) and the interior of the muscle (Fig. 3.14). The sarcolemma invaginates (enters) into the muscle to form the T-tubule (transverse tubule). On either side of the T-tubule there are two systems of tubules called the **sarcoplasmic reticulum** (L-tubules). The enlarged terminal part of L-tubule is called **terminal cistern.**

T- and L-tubules together form **sarcotubular system**.

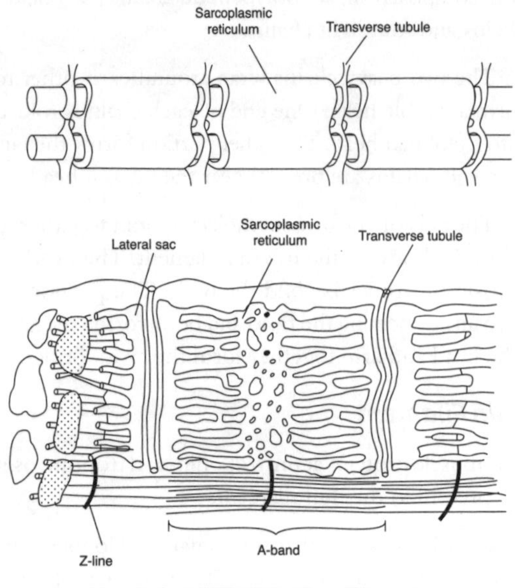

Fig. 3.14   Sarcotubular system.

Functions

- Helps in transmission of impulse from surface of the muscle to its interior.
- Stores calcium ions which are released during muscle contraction.

Excitation Contraction Coupling

The excitation contraction coupling comprises the electrochemical changes occurring in the nerve, neuromuscular junction, and muscle in response to a stimulus.

During this process, the electrical activity is transformed into the mechanical activity.

A threshold stimulus produces an action potential at the site of stimulation.

The impulse travels along the nerve fiber and crosses the neuromuscular junction.

This activates the motor end plate and generates the necessary signals to produce mechanical shortening of the muscle.

Mechanism of Muscle Contraction

- Stimulation of the motor nerve produces an impulse.

- This impulse travels through the nerve, crosses the neuromuscular junction, and activates motor end plate. (*Refer to the section Transmission across Neuromuscular Junction.*)

- Action potential is formed at the motor end plate.

- This action potential travels along the sarcolemma and enters the muscle through T-tubules.

- Action potential, on reaching the terminal vesicle of sarcoplasmic reticulum, releases calcium ions from it.

- Calcium ions bind to calcium-binding site on troponin molecule.

- This bondage of calcium with troponin weakens the link between troponin and tropomyosin. The change causes the tropomyosin to move away exposing the active binding site on actin molecule.

- Active site on the actin molecule attracts myosin.

- ATP molecule binds to the head of myosin.

- ATPase activity in the head of myosin cleaves ATP to ADP and phosphate with the release of energy.

- Energy liberated during chemical reaction helps in the sliding of thin filament over the myosin filament. This is called **power stroke**.

- Tilt of the head of myosin releases ADP and phosphate molecules from it.

- New ATP molecule binds to the head of myosin causing detachment of myosin from the active site on actin molecule.

- Cleavage of ATP molecule begins the next cycle, leading to new power stroke.

- Energy liberated during chemical reaction helps in the sliding of actin filament over the myosin filament. This is called power stroke.

- During relaxation, calcium ions are separated from troponin molecule and pumped back into terminal cistern. The changes that occur during contraction are reversed.

Troponin without the calcium ions allows tropomyosin to cover the active binding site on actin molecule.

The myosin cross-bridges reaching for the next active site on the actin molecule are blocked. Hence, the thin filaments are no longer held or pulled by the thick filament.

The muscle fiber remains at its contracted length. But the external forces restore the muscle to its resting length (Figs. 3.15a and 3.15b).

When myosin gets attached to the active site of actin there is a swiveling movement of the head of myosin that draws actin filament toward the center of the sarcomere. This movement or tilt of the myosin head is called the **power stroke**. Immediately after tilting, a new ATP binds to the myosin head and the head automatically breaks away from the active site and returns to its original position. Here it combines with a new binding site on actin and causes a new power stroke. Many such repeated power strokes produce successive shortening of the sarcomere resulting in muscle contraction.

Since this process involves sliding of actin filament over myosin filaments it is called **sliding filament theory** (Ratchet theory).

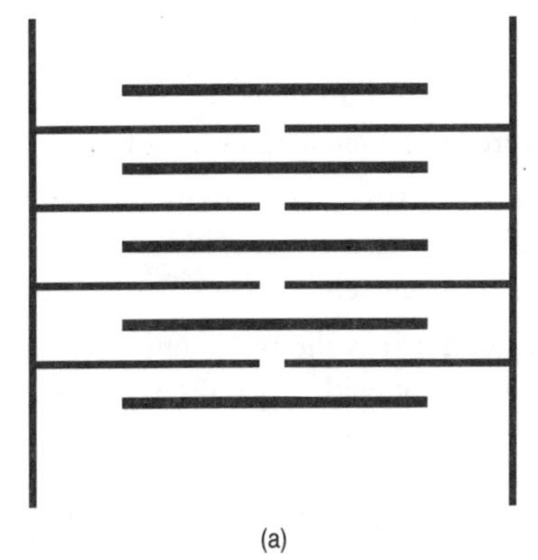

(a)

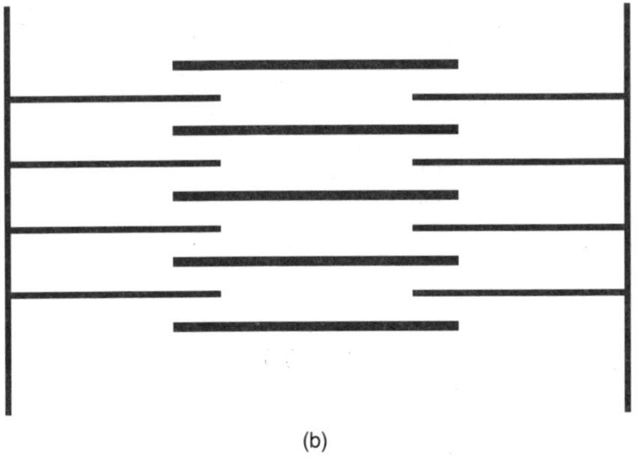

(b)

Fig. 3.15 Sarcomere: (a) contracted state and (b) relaxed state.

Energy Sources for Muscle Contraction

The energy needed for muscle contraction is obtained by hydrolysis of ATP. The energy is provided by breakdown of high-energy bonds present in ATP. The energy is necessary for the movement of thin filament over thick filament during contraction. ATP is resynthesized regularly from another high-energy compound creatine phosphate as the muscle can store only small quantity of ATP. Energy for the synthesis of both ATP and creatine phosphate comes from catabolism of food.

The efficient metabolism of nutrients by muscle requires glucose and oxygen. Glucose is a nutrient molecule containing chemical bonds. The energy contained in these chemical bonds is released during catabolic reaction and transferred to ATP and creatine phosphate. The muscle fibers maintain uninterrupted supply of glucose by storing it in the form of glycogen. The oxygen is needed for the metabolic process and aerobic respiration. The oxygen is stored in the muscle bound to a large protein molecule myoglobin.

Myoglobin is an iron-containing pigment similar to hemoglobin. It readily releases oxygen when the oxygen concentration decreases in the muscle. A gross reduction in the concentration of oxygen shifts the catabolic activity in the muscle to anaerobic respiration. Anaerobic respiration rapidly reforms ATP without the utilization of oxygen but it produces incompletely catabolized molecule called **muscle lactic acid**. The metabolic process of the cell is not 100% efficient. Some amount of energy is lost as heat.

Skeletal Muscle

Development

The skeletal muscle fibers develop from the cell of the embryonic mesoderm. These myogenic precursors (myoblasts) are formed from somites. The somites are tissue blocks adjacent to developing brain and spinal cord. The myoblasts migrate from somites to different parts of the body. They fuse with other cells in the new location to form multinucleated muscle fiber. The number of fibers in skeletal muscle appears to be genetically determined. However, the expression of their full genetic capacity depends on the development of the nerve supply to the muscle. The specific messengers, the **myogenic regulatory factors**, released by the motor nerves influence the development of the muscle fibers innervated by them.

Physiological Properties

Simple Muscle Twitch

It is the response of the muscle to a single stimulus (Fig. 3.16).

It consists of the following phases:

1. **Latent period (0.01 s):** It represents the time interval from application of stimulus to actual commencement of the response. The various electrical and mechanical changes occurring in the nerve and muscle after stimulation account for the latent period. First half of the latent period corresponds to the absolute refractory period. The second half corresponds to relative refractory period.

2. **Contraction period (0.04 s):** It represents the time from the commencement of contraction to reach maximum contraction.

3. **Relaxation period (0.05 s):** It is the period from the peak of contraction to the point of complete relaxation. In ideal condition, the contraction period is shorter than relaxation period. This is explained on the basis of release and reuptake of calcium ions.

4. During contraction, the calcium ions are released from the sarcoplasmic reticulum rapidly. But during relaxation, the calcium ions are pumped back into the sarcoplasmic reticulum. Pumping back of calcium takes a longer time. This accounts for a longer relaxation period.

5. **Total twitch period (0.10 s).**

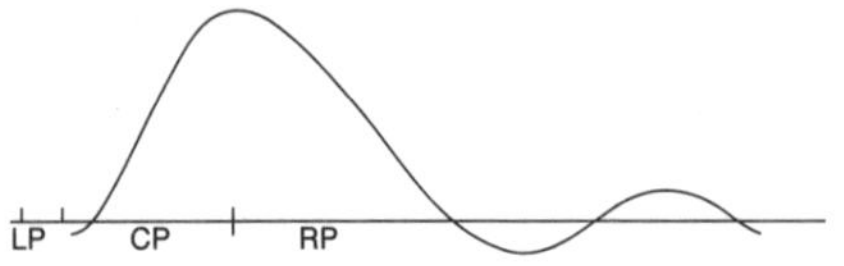

Fig. 3.16 Simple muscle twitch. LP, latent period; CP, contraction period; RP, relaxation period.

Excitability

- **Stimulus:** It is a sudden and significant change in the environment brought about by release of energy.

The types of stimuli are

(a) electrical,
(b) chemical,
(c) mechanical, and
(d) thermal.

Electrical stimuli are normally preferred as they can be measured accurately and their quantum can be regulated.

The stimulus has two variables, strength and duration.

Strength–duration curve is the relationship between the strength of the stimulus and the duration for which it is to be given to excite a tissue (Fig. 3.17).

- **Rheobase:** It is the minimum strength of current delivered indefinitely to excite a tissue.

- **Utilization time:** It is the minimum time required to excite a tissue with a single rheobasic strength of current.

- **Chronaxie:** It is the minimum time required to excite a tissue with twice the rheobasic strength of current.

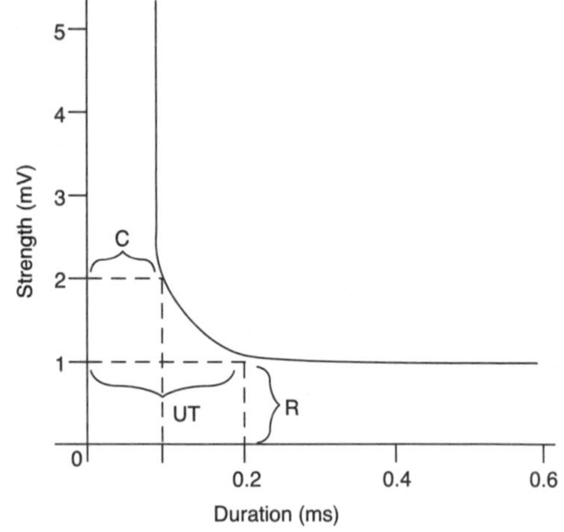

Fig. 3.17 Strength–duration curve. C, chronaxic, R, rheobase; UT, utilization time.

Contractility

The muscle contracts when it is stimulated. The force generated during contraction is dependent on initial length of the muscle.

1. Length–tension relationship
   - **Initial length:** It is the length of muscle fiber just before the contraction.
   - **Resting length:** It is the length of the muscle in relaxed state with its attachment intact.
   - **Equilibrium length:** It is the length of the muscle in relaxed state when it is cut off from its attachments.
   - **Optimal length:** It is the length of the muscle at which maximum tension is generated during contraction.
2. Length–force relationship
   - **Starling's law:** The force of contraction is directly proportional to the initial length of the muscle fiber within physiological limits.

     Molecular basis for Starling's law:

     (a) When the muscle fiber is stretched, more and more active binding sites on actin molecule are exposed. This helps in the formation of greater number of cross-bridges.

     (b) Stretch of the muscle increases resting metabolism producing heat. Increased temperature brings about better enzymatic activity. Increase of enzymatic activity enhances the force of contraction.

All-or-None Law

When a single skeletal muscle fiber or whole of the cardiac muscle is stimulated with an adequate stimulus, it responds to its maximum. If stimulus is not adequate, it does not respond at all.

Latent Period

It is the time interval between the application of stimulus and the onset of contraction.

Refractory Period

It is of two types:

1. **Absolute refractory period:** It is the period during which a second stimulus of any magnitude fails to produce a response. It corresponds to the first half of the latent period during muscle contraction.
2. **Relative refractory period:** It is the phase during which a second stimulus of greater intensity produces a response. It corresponds to the second half of the latent period during muscle contraction.

In the case of cardiac muscle, the entire phase of the cardiac contraction is in absolute refractory period. Hence, the cardiac muscle cannot be tetanized.

Fatigue

It is temporary inability of the muscle to respond satisfactorily after being repeatedly stimulated. (It is temporary state of inexcitability of the muscle.)

Causes

1. Depletion of acetylcholine at the nerve terminal.
2. Exhaustion of source of energy, ATP.
3. Accumulation of metabolic end products like lactic and pyruvic acid.

Site

1. In an isolated preparation, the site of fatigue is in neuromuscular junction.
2. In an intact animal, the site of fatigue is in synapse.

Tone

Tone is a state of partial contraction of the muscle at rest. It is also defined as the resistance offered by the muscle to its passive movement.

Effect of Increasing Strength of Stimulus

The contractile response of the muscle depends on the intensity of stimulation.

Motor Unit

It is a single motor nerve innervating a group of muscle fibers. The number of muscle fibers in a motor unit is about 20–50.

Quantal Summation

A gradual increase in the strength of stimulus increases the force of contraction. It is due to the activation of more and more motor units. This phenomenon is termed the **recruitment of motor unit.** The summated response is the **quantal summation.**

Temporal Summation

When the frequency of stimulation is increased, the stimuli add up and therefore the total strength of contraction is increased. This is termed the **temporal summation.**

Heat Production in the Muscle

Resting heat: It is heat given off by the muscle at rest. It measures the basal metabolic rate of the muscle.

Activation heat: It is heat produced by the muscle when it is contracting.

Shortening heat: It is heat generated because of the shortening of the muscle. It is due to the structural changes.

Recovery heat: It is heat liberated during recovery of the muscle to its precontraction state.

Types of Muscle Contractions

Isotonic Contraction

In the isotonic contraction, tension in the muscle remains constant but the length of the muscle changes. Effective work is done in this type of contraction. A part of energy is converted to useful work and the remaining is converted to heat, e.g., lifting a small weight from the ground.

Isometric Contraction

In this type of contraction, there is a change of tension in the muscle fiber but there is no change in the length. There is no effective work done. Energy is converted to heat, e.g., trying to lift a heavy object, which cannot be moved.

Effect of Load on Muscle Contraction

The load acting on the muscle before or during contraction alters its contractile response.

1. **Free load:** If the weight is acting on the muscle before the commencement of contraction, it is said to be free-loaded. This increases the initial length of the muscle and hence the force of contraction.

2. **After load:** The muscle is said to be after-loaded if weight is acting on the muscle during contraction.

Effect of Two Successive Stimuli

When a second stimulus is given immediately after the first, it potentiates the effect of the first stimulus.

Beneficial Effect   A second stimulus is applied to the muscle immediately after its relaxation following the first contraction. The second contraction has greater amplitude. This is termed the **beneficial effect.**

It is due to

-   calcium ions released during first contraction add to calcium released during second contraction to potentiate the effect;

-   reduction in viscosity of the muscle;

-   increase in the temperature of muscle, hence an enhanced enzyme activity and a better contraction.

Summation of Contractions (Fig. 3.18)

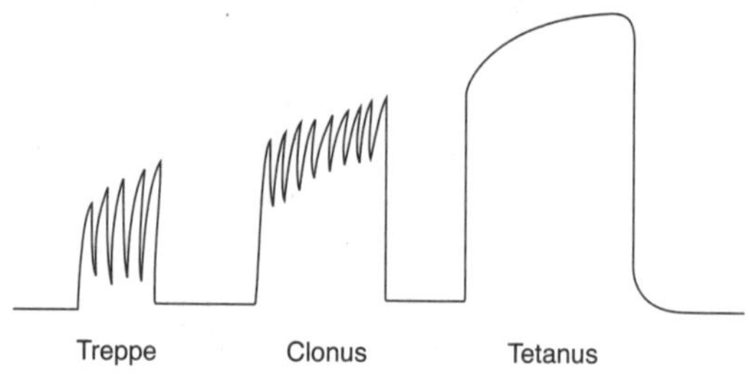

Fig. 3.18   Summation of contractions.

Treppe   When series of stimuli are given to the muscle in rapid succession, it increases the force of contraction gradually. This is **treppe** or **staircase phenomenon.**

Tetanus   A series of stimuli delivered to the muscle with a very short time interval between them results in a state of sustained contraction. This is termed **tetanus.**

Tetanizing frequency for frogs muscle is 30/s and for human muscle it is over 60/s.

Clonus   If the frequency of stimuli is less than tetanizing frequency, it results in clonus. The clonus is an incomplete tetanus.

Applied Physiology

Tone of the muscle can be altered in different conditions.

Hypertonia

It is a state of the muscle where tone is increased. It is described as the **rigidity** or **spasticity**.

Hypertonia is seen in upper motor neuron lesions and Parkinsonism.

Hypotonia

The reduction in tone of the muscle is termed **hypotonia**. It is clinically identified as **flaccidity**. Total absence of tone is **atonia**.

Hypotonia is seen in lower motor neuron lesion.

Muscle Cramps

Involuntary tetanic contractions of muscle produce muscle cramps. It is caused due to electrolyte imbalance surrounding the muscle.

Duchenne's Muscular Dystrophy

It is a genetic disorder common in males caused by a missing fragment in the X chromosome. It is a degenerative disease that leads to progressive wasting of the muscle and loss of ability to contract. The muscle is replaced by fat and fibrous tissue. It is seen in skeletal muscles. The condition is also called pseudohypertrophic muscular dystrophy.

Rigor mortis

Rigor mortis is a state of rigidity or stiffness developed in the muscle after death. Rigor mortis begins within 3–4 h and continues up to 24 h. However if the person or animal is killed in action, rigor mortis begins in about 30 min.

After death, there is exhaustion of ATP.

Actomyosin complex is formed in an abnormal, irreversible, and resistant way to produce the rigidity.

Changes during Rigor Mortis

- Muscle looses its excitability and shortens in length.
- It becomes more viscous.
- The glycogen stores disappear.
- It becomes acidic and liberates carbonic acid.

Importance:

Helps to determine time and cause of death.

Denervation Hypersensitivity

When a motor nerve supplying the muscle is cut, muscle degenerates and undergoes atrophy. It exhibits abnormal excitability responding to circulating acetylcholine. This is denervation hypersensitivity.

Denervated skeletal muscle shows fine, irregular contractions of the individual fibers termed **fibrillation**. Fibrillation is due to instability of membrane potential.

This response is due to the formation of more number of acetylcholine receptors on the surface of the muscle. The resting membrane potential decreases.

As a delayed response, muscle looses its capacity to develop tension on stimulation, change in enzymatic composition, and decrease in diameter of the fiber (**atrophy**).

Electromyogram

It is recording of electrical activities of the muscle. Activation of motor units can be studied by this recording. Small metal electrodes are placed over the skin overlying the muscle. These electrodes are used for recording the electrical activity.

Alternatively, hypodermic needles can also be used for recording. By using the needle electrodes, it is possible to record the activity from a single muscle fiber.

Red (Slow) Muscle	White (Fast) Muscle
Responds slowly	Responds rapidly
Has a long latency	Has a short latency
Is postural muscle, e.g., long muscles of back	Performs fine, skilled m ovements, e.g., extraocular muscles
Myoglobin content is more	Myoglobin content is less
Mitochondria are more in number	Mitochondria are less in number

Smooth Muscles

The smooth muscles are involuntary in function (Fig. 3.19). They do not exhibit the alternate light and dark bands. They are different from skeletal muscles by the following features:

- Z-line is not well defined.
- Actin and myosin are attached to dense bodies which replace Z-line.
- Sarcoplasmic reticulum is not well developed.
- Regulatory protein troponin is absent.
- Arrangement of actin and myosin does not follow a regular pattern.

Smooth muscles have an unstable membrane potential capable of contracting without nerve supply. They show continuous, irregular contractions. This partial contracted state is called **tonus** or **tone**. The membrane potential does not show a true resting value. It is low when the tissue is active and high when it is inhibited. During the period of quiescence the average resting membrane potential is about −50 mV.

Smooth muscles are of two types:

1. **Visceral smooth muscle (single unit):** It consists of thousands of muscle fibers functioning as a single unit. It is present in intestine, uterus, and ureter.

2. **Multiunit smooth muscle:** Each muscle is made up of discrete individual fibers. Each fiber has a separate innervation. The individual fiber can contract independently. It is present in the iris and ciliary muscle of the eye.

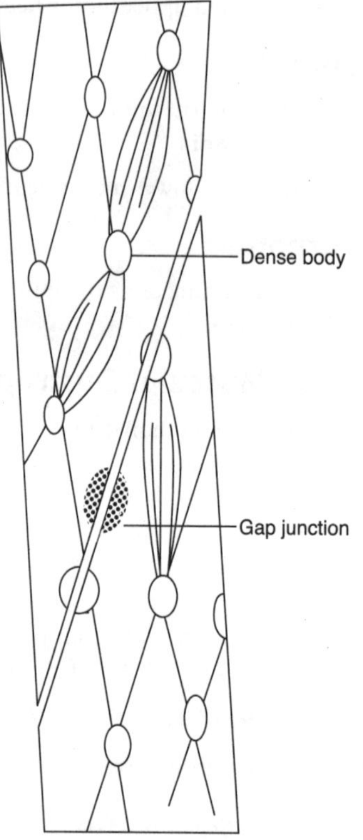

Fig. 3.19   Smooth muscle.

Molecular Basis of Smooth Muscle Contraction

- Stimulation of smooth muscle causes entry of calcium ions from the ECF.
- Calcium binds to the calcium-binding protein calmodulin.
- Calcium–calmodulin complex activates the enzyme myosin light-chain kinase, phosphorylating myosin.
- Phosphorylation reaction activates myosin ATPase releasing energy for the process of contraction. Actin slides on the myosin producing contraction (shortening).
- During relaxation, myosin is dephosphorylated by myosin light-chain phosphatase.

- However dephosphorylation does not lead to complete relaxation of the smooth muscle. The initial length is not restored immediately due to the presence of **latch bridges**.

Plasticity: Length–Tension Relationship

The special character of smooth muscle is variability of the tension at a given length.

Stretch of the smooth muscle results in contraction initially. However if the muscle is stretched further, it relaxes. This is termed **plasticity**.

Nerve Supply to Smooth Muscle

The visceral smooth muscles are supplied by two divisions of the autonomic nervous system. The function of these nerves is to modify activity in the muscle rather than to initiate the action.

The stimulation of one division of autonomic nervous system usually increases activity in the smooth muscle whereas stimulation of other division reduces the activity.

Sports and Exercise Physiology

Exercise is a stressful condition that calls for adjustment in functioning of the various systems.

Exercise is graded as

- mild,
- moderate, and
- severe.

Depending on the degree of exercise, there are adjustments in the body.

Performance of an athlete depends on the extent of training and adjustments of various systems.

Role of Muscle in Exercise

Critical factors that determine the performance of the muscle are as follows:

- **Strength:** It is the maximal contractile force that depends on cross-sectional area of the muscle.
- **Endurance:** It is the ability of the muscle to perform a sustained action. This depends on the nutrition of muscle.
- **Power:** It is the quantum of work done by the muscle in unit time. Training influences the power of the muscle.

Muscle derives the energy for its metabolic activities from

1. adenosine triphosphate,
2. phosphocreatine–creatine system, having the high-energy phosphate bond; energy derived used to replenish ATP;
3. glycogen–lactic acid system—glycogen in this system is broken down to glucose, which is used for the energy.
4. Aerobic system—foodstuff gets oxidized in mitochondria to provide energy.

Glycogen used during exercise is resynthesized from carbohydrates and fats taken in the diet.

After the completion of exercise, oxidative metabolism of aerobic system replenishes energy-providing systems of the body.

Training of the muscle increases its bulk and it undergoes hypertrophy. Exercise-induced hypertrophy increases the efficiency of the muscle.

Respiratory Changes

The demanding condition like exercise increases oxygen consumption and pulmonary ventilation. However, pulmonary ventilation is not the limiting factor for exercise.

The rate of oxygen usage under maximal aerobic metabolism (VO_{2max}) increases with training of the athlete.

Diffusing capacity of oxygen through the respiratory membrane increases with training.

The blood gases do not show significant variation in its concentration even in severe exercise.

Oxygen Debt

Muscular exercise increases demand for the supply of oxygen. Initially, the increased demand is met by enhanced flow of blood due to local vasodilatation. With the progress of exercise, oxygen demand increases and the energy requirement is satisfied by anaerobic mechanism. The extra amount of oxygen consumed by tissue during its increased activity is termed **oxygen debt**.

Cardiovascular Changes

The exercising muscle needs more oxygen and nutrients. This increased demand warrants increase in blood flow to the muscle.

The normal blood flow of resting skeletal muscle is 2–4 mL/100 g/min. During muscle contraction blood flow increases 30-fold. This is accomplished by increasing the cardiac output. However, the actual contractile process reduces the blood flow by compressing the blood vessels.

The force of compression on the blood vessel is overcome by vasodilatation caused by accumulation of metabolites locally and by increase in the systolic blood pressure. As the intensity of exercise increases, the blood flow to the muscle increases. The vasodilatation in the muscle decreases the peripheral resistance reducing the diastolic blood pressure.

In an untrained person, the cardiac output increases fourfolds, whereas in a trained individual it can increase up to sixfolds.

Exercise training causes hypertrophy of the cardiac muscle and hence increases its pumping capacity.

There is also demonstrable increase in the stroke volume during exercise and even at rest.

Heat Generation during Exercise

The muscle under ideal condition converts 20–25% of energy input to useful work. The remaining energy is utilized for the production of heat.

Although a small percentage of heat is used to overcome viscous resistance and friction of blood flow, a major part of heat is injected into core of the body.

Increase in body temperature stimulates hypothalamic center that regulates heat-dissipating mechanism. There is a marked increase in the sweat secretion; the vaporization of this sweat results in heat loss.

During severe exercise, normal heat loss mechanisms fail to lose the heat generated.

Reduction in heat loss when compared to its generation can increase the body temperature significantly to result in **heat stroke**.

Fluid and Electrolyte Balance

The heat generated during exercise is lost with excessive sweating. There is associated electrolyte loss. The loss of fluid and electrolytes can adversely affect the performance.

If an athlete gets acclimatized to heat, formation of sweat reduces. There is secretion of aldosterone, which reabsorbs sodium before it is excreted by sweat. However, there could be potassium loss in such conditions. Thus, exercise could result in fluid and electrolyte imbalance.

Effect of Training

Strenuous exercise training produces hypertrophy of the muscle fibers. Endurance exercise training increases capacity for oxidation of pyruvates and long-chain fatty acids. This is due to an increase in the density of mitochondria and the enzymes needed for oxidation of long-chain fatty acids.

There is an increase in capillary density and myoglobin. These modifications enhance diffusion of oxygen from cell membrane to mitochondria.

Trained individuals have increased intramuscular stores of triglycerides and lower serum triglycerides. Their muscle can use lipids directly from blood.

During submaximal exercise, they derive more energy from fats than carbohydrates.

The liver and muscle glycogen stores are better maintained during exercise.

During exercise, greater proportion of oxygen is extracted from the blood supplying active muscle.

Effect of Aging

The size, speed, and strength of skeletal muscle decrease with age. The age-related reduction in skeletal muscle mass is termed **sarcopenia**. The muscle fibers undergo denervation with aging. Few of the denervated fibers die and the remaining fibers get reinnervated by nerve fibers from the nearby motor unit. Thus, there is a decrease in the number of motor units but the size of individual motor unit increases. This results in overall slowing of muscle contraction. The potency of synaptic transmission also decreases due to structural changes at the neuromuscular junction.

Effect of Damage to the Muscle

Damaged muscle fibers do not divide and they lack the capacity for regeneration. The damage is repaired by activation of satellite cells present beneath the basal lamina of muscle fiber. These are special generation of myoblasts that migrate from somite during development. Appropriate stimulus triggers them to undergo mitosis, increase in number, and finally fuse to form multinucleated muscle fibers.

CHAPTER 4

Cardiovascular System

The cardiovascular system consists of heart and blood vessels. The heart acts as a pump and the blood vessels are channels carrying blood.

The heart is covered by an outer fibrous pericardium and inner serous pericardium. The space between these two layers is termed the **pericardial cavity**. The fluid present in the pericardial cavity ensures smooth movement of the heart by acting as a lubricant.

The human heart consists of four chambers, two atria and two ventricles. The opening between the right atrium and the right ventricle is guarded by the **tricuspid valve**. The opening between the left atrium and the left ventricle is guarded by **bicuspid valve** (mitral valve). These valves present between the atrium and the ventricle on both the sides are together called the **atrioventricular** (AV) valves. The AV valves permit the flow of blood from the atrium to the ventricle and prevent the blood from flowing in the opposite direction.

The opening and closing of the AV valves is passive. It depends on the pressure changes in atrium and ventricle. When the pressure increases in the atrium, the valves are pushed open and the blood flows from the atrium to the ventricle.

The contraction of the ventricles increases the AV pressure. This in turn closes the AV valves. The closure of the AV valves prevents the backward flow of blood from the ventricle to the atrium.

The AV valves are held in position by the **papillary muscles** arising from the walls of the ventricle.

The papillary muscles are attached to the free margins of AV valves with the help of fibrous strands termed **chordae tendinae**.

The papillary muscles prevent the bulging of AV valves into the atrium during ventricular contraction. These muscles do not help in opening or closing of the valves.

The pulmonary artery arises from right ventricle and aorta arises from left ventricle. The blood flow through these vessels is regulated by the pulmonary and aortic **semilunar valves**.

The arteries carry blood away from the heart and the veins carry blood toward the heart. All the arteries carry oxygenated blood except pulmonary artery. All the veins except pulmonary vein. Carry deoxygenated blood.

Structure of Heart (Fig. 4.1)

The wall of the heart has three layers:

1. epicardium,
2. myocardium, and
3. endocardium.

Epicardium is a serous layer covering the heart.

Myocardium is made up of cardiac muscle cells which are involuntary.

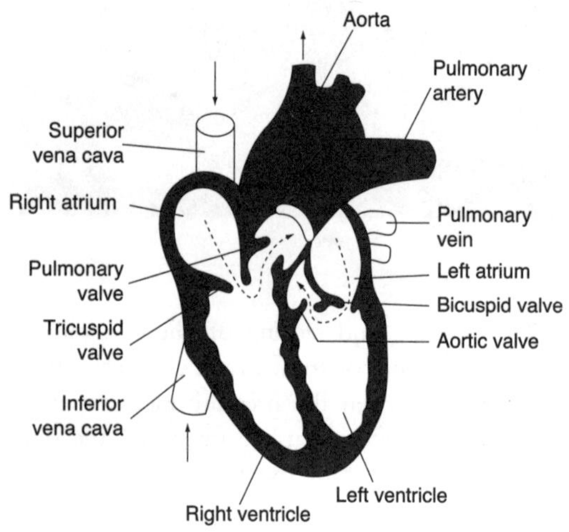

Fig. 4.1 Structure of heart.

Endocardium is a single layer of endothelial cells lining the inner surface of the heart.

The cardiac muscles have branching fibers with centrally located nucleus. The adjacent fibers are connected by intercalated disks. These are cell membranes that separate cardiac muscle cells from one another. The electrical resistance through the intercalated disk is 1/400th of the cardiac cell membrane. The intercalated disks contain gap junctions. The gap junctions (specialized intercellular connections) between the adjacent fibers offer low resistance to the passage of ions. Because of the presence of low-resistance bridges, cardiac muscle fibers contract as a single unit. It is termed **functional syncytium**.

The desmosomes (a cell structure specialized for cell-to-cell adhesion) in the disk provide site for adhesion between two cardiac muscle cells. These adhesions help to transmit the tension developed in one cell to the other during contraction.

Two atria or two ventricles contract simultaneously as a single unit.

The cardiac muscle has the contractile proteins actin and myosin arranged in a sarcomere (Fig. 4.2). It has the characteristic A-, I-, and H-bands with M- and Z-lines. In the cardiac muscle, the sarcoplasmic reticulum is not well formed. T-tubule is wider and located at the Z-line unlike the A–I junction in the skeletal muscle.

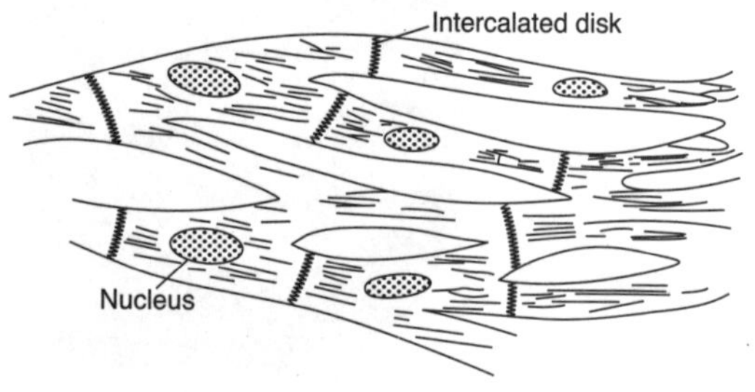

Fig. 4.2 Cardiac muscle.

Nerve Supply to Heart

The heart is supplied by the sympathetic and parasympathetic nerves.

Sympathetic Innervation

The sympathetic nerves to the heart are from the first five thoracic segments of the spinal cord. The sympathetic preganglionic fibers arise from the thoracic segments. They reach superior, middle, and inferior cervical ganglion located in the sympathetic chain. The postganglionic fibers arising from these ganglions innervate the heart. The sensations from the heart are also carried by the sympathetic nerves. Stimulation of sympathetic nerves to the heart increases the rate and force of contraction.

Parasympathetic Innervation

The parasympathetic nerve supply is through the vagus nerve. The preganglionic parasympathetic fibers arise from the vagal nucleus. They pass through the cardiac nerve and end in the parasympathetic ganglion in the heart. The postganglionic fibers arise from the ganglion to innervate the heart. The right vagus supplies the sinoatrial (SA) node and the left vagus supplies the atrioventricular (AV) node. The stimulation of parasympathetic nerve reduces rate and force of contraction.

The stimulation of the left vagus delays the conduction of the impulse through the AV node. The ventricles do not have parasympathetic supply.

Blood Circulation

The blood pumped out from the left side of the heart passes through

- **large-sized arteries**, e.g., aorta;

- **medium-sized arteries**, e.g., femoral artery;

- **small-sized arteries**;

- **arterioles** (resistance vessels)—the precapillary sphincter offers resistance to the flow of blood and hence they are termed resistance vessels;

- **capillaries** (exchange vessels)—the capillaries have a thin wall. They participate in exchange of substances and gas across its wall. The blood returns to the heart through venous system;

- **venules** (capacitance vessels)—they are capable of storing a reasonable quantity of blood when it is not in circulation and release the same when it is needed most;

- **major veins**, e.g., superior and inferior vena cava, return blood to right side of the heart.

Blood Vessel

Structure

The blood vessels except the capillaries have distinct layers in their wall. The layers from outside to inside are

- tunica adventitia (externa),

- tunica media, and

- tunica intima (interna).

The tunica adventitia is made up of elastic and collagen fibers. It has great tensile strength and maintains integrity of the vessel.

The tunica media is made up of vascular smooth muscles and elastic fibers. The muscle fibers are arranged in concentric layers and they help to maintain the size of the blood vessel.

Tunica intima is further made up of three layers:

1. internal elastic lamina,
2. lamina propria, and
3. endothelial layer.

Internal elastic lamina has pores. It allows the passage of various substances.

Lamina propria has elastic fibers, areolar tissue, and lipid deposits.

Endothelial lining is smooth. The smooth surface prevents clotting within the blood vessels. The endothelial lining is considered as the largest endocrine gland. It secretes various hormones and physiologically useful substances. Nitric oxide and endothelium-derived relaxing factor are produced by lining of the blood vessel.

Vascular Smooth Muscle

It responds to circulating vasoconstrictor, vasodilator substances, and stimulation of autonomic nerves.

Vasoconstrictor substances cause contraction of vascular smooth muscle. This results in narrowing of the blood vessel (vasoconstriction).

Vasodilator substances produce relaxation of the smooth muscle resulting in dilatation of the blood vessel (vasodilation).

Normal size of the blood vessel is maintained by tone in the vascular smooth muscle.

Contraction of Vascular Smooth Muscle

Calcium ions are needed for contraction of the vascular smooth muscle. The sequence of events occurring in contraction of the vascular smooth muscle is similar to contraction of the smooth muscle elsewhere in the body.

Calcium ion channel blockers prevent contraction of the vascular smooth muscle resulting in relaxation. These blockers are used in the management of hypertension.

Arteries

The arteries carry blood away from the heart toward the various body tissues. They carry oxygenated blood, except pulmonary artery which carries deoxygenated blood. They contain all the three layers seen in the blood vessels. The tunica media is well formed with vascular smooth muscle. The larger arteries exhibit Windkessel effect.

Windkessel Effect

Blood is pumped into the blood vessels during systole. When blood is pumped into large- and medium-sized arteries, they expand to accommodate the sudden rush of blood. The expansion of blood vessel is possible due to the presence of plenty of elastic and collagen fibers in their walls.

During diastole, blood is not pumped from the heart. The walls of the blood vessel undergo elastic recoil and push the blood forward. The potential energy stored in the walls of the blood vessel during systole is converted to kinetic energy to propel the blood during diastole.

Windkessel effect helps in converting intermittent pulsatile flow from the heart to continuous flow through arteries.

It prevents excessive increase in pressure during systole.

As the age advances, walls of the blood vessel become harder due to the loss of elasticity. This causes an increase in systolic blood pressure, termed **systolic hypertension**.

Arteriole

The arterioles are smaller sized blood vessels with narrower lumen. They have less of elastic fibers but are rich in vascular smooth muscles.

The arterioles offer maximum resistance to the flow of blood due to lack of elasticity. This high resistance reduces the blood pressure as blood flows through the arterioles. The pulsatile flow is converted into a continuous steady flow.

The vascular smooth muscles present in the arterioles respond to vasoconstrictor substances. The arteriolar constriction increases the systemic arterial blood pressure but reduces pressure in the capillaries.

Adjustment in the size of the arteriole regulates

- blood flow through the tissues and
- movement of fluid across the walls of capillaries.

Capillaries

The capillaries are thin-walled blood vessels. They have a single layer of endothelial cells on the basement membrane. The capillary walls have pores.

The capillary network provides a large cross-sectional area. The blood flows slowly through the capillaries. It provides ideal condition for the exchange of gases and other substances between the blood and the interstitial fluid.

The fluid that leaks across the capillary wall is returned to systemic circulation through the lymphatic system.

Veins

The veins are thin-walled blood vessels; they are larger in size as compared to arteries. The veins also have three layers in their walls and respond to vasoactive substances. They can hold large quantity of blood without a significant increase in pressure.

The veins have valves formed from the intima layer of the blood vessel. These valves permit the passage of blood only toward the heart. They transport blood at low pressures.

Systemic Circulation (Major or Greater Circulation)

The oxygenated blood from the left ventricle reaches different tissues of the body passing through the aorta. The deoxygenated blood from these tissues reaches the right atrium through the superior and inferior venae cavae. This circulation is called **systemic circulation** (Fig. 4.3).

Left ventricle
| Aorta
Tissues
SVC | IVC
Right atrium

Pulmonary Circulation (Lesser or Minor circulation)

The deoxygenated blood from the right ventricle reaches the lungs through the pulmonary artery. The oxygenated blood comes back to the left atrium through the pulmonary vein. This is calle **pulmonary circulation** (Fig. 4.3).

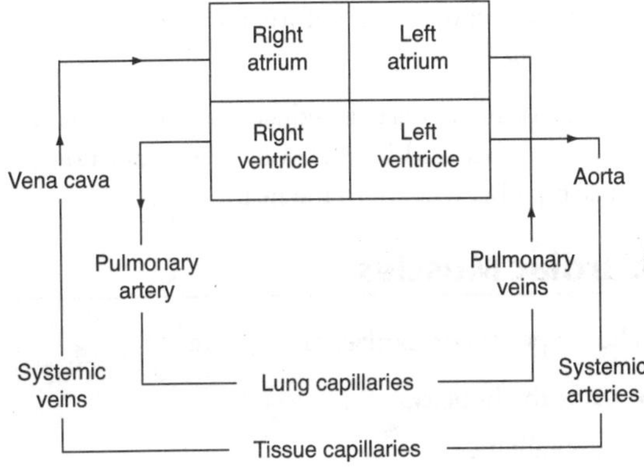

Fig. 4.3   Systemic and pulmonary circulation.

Right ventricle
| Pulmonary artery
Lungs
| Pulmonary veins
Left atrium

Conducting System of the Heart (Junctional Tissue)

The conducting system of the heart (Fig. 4.4) consists of

- sinoatrial node (SA node),
- atrioventricular node (AV node),
- bundle of His,
- right and left bundle branches, and
- purkinje fibers.

Sinoatrial Node

The SA node is a specialized cardiac tissue present at the junction of the superior vena cava and the right atrium. It generates maximum number of impulses (70–80/min) and sets the pace for the heart. Hence, it is called **pacemaker** of the heart.

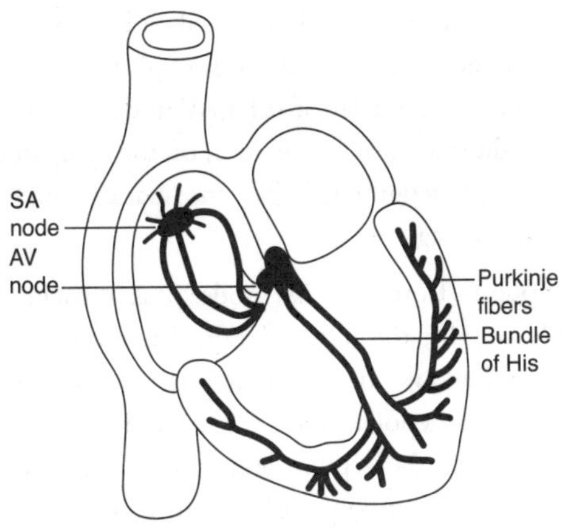

Fig. 4.4   Conducting system of the heart.

Atrioventricular Node

The AV node is present between the atrium and the ventricle close to the AV opening. It can produce 50–60 impulses/min. It is connected to the SA node by mean of internodal pathways (anterior: Bachman, middle: Wenckebach, and posterior: Thorel). It conducts the impulse generated by the SA node.

Bundle of His

The AV node continues as the bundle of His. It gives out a left bundle branch and continues as the right bundle branch. The left bundle branch divides into the anterior and posterior divisions. It supplies the left ventricle and interventricular septum. The right bundle branch supplies the right ventricle.

Purkinje Fibers

These are specialized myocardial cells with gap junctions. They form network in both the ventricles and transfer impulses from the bundle branches to the working myocardium. Purkinje fibers can generate about 15–40 impulses/min.

Origin and Spread of Cardiac Impulse

The cardiac impulse originates at the SA node.

It spreads over the atria through the atrial musculature. The depolarization of atria is completed in 0.1 s.

It passes through the internodal pathway to reach the AV node. The conduction through the AV node is slow. There is a delay of 0.1 s(AV nodal delay). The delay is shortened by stimulation of the sympathetic nerves and lengthened by the parasympathetic stimulation (vagi).

Impulses from the AV node pass through the bundle of His, the left and right bundle branches, and the Purkinje fibers to activate the ventricles. The wave of depolarization for the ventricles begins at the base of the septum and spreads to the other parts through Purkinje fibers in 0.08–0.1s. The wave of depolarization commencing on the left side of the interventricular septum moves to the right side across the midportion of the septum. Later, it spreads to the apex down the septum. It returns to the AV groove passing along the ventricular wall. The wave moves from the endocardial to the epicardial surface.

Depolarization of Ventricles

The impulse spreads through the interventricular septum and reaches the apex of the heart. It turns backward to finally depolarize the posterobasal part of the ventricles.

Velocities of conduction in different cardiac tissues are as under:

SA node	0.05 m/s
AV node	0.05 m/s
Atrial pathways	1.00 m/s
Bundle of His	1.00 m/s
Purkinje system	4.00 m/s
Ventricular muscle	1.00 m/s

AV Nodal Delay

The delay occurring at AV node before excitation spreads to the ventricle is termed **AV nodal delay**. The normal delay is 0.1 s. This is due to small size of the fibers, long refractory periods, and low resting membrane potential.

Importance

The AV nodal delay allows contraction of the atria to be completed before the ventricle starts contracting.

The AV nodal delay is reduced by the stimulation of sympathetic and increased by the stimulation of parasympathetic nerve to the heart.

Cardiac Muscles

The properties of cardiac muscles are

- autorhythmicity,
- excitability,
- conductivity,
- contractility,
- all-or-none law,
- staircase phenomenon,
- refractory period, and
- tone.

Autorhythmicity

The junctional tissue of the heart is capable of generating its own impulses without external stimulation. The ability of the cardiac muscles to generate their own impulses is called **autorhythmicity**. This is due to unstable membrane potential in the junctional tissues.

Applied Physiology

Artificial Pacemakers (Implanted Pacemakers)

These are external electronic devices implanted when the patient has severe bradycardia due to defective functioning of natural pacemaker or conducting system of the heart.

Heart Block

Damage to the conducting system of the heart hampers impulse transmission. This results in heart block. Depending on the site and extent of damage, it is categorized as first-, second-, and third-degree heart block.

Pacemaker Potential (Fig. 4.5)

- It is a potential generated in the pacemaker tissue of the heart.
- Sodium and potassium ions move in and out of the cell through leak channels at rest in an excitable tissue.
- In the pacemaker tissue, permeability of membrane to potassium ions decreases spontaneously.
- The efflux (exit) of potassium is reduced resulting in a depolarizing change.
- This initial depolarizing change causes the opening of the **transient calcium channels** and entry of calcium. This produces the prepotential.
- Later, **long-lasting calcium channels** open, facilitating the rapid entry of calcium. This produces depolarization.
- At the end of depolarization, the calcium channels close and the potassium channels open.
- Efflux of the potassium ions results in repolarization. Thus, an impulse is generated.
- The impulse generated spreads over the cardiac muscle.

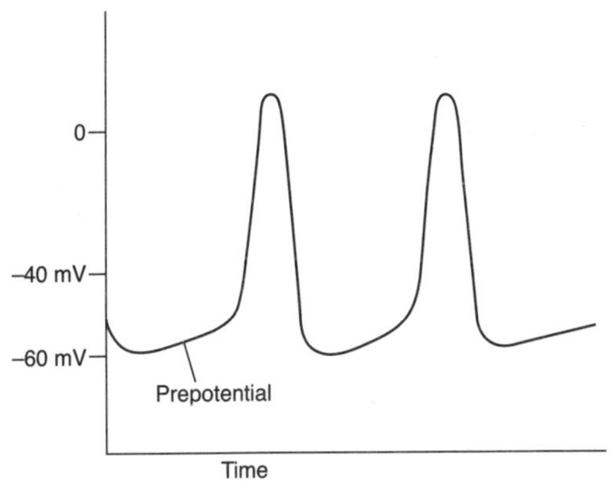

Fig. 4.5 Pacemaker potential.

The action potentials produced in SA and AV nodes are due to the calcium ions with little contribution from the sodium ions.

The stimulation of the vagus nerve supplying the nodal tissue results in hyperpolarization of the membrane. The slope of prepotential decreases, reducing the heart rate. The action is mediated through the muscarinic receptors.

The stimulation of the sympathetic fibers causes a rapid decline in the membrane potential increasing the rate of spontaneous discharge. This increases the slope of prepotential and hence the heart rate.

Excitability

Action Potential in a Ventricular Muscle

Excitability is the responding property of the tissue to a stimulus. In the cardiac muscle, it occurs in the following phases:

- Resting membrane potential in a normal cardiac muscle is about −80 to −90 mV.
- **Phase 0:** Excitation of cardiac muscle causes the entry of *sodium ions* resulting in depolarization.
- **Phase 1:** There is slight repolarization after a rapid depolarization. It is due to sudden closure of sodium channels associated with transient efflux of potassium ions.
- **Phase 2:** The state of depolarization is maintained by delayed and sustained entry of **calcium ions**. This phase is called *plateau*.
- **Phase 3:** The exit of *potassium ions* coupled with the closure of calcium channels results in the phase of repolarization.
- **Phase 4:** Restoration of resting membrane potential constitutes Phase 4. The ionic balance is restored by sodium–potassium and sodium–calcium ATPase pump.

The duration of cardiac muscle action potential is about 200–250 ms (Fig. 4.6).

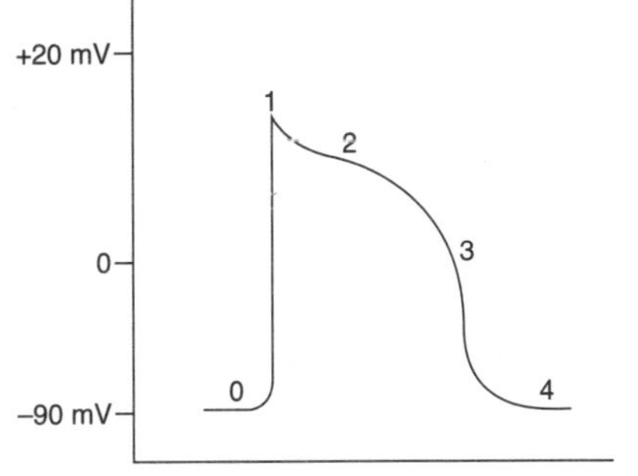

Fig. 4.6 Cardiac muscle action potential.

Action Potential in Atrial Muscle

The ionic basis of action potential in atrial muscle is the same as in ventricular muscle. In atrial muscle action potential, duration of plateau phase (Phase 2) is shorter. Therefore the repolarization phase (Phase 3) is prolonged.

Conductivity

The impulses generated by the pacemaker tissue spread to the entire cardiac muscle with the help of the **conducting system** or the **junctional tissue** of the heart.

The presence of gap junctions between the cardiac muscle fibers hastens the movement of ions. This helps in rapid spread of impulse in the cardiac muscle.

Refractory Period

The absolute refractory period is the period during which second stimulus of any intensity fails to produce a response. It corresponds to a major part of the cardiac muscle action potential. The cardiac muscle cannot be tetanized because of a long absolute refractory period.

The relative refractory period is the period during which second stimulus of greater intensity produces a response. It corresponds to the last part of repolarization.

All-or-None Law

When the cardiac muscle is stimulated with threshold stimulus, it responds to its maximum. However, if the stimulus is subthreshold, the muscle does not show any response.

All-or-none law applies to the entire cardiac muscle.

Tone

Tone is a partial contracted state of myocardium without an external stimulus.

Contractility

The chemical changes and mechanical shortening of the muscle in response to a stimulus is contractility. The molecular basis for the cardiac muscle contraction is similar to that of the skeletal muscle contraction.

Staircase Phenomenon

The heart is stopped by stimulation of the vagus nerve. Later, the heart is allowed to beat again by withdrawing the vagal stimulation. Initial few contractions show an increase in the amplitude of contractions. This is termed **staircase phenomenon**.

It is due to

- accumulation of calcium ions released during the previous contraction potentiating the effect of subsequent contractions,
- decrease in the viscosity of the muscle, and
- increase in the temperature of the muscle, which enhances the enzymatic activity and hence improves contraction.

Starling's Law

The force of contraction is directly proportional to the initial length of the muscle fiber within physiological limits. With respect to the heart, it is stated as greater the preload, greater is the force of contraction within physiological limits.

Importance

- It helps to maintain the cardiac output equally on both right and left sides of the heart.
- In cases of heart failure, heart pumps out excess blood which has accumulated during earlier contractions to reduce load on the heart.

Molecular Basis

- When the muscle is stretched, actin and myosin are separated exposing active binding sites on the actin molecule. This increases the number of cross-bridges formed. Greater the number of cross-bridges formed, greater is the force of contraction.
- Actin filament moves a longer distance in a stretched muscle during contraction. This increases the force of contraction.
- When the muscle is stretched, resting metabolism increases. There is increase in the temperature of the muscle resulting in better enzymatic activity. This enhances the force of muscle contraction.

Cardiac Cycle

The cardiac cycle is the cyclical repetition of various changes in the heart from beat to beat.

The contraction of the heart is called **systole**. During systole, blood is ejected from contracting chamber of the heart.

The relaxation of heart is termed **diastole**. During diastole, blood collects in chambers of the heart.

The normal duration of cardiac cycle is 0.8 s when the heart rate is 75 beats/min.

The duration of each cardiac cycle depends on the heart rate. Increase in the heart rate decreases the duration of the cardiac cycle.

Two atria or two ventricles contract simultaneously, but the atrial and ventricular contractions never overlap.

Mechanical Events (Fig. 4.7)

Atrial Events

Atrial systole	0.1 s
Atrial diastole	0.7 s

Ventricular Events

Ventricular systole	0.3 s
Ventricular diastole	0.5 s

Ventricular Systole

1.	Isovolumetric contraction phase	0.05 s
2.	Rapid ejection phase	0.10 s
3.	Reduced ejection phase	0.15 s

Ventricular Diastole

1.	Protodiastolic phase	0.04 s
2.	Isovolumetric relaxation phase	0.06 s
3.	First rapid-filling phase	0.10 s
4.	Slow-filling phase or diastasis	0.20 s
5.	Last rapid-filling phase	0.10 s

Atrial Systole and Diastole

During major part of cardiac cycle, the atrium is relaxing. Atrial systole lasts for 0.1 s and its diastole for 0.7 s.

Ventricular Systole

1. **Isovolumetric contraction phase:** At the beginning of ventricular systole, AV valve is open and the semilunar valve is closed. Due to ventricular contraction, intraventricular pressure increases and the blood tries to enter the atrium. This is prevented by closure of AV valve producing the *first heart sound.* Now ventricle becomes a closed cavity containing blood. It continues to contract. As the volume of ventricle does not change, this phase is called isovolumetric contraction phase. However, the intraventricular pressure increases due to continued ventricular contraction.

2. **Rapid ejection phase:** When the intraventricular pressure increases above the pressure in the aorta and pulmonary artery, the semilunar valves open. This forces the blood into these vessels rapidly.

3. **Reduced ejection phase:** The continued contraction of the ventricles pushes the remaining blood into the pulmonary artery and the aorta slowly. At the end of this phase, the ventricles begin to relax.

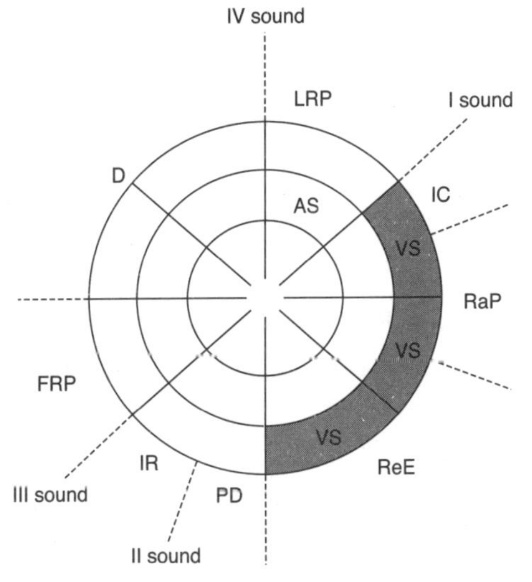

Fig. 4.7 Mechanical events during a cardiac cycle. IC, isovolumetric contraction; RaP, rapid ejection; ReE, reduced ejection; PD, protodiastole; IR, isovolumetric relaxation; FRP, first rapid filling; D, diastasis; LRP, last rapid filling; AS, atrial systole; VS, ventricular systole.

Ventricular Diastole

1. **Protodiastolic phase:** During this phase, the ventricles begin to relax. The AV valve is closed and the semilunar valve is still open.

As the intraventricular pressure decreases below the pressure in the aorta and pulmonary artery, blood tries to come back into the ventricle. This is prevented by closure of the semilunar valve producing the *second heart sound.*

2. **Isovolumetric relaxation phase:** Now, the ventricle is again a closed cavity, which is relaxing. During this phase, the intraventricular pressure goes below the atrial pressure.

3. **First rapid-filling phase:** The reduced intraventricular pressure causes the opening of AV valves and there is sudden rush of blood. Turbulence to the flow of blood through narrow opening produces the *third heart sound.*

4. **Slow-filling phase or diastasis:** During this phase, both atria and ventricles are relaxing. The AV valve is open. Blood entering the atria fills the ventricles passively.

5. **Last rapid-filling phase:** This phase coincides with atrial contraction. The atrial systole forces the blood from the atria to the ventricle. Turbulence produced due to a rapid rush of blood produces the *fourth heart sound.*

Pressure Changes (Fig. 4.8)

The chambers of the heart show different pressures during different phases of the cardiac cycle. Generally, both atria and right ventricle have low pressure when compared to left ventricle, which has a high pressure.

Ventricular Pressure Changes

In a normal individual, pressure in the left ventricle reaches a maximum of 120–140 mm Hg during the rapid ejection phase. The pressure in the right ventricle during the corresponding period is about 25–30 mm Hg. During diastole, left ventricular pressure drops to about 15–20 mm Hg and right ventricular pressure reaches 0 mm Hg.

Aortic Pressure Changes

It is around 120 mm Hg at the beginning of the rapid ejection phase of the ventricle and about 80 mm Hg at the beginning of the ventricular diastole.

Pulmonary Artery Pressure Changes

It reaches a maximum of 25–30 mm Hg during ventricular systole and reduces to 0 mm Hg during ventricular diastole.

Atrial Pressure Changes

The atrial pressure varies between 0 mm Hg when it is relaxing and a maximum of 15–20 mm Hg during its contraction.

The atrial systole starts after the P-wave of ECG; the ventricular systole starts near the end of R-wave and is completed after the T-wave.

Volume Changes (Fig. 4.8)

The ventricular volume changes are studied during different phases of the cardiac cycle.

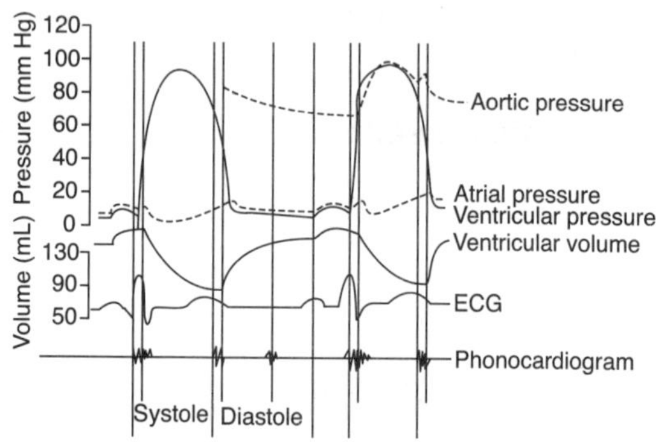

Fig. 4.8 Pressure and volume changes during cardiac cycle.

- During atrial contraction, blood enters the ventricles. As a result of the entry of blood, there is a slight increase in the ventricular volume.

- The atrial contraction is followed by commencement of the ventricular contraction.

- The beginning of ventricular contraction is marked by the closure of AV valves.

- The ventricle is now a closed cavity that is contracting. There is no change in the volume of the ventricle which is under isovolumetric contraction phase.

The atrial systole starts after the P-wave of ECG; the ventricular systole starts near the end of R-wave and is completed after the T-wave.

- The isovolumetric contraction phase is terminated by opening of the semilunar valves.

- It is followed by the rapid ejection phase. As substantial quantity of blood contained in the ventricle is ejected out rapidly during this phase, there is a sharp fall in the ventricular volume.

- The ventricles continue to contract ejecting the blood relatively slowly. This is reduced ejection phase. During this phase, ventricular volume decreases slowly.
- The reduced ejection phase is followed by the ventricular diastole.
- During the protodiastolic phase there is no change in the ventricular volume.
- The protodiastolic phase ends with the closure of semilunar valves.
- Now ventricles are closed cavities, relaxing.
- During the isovolumetric relaxation phase, there is no change in the ventricular volume.
- Decrease in the intraventricular pressure causes the opening of the AV valves.
- Opening of the AV valves marks the beginning of first rapid-filling phase. During this phase, there is significant increase in the ventricular volume

due to a sudden rush of blood from the atrium.

- There is a slow increase in the ventricular volume during diastasis (slow-filling phase) which follows the first rapid-filling phase.
- The slow-filling phase is followed by the last rapid-filling phase due to contraction of the atrium.

Heart Sounds

There are four heart sounds. These sounds are produced due to the closure of valves or turbulence to the flow of blood during different phases of the cardiac cycle.

The heart sounds are produced due to vibrations set up by the closure of valves and the vibrations of walls of the heart, blood vessel, and column of blood in the vessel.

Applied Physiology

Cardiac Catheterization

It is a technique in which a multichannel catheter is passed into a chamber of the heart through antecubital vein or femoral artery.

It is useful to

- study pressure changes in the chambers of the heart;
- measure electrical activities of the heart;
- detect source of normal and abnormal cardiac sounds;
- perform coronary angiography;
- analyze gas content of the blood in different chambers;

Echocardiography

Echocardiography is a noninvasive technique to evaluate the cardiac function.

The pulses of ultrasonic waves are emitted toward the organ and reflected waves are analyzed. The change in the acoustic impedance and recording of echoes provide information about the movement of wall of the heart, valves, and septum.

Echocardiography uses the reflected ultrasound to study the following:

- blood flow,
- structure of the heart,
- movement of valves, and
- cardiac muscle.

It is also used to measure the velocity and volume of blood flow.

Ultrasound is reflected at interfaces between blood and solid tissues. This is helpful in measuring the anatomic dimensions.

The first and second heart sounds are heard by using the stethoscope. The other sounds are demonstrated by the **phonocardiogram.**

The heart sounds are auscultated in the following areas:

- **Mitral area:** It is located in the left fifth intercostal space half an inch medial to midclavicular line.
- **Tricuspid area:** It is located at the left border of sternum in the fifth intercostal space.
- **Aortic area:** It is located in the second intercostal space at the right border of sternum.
- **Pulmonary area**: It is located in the second intercostal space at the left border of sternum.

Both first and second heart sounds are heard in all the four areas. However, first heart sound is heard better in the mitral and tricuspid areas; second heart sound is better heard in the aortic and pulmonary areas.

During prolonged inspiration, second heart sound is split due to asynchronous closure of the aortic and pulmonary semilunar valves.

Murmurs

These are abnormal sounds produced due to turbulence in the flow of blood. They are appreciated when blood flows through a narrow opening as in mitral stenosis or through a defective valve as in aortic regurgitation. The murmur heard between the first and second heart sounds is **systolic murmur.** Systolic murmur is heard in aortic stenosis and mitral regurgitation.

Diastolic murmur is heard between second and first heart sounds of the next cardiac cycle. It is heard in mitral stenosis and aortic regurgitation.

	First Heart Sound	**Second Heart Sound**
Cause	Closure of AV valves	Closure of semilunar valves
Duration	0.09–0.15 s	0.10 s
Character	Prolonged, loud	Short, sharp (high pitch)
Heard as	Syllable LUBB	Syllable DUP
Heard best in	Mitral and tricuspid areas	Aortic and pulmonary areas
ECG	Coincides with R-wave	Coincides with end of T-wave

Pulse

The pulse is an expansile impulse arising from the base of the heart traveling along the walls of the blood vessel.

The pulse is also defined as the expansion and elongation of the arterial wall traveling along the walls of the blood vessel.

Types of pulsations are

1. arterial and
2. venous.

Radial artery is commonly used to examine arterial pulse.

Venous pulsations are observed in the jugular vein.

Arterial pulsations are felt better and venous pulsations are seen better.

Arterial Pulse

The arterial pulse tracing (Fig. 4.9) is called the **sphygmogram.** It is recorded by using the instrument **sphygmograph.** The normal pulse is a catacrotic pulse. (Dicrotic notch is in the descending limb of pulse tracing.) Normal pulse rate is 60–90 beats/min. A decrease in pulse rate is bradysphygmia and an increase is tachysphygmia. The heart rate and pulse rate are equal in a normal individual. In some pathological conditions, pulse rate is less than heart rate. It is called **pulse deficit.**

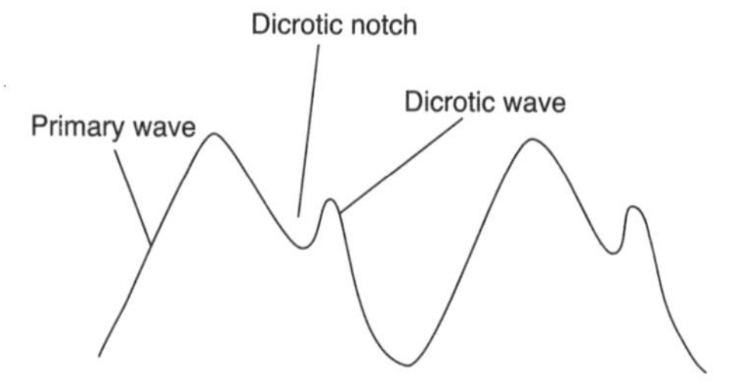

Fig. 4.9   Arterial pulse tracing.

Pulse tracing has the following

- **Primary wave,** or a percussion wave, is produced due to ventricular systole.
- **Dicrotic notch** is present in the descending limb of the pulse tracing. It is produced due to the

rolling back of blood in aorta at the beginning of ventricular diastole.

- **Dicrotic wave** follows the dicrotic notch. It is due to the sudden closure of semilunar valves.

Arterial pulse is examined under the following headings:

1. **Rate:** Number of beats per minute counted for one complete minute

2. **Rhythm:** Regularity of the occurrence of pulse wave (regular/irregular)

3. **Volume:** Extent of displacement of the palpating finger (normal/high/low volume)

4. **Character of the vessel wall:** Thickened and palpable/soft and not palpable

5. **Character of the pulse:** Anacrotic/catacrotic

6. **Equality of the pulse:** Equal/unequal in volume in both the upper limbs

7. **Comparison of volume:** Comparison of volume of upper and lower limb pulse.

Jugular Venous Pulse (JVP; Fig. 4.10)

The examination of venous pulse gives an indication about the functioning of the right side of the heart. A recording of venous pulsation has the following waves:

- Positive waves
  1. *a*-wave: It is produced due to atrial systole.
  2. *c*-wave: It is pruduced due to ventricular contraction (isovolumetric contraction) causing AV valve to bulge into the atrium.
  3. *v*-wave: It is pruduced due to increased intra-atrial pressure during the filling of atrium.

Applied Physiology

Tachycardia (Tachysphygmia)

It is an increase in pulse rate above 90 beats/min. Physiologically, it occurs during muscular exercise. Pathologically, it is seen in fever, circulatory shock, and thyrotoxicosis.

Bradycardia (Bradysphygmia)

Bradycardia is a decrease in pulse rate below 60 beats/min. Physiologically, it is seen in athletes and during sleep. Pathologically, it is observed in myxedema and heart blocks.

High-Volume Pulse

Physiologically, it is seen during exercise. Pathologically, it is seen in hyperdynamic states like fever, thyrotoxicosis, and aortic regurgitation (water hammer pulse or Corrigan's pulse or collapsing pulse).

Low-Volume Pulse

Physiologically, it is seen during sleep, and pathologically, observed during shock.

Pulse Deficit

It is a condition in which pulse rate is less than the heart rate.

Pulses Paradoxus

In pulses paradoxus, volume of the pulse increases during expiration and decreases during inspiration. It is the reverse of normal variation in the volume of pulse.

Pulses Alternans

In this condition, there are alternate strong and weak pulsations. It is due to alteration in the stroke volume in successive beats. It is seen in severe myocardial infarction and cardiac failure.

- Negative waves
    1. **x-wave:** It is caused due to fall in intra-atrial pressure during diastole.
    2. **x_1-wave:** It is caused due to distension of atria as the AV ring is pulled down by ventricular contraction.
    3. **y-wave:** It is due to fall in intra-atrial pressure due to opening of AV valve.

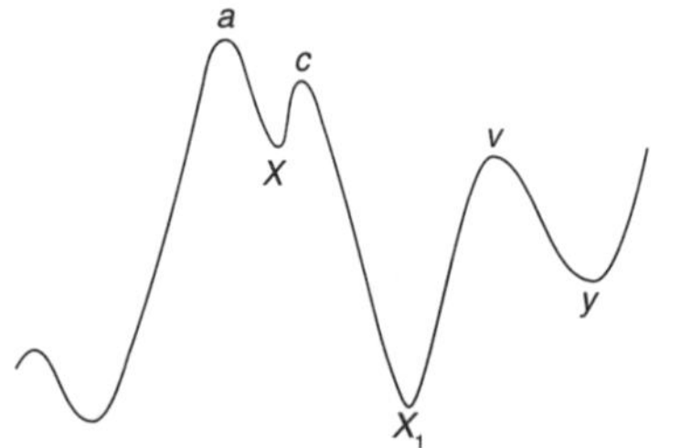

Fig. 4.10   Jugular venous pulse.

Regulation of Heart Rate

The normal heart rate ranges from 60 to 90 beats/min. The average heart rate is 72 beats/min.

Heart rate is regulated by the neural and chemical mechanisms. The vasomotor center plays a key role in the neural regulation. The chemical regulation is brought about by general, local hormones and metabolites. Autoregulation also has a role in the control of heart rate.

Vasomotor Center

Vasomotor center (VMC) is present in the ventrolateral part of the medulla.

It is concerned with the regulation of heart rate and blood pressure. The neurons regulating heart rate and blood pressure project directly to the preganglionic sympathetic fibers. VMC has intrinsic ability to generate impulses without external stimulation.

VMC has three areas:

1. vasodilator area,
2. vasoconstrictor area, and
3. sensory area.

Vasodilator Area

This is present in the medial portion of VMC. It decreases the heart rate acting through vagus nerve.

Vasoconstrictor Area

This is present in the lateral portion of VMC. It increases the heart rate through sympathetic stimulation.

Sensory Area

It lies in the nucleus of tractus solitarius. It receives sensory information from periphery through IX and X cranial nerves.

Heart rate is regulated by

- stimulation of the autonomic nervous system,
- reflexes arising from outside the heart,
- reflexes from within the heart, and
- other reflexes.

Stimulation of Autonomic Nervous System

Stimulation of the sympathetic nerve fibers increases the heart rate and produces vasoconstriction.

Stimulation of the parasympathetic fibers decreases the heart rate and produces vasodilation.

Reflexes from Outside the Heart

Baroreceptor Mechanism

The baroreceptors are specialized cells capable of sensing changes in the blood pressure. They are present in the carotid sinus and the arch of aorta.

Increase of blood pressure stimulates baroreceptors.

This inhibits VMC and stimulates vagal nucleus.

These changes decrease the heart rate (also produce vasodilation, reduced cardiac output, and blood pressure).

Chemoreceptor Mechanism

The chemoreceptors are present in the carotid body and the arch of aorta. They are capable of recognizing changes in the chemical nature of blood.

- Reduction in the blood flow causes local accumulation of carbon dioxide and lack of oxygen at the chemoreceptors.

- These changes stimulate the chemoreceptors. This in turn activates VMC and inhibits vagal nucleus.
- These changes increase the heart rate (also produce vasoconstriction).

Vasomotor Center

Ischemia (reduced blood flow) of vasomotor center

- stimulates vasomotor center;
- increases heart rate by intrinsic activation;
- produces vasoconstriction.

Reflexes Arising from within the Heart

Bainbridge Reflex

Accumulation of blood in superior and inferior venae cavae causes stretch of these vessels and activation of receptors in them. This increases the heart rate. The reflex response is called **bainbridge reflex**.

Right Atrial Stimulation

Stretch of right atrium stimulates A and B receptors. Impulses from these receptors pass through the vagus nerves. The efferent pathway is through both sympathetic and parasympathetic nerves. This reflex results in increased heart rate. It helps to reduce the load on right side of the heart by removal of blood.

Role of Atrial Natriuretic Peptide

Distension of atrium causes the release of hormone atrial natriuretic peptide (ANP). It reduces cardiac congestion by increasing the sodium and water excretion. This hormone also produces vasodilation.

Left Ventricular Stimulation

The left ventricle has stretch receptors. Stimulation of these receptors decreases the heart rate and produces vasodilation.

Bezold–Jarisch Reflex

Injection of veratrum alkaloids results in decreased heart rate. The receptors for this reflex are present in left ventricle.

Other Reflexes Regulating Heart Rate

- Stimulation of limbic system, hypothalamus, and cerebral cortex increases the heart rate.
- During inspiration, there is an increase in heart rate, and during expiration, there is a decrease in heart rate. This is called **sinus arrhythmia**. During inspiration, the intrathoracic pressure decreases. This increases the venous return. Activation of bainbridge reflex increases the heart rate.
- An increase of body temperature as in fever increases heart rate by enhancing the activity of the pacemaker. For every degree Fahrenheit rise in body temperature, the heart rate increases by about 10 beats/min.
- Muscular exercise increases the heart rate by stimulation of sympathetic system.
- Advanced stages of pregnancy are associated with an increase in the heart rate.
- Hormones like epinephrine and thyroxine increase the heart rate. (Thyroxine increases the metabolism of SA node.)
- Pathological conditions like fever, heart failure, and shock are associated with tachycardia (increased heart rate).
- Sleep decreases the heart rate due to reduced metabolism.
- Athletes have a low heart rate due to increased vagal tone.
- Heart blocks and myxedema produce bradycardia (decreased heart rate).
- Pain increases the heart rate by sympathetic stimulation. However pain produced by a blow to abdomen or testis reduces the heart rate by intense vagal stimulation.

Marey's Law

Marey's law states that heart rate and blood pressure are inversely related:

$$\text{Heart rate } \alpha \frac{1}{\text{Blood pressure}}.$$

Exception: During exercise, both heart rate and blood pressure are increased.

Hemodynamics

The normal flow of fluid in a tube is **laminar** or **streamline**. The movement of blood in blood vessels follows the same pattern. The blood cells move in the same direction in concentric layers. The velocities of motion of these layers are different. The central lamina has maximum velocity. It is lowest in the outermost lamina which is in contact with the vessel wall. When the fluid follows a laminar flow pattern it does not produce any sound. Hence, no sound is heard when normal artery is auscultated.

Turbulent Flow

The loss of laminar pattern of flow results in turbulence. The molecules move randomly in different directions and collide with each other. When the flow pattern is turbulent it becomes noisy.

Reynold's Number

It is a number to evaluate whether the flow pattern is turbulent or laminar.

If the number is less than 2000, flow is not turbulent. A value of more than 3000 indicates that the flow is turbulent. The velocity at which the flow becomes turbulent is called **critical velocity**.

Reynold's number is calculated by using the formula

$$Re = \frac{\rho V D}{\eta}.$$

where ρ is density of fluid, V velocity of flow, D diameter of the tube, and η viscosity of the fluid.

Blood Pressure

It is the lateral pressure exerted by a column of blood on the walls of blood vessel through which it flows.

Systolic Blood Pressure

Systolic blood pressure (SBP) is the maximum pressure exerted during ventricular systole.

It ranges from 100 to 140 mm Hg with an average of 120 mm Hg.

Diastolic Blood Pressure

Diastolic blood pressure (DBP) is the minimum pressure during ventricular diastole. It ranges from 60 to 90 mm Hg with an average of 80 mm Hg. It is the measure of peripheral resistance.

Pulse Pressure

Pulse pressure (PP) is the difference between systolic and diastolic blood pressure:

Pulse pressure = Systolic BP – Diastolic BP.

Mean Arterial Pressure

Mean arterial pressure (MAP) is the average pressure present throughout the cardiac cycle.

It is around 93 mm Hg.

It is equal to diastolic pressure plus one-third of pulse pressure:

$$MAP = DBP + \tfrac{1}{3}\,PP.$$

Methods of Recording Blood Pressure

Blood pressure is recorded by

1. direct method and
2. indirect method.

Applied Physiology

Tachycardia

Increase in heart rate >90 beats/min

Causes

Physiological: Exercise, anxiety, and emotional disturbances

Pathological: Fever and thyrotoxicosis

Bradycardia

Decrease in heart rate <60 beats/min

Causes

- Physiological: During sleep and in athletes
- Pathological: Myxedema and heart blocks

In direct method, artery is cannulated and pressure is recorded by using a manometer. This type of recording is done in experimental animals.

In human beings, blood pressure is recorded by indirect method. The instrument used for recording is called sphygmomanometer.

The parts of sphygmomanometer are

- arm cuff,
- rubber bulb, and
- mercury/aneroid manometer.

The methods for recording blood pressure are

1. palpatory method,
2. auscultatory method, and
3. oscillatory method.

Palpatory Method

The arm cuff is tied around the arm, 1 inch above the cubital fossa. The sphygmomanometer is kept at the level of subject's heart. The radial artery pulsations are felt. The arm cuff is inflated by pressing the rubber bulb. The pressure at which pulse disappears is systolic pressure. This is confirmed by noting the reappearance of pulse when pressure is decreased in the arm cuff.

The palpatory method gives an approximate idea about SBP.

Auscultatory Method

The pressure in the arm cuff is increased 20 mm above the systolic pressure recorded by the palpatory method. The pressure is gradually reduced. The brachial artery is auscultated for any sound. The pressure at which the first heart sound is heard corresponds to the SBP. As the pressure is decreased, the character of sound changes and finally disappears. The pressure corresponding to the disappearance of sound is DBP.

These sounds are **Korotkoff's sounds**, named after a Russian scientist who described them. These sounds are produced due to turbulence in the flow of blood.

Silent Gap (Auscultatory Gap)

Silent gap is observed sometimes in people with high blood pressure.

During blood pressure recording, following initial tapping sound, there is a period of silence during which no sounds are heard. The sounds reappear after sometime. This gap is called **silent gap**. Because of the silent gap, a systolic pressure lower than normal can be recorded.

Factors Influencing Blood Pressure

- **Age:** Blood pressure increases with age. In infants, BP is around 70/50 mm Hg. In a young healthy adult, it is around 120/80 mm Hg. Blood pressure of 140/90 mm Hg or more at any age is considered abnormal.
- **Sex:** Females (before menopause) have slightly lower BP than males.
- **Sleep:** There is a decrease in BP during sleep.
- **Meals:** Blood pressure rises after meals.
- **Emotions:** Fear or anger increases BP.
- **Exercise:** Systolic blood pressure increases during exercise.
- **Build:** Obese persons have higher BP.
- **Posture:** Blood pressure varies with posture. It is least in lying-down posture.
- **Respiration:** It varies with different phases of respiration. It increases during inspiration and decreases during expiration.
- **Diurnal variation:** It is lowest in the mornings; it is higher in late afternoon and evenings.

Factors Controlling Blood Pressure

The systemic arterial blood pressure depends on the stroke volume, heart rate, and peripheral resistance. The blood pressure is controlled by alteration in the following variables:

- **Cardiac output:** Cardiac output depends on stroke volume and heart rate. Systolic blood pressure increases as the stroke volume increases. Increase in heart rate increases the DBP.
- **Heart rate:** Mild to moderate increase in the heart rate does not significantly alter the BP. However, a marked increase in heart rate decreases the BP by reducing the diastolic filling time and stroke volume.
- **Peripheral resistance (PR) and elasticity of blood vessel:** Peripheral resistance varies in-

versely as the elasticity of the vessel wall. Further, DBP varies directly as the PR. Vasodilation reduces the PR and hence the diastolic pressure decreases. Diastolic pressure increases due to enhanced PR following vasoconstriction.

- **Viscosity of blood:** Viscosity of blood increases frictional resistance. Increase in viscosity increases the arterial blood pressure.

- **Velocity of blood flow:** Increase in velocity of the blood flow increases the resistance and in turn enhances blood pressure.

- **Diameter of blood vessel:** Blood pressure is inversely proportional to the diameter of the blood vessel.

Regulation of Blood Pressure

Short-Term Regulation

This type of regulation works for a few seconds to few minutes:

1. **Baroreceptor mechanism (sinoaortic mechanism; Fig. 4.11):** Whenever the blood pressure increases, baroreceptors present in carotid sinus and the arch of aorta are stimulated. This inhibits the VMC and stimulates the vagal nucleus. As a result, the heart rate decreases associated with vasodilation (decrease of peripheral resistance). These changes bring about a reduction in BP.

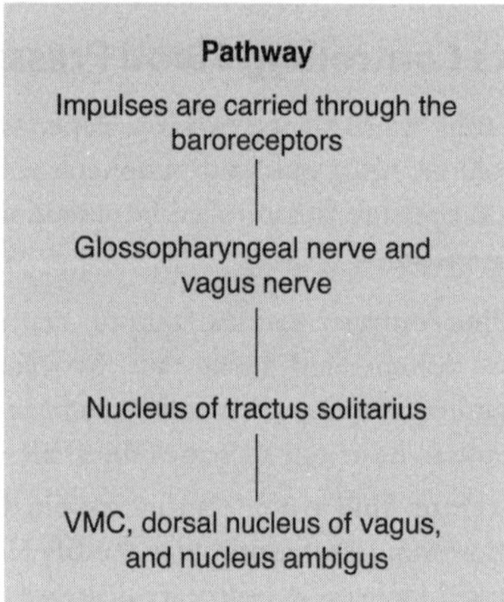

IX and X cranial nerves help in the regulation of blood pressure. Hence, they are called **buffer nerves.**

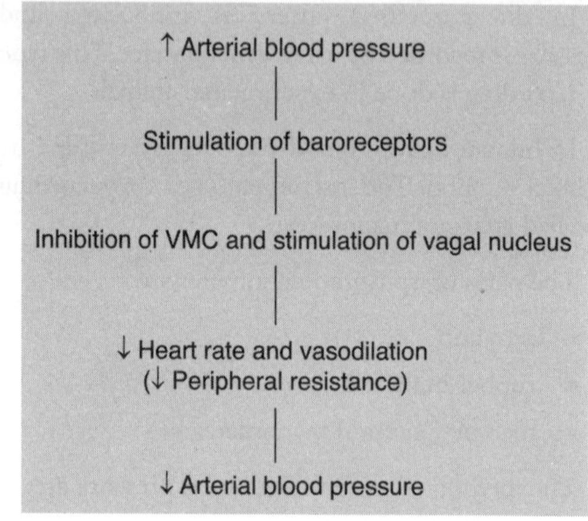

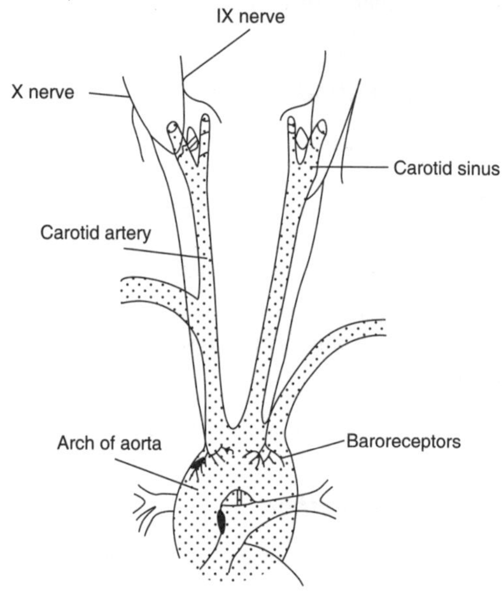

Fig. 4.11   Arterial baroreceptors.

2. **Chemoreceptor mechanism (Fig. 4.12):** A decrease in BP reduces blood flow to chemoreceptors present in the carotid body and the arch of aorta. Reduced oxygen supply stimulates the chemoreceptors. This stimulates the VMC increasing the heart rate and peripheral resistance by vasoconstriction. These changes result in increase of blood pressure.

3. **Vasomotor Center Mechanism:** The reduced blood flow to VMC causes its ischemia. This stimulates the VMC causing an increase in heart rate and peripheral resistance. The net effect of these changes is an increase in BP.

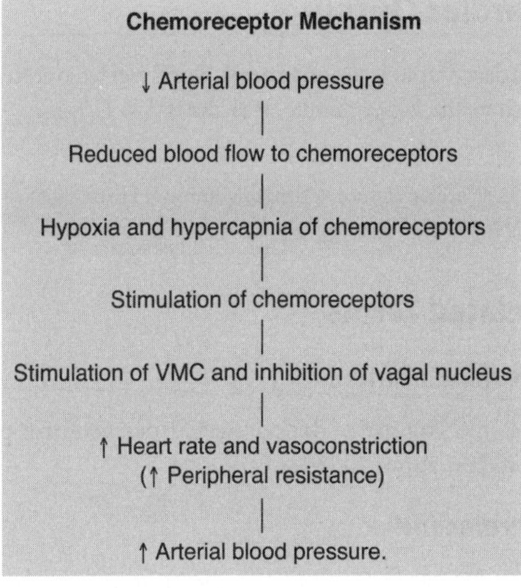

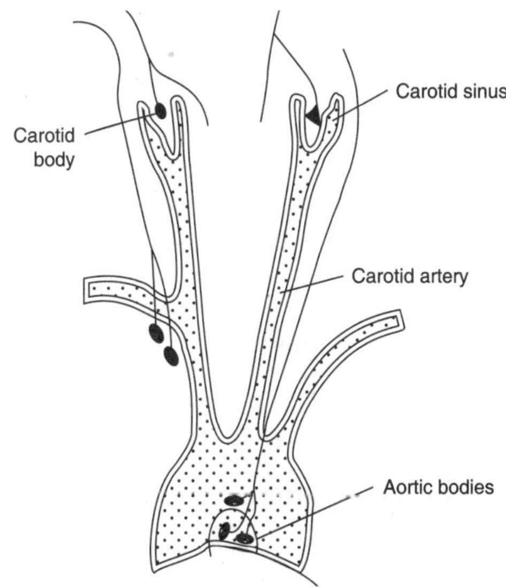

Fig. 4.12   Arterial chemoreceptors.

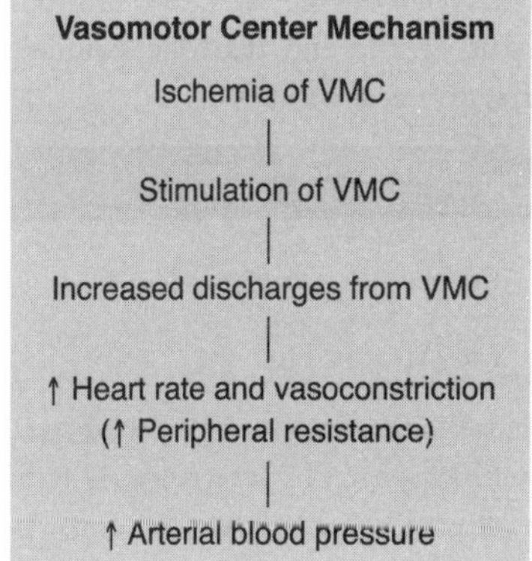

Cushing's Reflex

An increase in the intracranial pressure decreases blood flow to the VMC. Hypoxia and hypercapnia at the VMC increase the discharge from it. This enhances BP. Increased BP overcomes the raised intracranial pressure. Thus, blood flow to the intracranial structures is restored. Increase in systemic arterial BP reduces the heart rate by acting through baroreceptors.

Intermediate-Term Regulation

This mechanism works from few minutes to few hours.

1. **Stress relaxation:** Increased BP exerts a greater force on the walls of blood vessel. This stretch of blood vessel causes initial contraction of the smooth muscle in its walls followed by relaxation. The relaxation of the vessel wall brings down the BP.

2. **Fluid shift mechanism:** Increased BP increases the hydrostatic pressure. This pushes fluid out of blood vessel into the interstitial space. Loss of fluid from the blood vessel reduces the blood volume. There is a reduced venous return and hence a decrease in BP.

3. **Renin angiotensin mechanism:** Reduced BP decreases blood flow to the kidney. This causes the juxtaglomerular apparatus of the kidney to produce renin.

   Renin acts on the plasma substrate, angiotensinogen, to form angiotensin I.

   Angiotensin I is converted to angiotensin II by angiotensin converting enzyme (ACE) present in the lungs. ACE inhibitors prevent the conversion of angiotensin I to angiotensin II.

   Angiotensin II causes peripheral vasoconstriction and increases peripheral resistance. Increase in peripheral resistance restores the blood pressure.

Long-Term Mechanism

Renin–Angiotensin–Aldosterone Mechanism

Angiotensin II produced during the intermediate-term regulation stimulates the adrenal cortex to produce aldosterone as a delayed effect.

Aldosterone increases sodium reabsorption. Water is retained along with sodium. This helps to increase fluid volume. Increased fluid volume increases venous return to the heart and therefore the blood pressure increases.

It stimulates hypothalamus and posterior pituitary to release ADH (antidiuretic hormone). ADH helps in water retention.

This mechanism also activates thirst, enhancing the fluid intake.

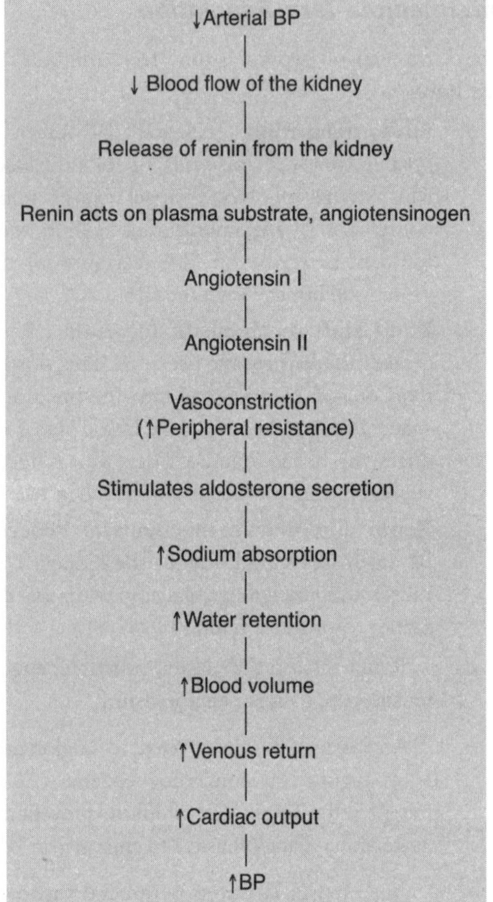

Cardiac Output

Cardiac output is the volume of blood ejected out from each ventricle per minute. It is about 5–6 L/min.

$$\text{Cardiac output} = \text{Stroke volume} \times \text{Heart rate}$$

$$= 70 \text{ mL} \times 72 \text{ beats/min.}$$

Related Terms

Stroke Volume

It is the volume of blood ejected per ventricle per beat. It is about 70–80 mL.

Cardiac Index

It is the cardiac output per meter square of body surface area:

$$\text{Cardiac index} = \frac{\text{Cardiac output}}{\text{Body surface area}}.$$

Normal cardiac index is 3.1–3.3 L/m^2.

It is a better indicator to evaluate the efficiency of the heart.

End Systolic Volume

It is the volume of blood present in each ventricle at the end of systole. It is about 50 mL.

End Diastolic Volume

It is the volume of blood accumulated in the ventricle at the end of diastole. It is about 130 mL.

Ejection Fraction

It is that part (percentage) of blood ejected from the ventricle out of the end diastolic volume. Normal ejection fraction is about 65%.

Applied Physiology

Hypertension

It is a condition in which BP increases above the normal value of 140/90 mm Hg.

1. **Primary hypertension:** It is also termed essential hypertension. In about 90% of the patients with elevated BP, the cause for hypertension is not known. Essential hypertension is treatable but not curable. Effective lowering of BP can be achieved by the use of conventional antihypertensive drugs.

2. **Secondary hypertension:** Hypertension is secondary to a disease affecting the other systems. For example, pheochromocytoma, tumor of the adrenal medulla, or catecholamine-secreting tissue in other parts of the body can produce hypertension.

    - *Renal hypertension:* Constriction of the renal artery or compression of the kidney increases the blood pressure. Decreased ability of the kidney to excrete sodium ions can contribute to renal hypertension.

    - *Cushing's syndrome:* Hypertension is due to increased secretion of deoxycorticosterone and angiotensin.

3. **Malignant hypertension:** Chronic hypertension can show necrotic arteriolar lesion. The condition is associated with papilledema, cerebral manifestation, and renal failure. This syndrome is termed malignant hypertension. The condition can be reversed by suitable antihypertensive therapy.

Management

A persistent increase in BP can damage the internal organs. There is greater risk of cerebrovascular accidents. Hence, it is advisable to maintain the BP within normal range to reduce the risk of complication and improve survival.

Hypertension is managed by

(a) pharmacological methods and

(b) nonpharmacological methods.

Pharmacological methods use various drugs to manage hypertension.

The principle drugs used are

1. diuretics,
2. β-adrenergic receptor antagonists,
3. calcium channel blocker,
4. ACE inhibitors,
5. angiotensin II receptor blocker, and
6. vasodilators.

Diuretics reduce the fluid volume. This reduces the venous return and cardiac output, thus reducing the BP.

The cardiac muscles have β-adrenergic receptors. Blocking these receptors results in reduced cardiac output and hence reduces the BP.

The calcium channel blockers reduce the availability of calcium ions to myocardial cell. This reduces the myocardial contractility, cardiac output, and blood pressure.

ACE inhibitors prevent the conversion of angiotensin I to angiotensin II. This drug reduces BP by blocking the vasoconstrictor effect of angiotensin II.

Angiotensin receptor antagonists have action similar to that of ACE inhibitors. But they are free of side effects seen with the use of ACE inhibitors.

Vasodilators act directly on the smooth muscles of blood vessels. They produce vasodilation and reduce the blood pressure by decreasing the peripheral resistance.

Nonpharmacological methods for the management of hypertension include the followings:

- **Diet:** Correction of obesity by regulated intake of food. Reduce the consumption of alcohol. Decrease salt intake. Salt sensitizes the receptors to circulating norepinephrine.

- **Modification of risk factors:** Reduce smoking. Effective treatment of hyperlipidemia.
- **Relaxation and exercise:** Relaxation and regular exercise can lower the BP by improving physical fitness and reaction to stressful stimulus. Nonpharmacological management can be used as an adjuvant for pharmacological management.

Hypotension

A decrease in BP below the normal value of 90/60 mm Hg, e.g., circulatory shock.

Cardiac Reserve

It is the maximum volume of blood that can be pumped out of the heart in excess of the normal cardiac output.

Factors Regulating Cardiac Output

1. **Venous return:** Venous return is the flow of blood back to the heart. Venous return influences the initial length of the cardiac muscle. Whenever the venous return increases, cardiac muscle is stretched resulting in increased cardiac output. The venous return depends on the following factors:

    (a) *Respiration:* During inspiration, the intrathoracic pressure decreases and becomes negative, but there is an increase in the intra-abdominal pressure. These changes cause an increase in the blood flow to right atrium from lower parts of the body.

    (b) *Muscle pump:* When the skeletal muscles are contracting, they squeeze or compress the veins. This results in movement of blood toward the heart. (Flow of blood in the opposite direction is prevented by valves present in the veins.)

    (c) *Venomotor tone:* Veins are supplied by sympathetic nerves. When they are stimulated, veins undergo constriction mobilizing blood toward the heart.

    (d) *Gravity:* Standing or sitting increases blood flow from upper parts of the body toward the heart due to the effect of gravity.

    (e) *Force of pumping of the blood:* When the force of cardiac contraction increases, it improves cardiac output and velocity of circulation. This causes greater venous return. Force exerted by the column of blood from behind to move blood toward the heart is termed **vis-a-tergo**. At the right atrium the negative pressure created during diastole draws the blood toward it. This is termed **vis-a-fronte**.

2. **Contractility of the heart:** Cardiac output is directly proportional to the force of contraction. Force of contraction depends on diastolic filling time. Longer the diastolic period greater is the end diastolic volume. Increase in initial length of cardiac muscle fiber enhances the force of the contraction. Stimulation of sympathetic nerve or injection of epinephrine increases the contraction of cardiac muscle. Hence the cardiac output increases.

3. **Nutrition of heart muscle:** Whenever the cardiac activity increases, there is greater demand for oxygen and supply of nutrients. This demand is met by increasing the blood flow. If the cardiac activity increases without an increase in oxygen and nutrition supply, heart muscles get damaged reducing the cardiac output.

4. **Heart rate:** A moderate increase in heart rate (up to about 180 beats/min) shows an increase in the cardiac output. However if the heart rate increases to about 250–300 beats/min, cardiac output decreases.

Increase in heart rate decreases the diastolic filling time. There is reduction in the volume of blood collected in the ventricle at the end of diastole. Reduced end diastolic volume decreases the initial length of ventricular muscle. This reduces the force of contraction.

Heart rate and cardiac output are increased during exercise. The venous return is increased due to muscle and respiratory pump. Hence a shorter diastolic time is sufficient to ensure a good ventricular filling and a better cardiac output.

Estimation of Cardiac Output

Cardiac output is estimated by the following methods:

1. Fick's principle,
2. Hamilton's dye dilution method,
3. thermodilution method,
4. ballistocardiography, and
5. Doppler with echocardiography.

Fick's Principle

According to Fick's principle, the amount of substance taken up by an organ is equal to the arteriovenous difference of the substance times the blood flow.

Cardiac output can be determined by measuring the O_2 consumed by the body in 1 min and dividing this value by $A - V$ difference of oxygen.

Oxygen consumption = Blood flow × AV difference of O_2

$$\text{Cardiac output} = \frac{O_2 \text{ consumption (mL/min)}}{\text{Arterial } O_2 - \text{Venous } O_2}.$$

Hamilton's Dye dilution method

A known amount of the dye or radioactive isotope is injected into the arm vein. Concentration of the indicator is estimated in serial samples from the arterial blood. Cardiac output is equal to the amount of dye injected divided by its average (mean) concentration in the arterial blood after a single circulation through the heart.

Thermodilution method

Cold saline (indicator) is injected into the right atrium. Temperature change of the blood is recorded in pulmonary artery. The temperature change is inversely proportional to the volume of blood flowing through the pulmonary artery.

Electrocardiogram

Electrocardiogram (ECG) is the electrical activity of the heart recorded from the surface of the body (Fig. 4.13). ECG is recorded by using different electrodes.

The body acts as a volume conductor. The body fluids are good conductors of electricity. The summated effect of action potentials from cardiac muscle can be recorded from the surface. The record of these potential fluctuations during a cardiac cycle is the **electrocardiogram**.

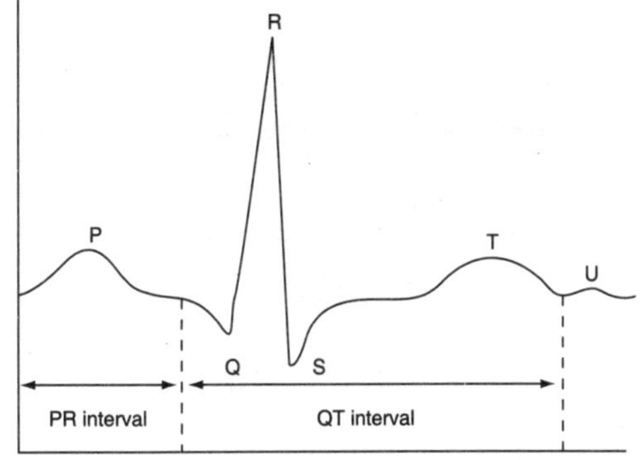

Fig. 4.13   Electrocardiogram.

ECG is recorded by using an **active** or **exploring electrode** and an **indifferent electrode** at zero potential (as in unipolar recording) or by using two active electrodes as in bipolar recording.

1. Bipolar limb leads left
   - **Lead I:** Between right arm (–ve) and left arm (+ve)
   - **Lead II**: Between right arm (–ve) and left leg (+ve)
   - **Lead III**: Between left arm (–ve) and left leg (+ve)

2. Augmented unipolar limb leads (Fig. 4.14)
   - **aVR:** Exploring electrode connected to right arm
   - **aVL:** Exploring electrode connected to left arm
   - **aVF:** Exploring electrode connected to left leg

   The indifferent electrode is kept at zero potential.

3. Chest leads
   - V_1: Fourth intercostal space at the right margin of sternum
   - V_2: Fourth intercostal space at the left margin of sternum
   - V_3: In between V_2 and V_4
   - V_4: Fifth intercostal space in midclavicular line

- **V_5:** Fifth intercostal space in anterior axillary line
- **V_6:** Fifth intercostal space in midaxillary line

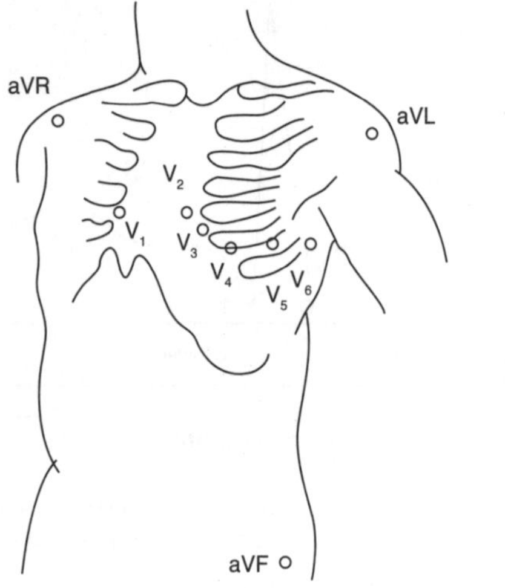

Fig. 4.14   ECG leads.

ECG Recording

ECG is recorded on a heat-sensitive paper. Time (duration) is measured on the X-axis and voltage is measured on the Y-axis. The paper has small boxes of 1 mm^2. Five small squares are demarcated by a thick line. Each small square on the X-axis corresponds to 0.04 s. A block of five small squares is equal to 0.2 s (0.04×5). Each of the small squares on Y-axis corresponds to 0.1 mV.

Calibration

Instrument has to be calibrated before recording the ECG. For normal recording, instrument has to be calibrated to show a displacement of 10 mm for 1 mV. Thus each mm corresponds to 0.1 mV.

Speed

The ECG paper can be moved at two different speeds depending on the type of recording. Normally a speed of 25 mm/s is used. The paper moves a distance of 1500 mm (25×60) in 1 min. A speed of 50 mm/s is used when the heart rate is high and a better view of different waves is required. At this speed, 3000 mm of the paper moves in 1 min.

Einthoven's Law

Einthoven's law states that voltage recorded in standard limb lead II is equal to the sum of voltages recorded in the other two leads:

$$\text{Lead II} = \text{Lead I} + \text{Lead III.}$$

This equation helps to check the proper placement of leads. Einthoven's law holds good for ECG recording done by using standard bipolar limb leads.

Einthoven's Triangle

It is an equilateral triangle with upper corners corresponding to right and left shoulders. The lower corner corresponds to pubic symphysis. The heart which is oriented downward and to the left is considered to be situated in the center of this triangle. The recording electrodes (leads) placed on right arm, left arm, and left foot are considered to be placed at the corners of this equilateral triangle.

In standard bipolar limb leads, the recordings are obtained between any two corners of the triangle. Fourth lead connected to the right limb serves as an earth (ground terminal).

In augmented limb leads, unipolar recording is obtained from one of the three corners of the triangle. Exploring electrode is placed at one corner and the other two corners are connected through a high resistance to function as indifferent electrode.

In augmented electrodes, recording shows an enhanced voltage (about 50% more) when compared to the voltage in standard limb leads.

In chest leads, unipolar exploring electrode is placed in one of the six locations on the chest. Left arm, right arm, and left foot are connected together through a high resistance to form the indifferent electrode.

Waves of ECG

P-Wave

It is produced due to atrial depolarization. Its normal duration is 0.1 s and voltage 0.1–0.12 mV.

It is an upright wave in all the leads except aVR. In this lead P-wave is inverted.

P-wave is inverted in nodal rhythm. In this condition impulses travel in the opposite direction, from AV node toward the SA node.

P-wave is absent when the SA node is not generating the impulses as in SA block.

QRS Complex

It is produced due to ventricular depolarization. Its duration is 0.08–0.1 s and voltage varies from 0.5 to 2 mV.

QRS complex in limb lead helps to determine the electrical axis of the heart.

T-Wave

It is produced due to ventricular repolarization. Its normal duration is 0.15 s and voltage 0.3 mV.

It is a positive wave in all the leads except aVR. Inverted T-wave in lead III is considered normal. Inversion of T-wave in other leads is considered abnormal. Inverted T-wave is seen in myocardial ischemia, infarction, and ventricular hypertrophy.

U-Wave

It is due to repolarization of the septum of ventricle and papillary muscle.

Atrial Repolarization Wave

Repolarization wave of atrium is submerged in QRS complex.

PR Interval

It is measured from the beginning of P-wave to beginning of QRS complex. It measures about 0.12–0.16 s with a maximum of 0.2 s. It indicates the time for atrial depolarization and conduction of impulse through AV node.

PR interval increases gradually beat after beat in Wenckebach phenomenon.

It is very short in Wolff–Parkinson–White syndrome.

QT Interval

It is from the beginning of Q-wave to the end of T-wave. It is the measure of ventricular electrical events (depolarization and repolarization). Its normal duration is 0.40–0.43 s.

QT interval is altered by drugs like quinidine.

ST Segment

- It is a segment between the end of S-wave and the beginning of T-wave. This segment is present on the isoelectric line. As the ventricle is completely depolarized, no potential difference is recorded in this segment.
- Ischemia of ventricular muscle causes the depression of ST segment.
- Myocardial infarction results in elevation of ST segment.
- In cases of ischemia or infarction, ventricular muscles are not completely depolarized. Hence a potential difference is recorded. This potential difference causes the shift of ST segment from isoelectric line.

Electrical Axis of the Heart

Mean electrical axis is the direction of largest vector in limb leads. It correlates with long axis of the heart. Mean electrical axis can be used to determine the orientation of heart.

Normal mean electrical axis is about 55° (range –30° to 110°). If the heart is rotated in anticlockwise direction, it is termed **left axis deviation**.

Hypertrophy of left ventricle results in left axis deviation.

Rotation of heart in clockwise direction beyond 110° is called **right axis deviation**.

Hypertrophy of right ventricle produces right axis deviation.

Tall and thin people with narrow thorax have vertical electrical axis.

A tall R-wave in lead II indicates a normal electrical axis of the heart.

In left axis deviation, R-wave becomes prominent in lead I.

When the R-wave is taller in lead III, it is suggestive of right axis deviation.

Cardiac Vectors

Cardiac muscle cells show electrical activity with waves of depolarization and repolarization. At any given time, these waves having different magnitudes are moving in different directions. The resultant electrical activity having both magnitude and direction constitutes the **cardiac vector.**

Depolarization of atria commences at SA node and spreads through atrial muscles to AV node. The resultant vector is directed downward and toward left (P-wave).

Later, the wave of depolarization spreads through ventricular muscle from inside to outside. Since the wall of left ventricle is thick, direction of vector is downward and left (QRS complex).

Activation of the last part of the ventricle (basal part) results in vector directed upward and toward right (QRS complex).

Wave of ventricular repolarization spreads from outer to inner surface of ventricular myocardium. Since it is opposite in direction to the wave of ventricular depolarization, it produces a vector in the same direction as that of ventricular depolarization, directed downward and toward left (T-wave).

When the vector is directed toward positive electrode (exploring electrode), a positive wave is recorded. When the vector moves away from positive electrode, a negative wave is recorded in ECG.

Uses of ECG

- Useful in calculating the heart rate in a regularly beating heart

- Detecting functional abnormalities of heart like heart blocks, arrhythmias, and myocardial infarction

Circulatory Shock

Shock is a state of circulatory failure. It is a condition characterized by insufficient cardiac output. The circulatory system fails to meet the oxygen and nutritional requirement of the tissues.

Types of shock are

1. hypovolemic shock,
2. distributive shock,
3. cardiogenic shock, and
4. obstructive shock.

Applied Physiology

In **myocardial infarction**, ST segment is elevated and T-wave is inverted. Isolated T-wave inversion in limb lead III is considered normal.

In **first-degree heart block**, PR interval is prolonged beyond 0.2 s.

Arrhythmias

These are abnormal rhythms of the heart. They include atrial, ventricular flutters, and fibrillations.

Stress ECG

ECG recorded at rest in some individuals does not give an indication about ischemia. If there are symptoms suggestive of ischemia, ECG is recorded during graded physical activity. The changes in stress ECG recording provide evidence for ischemia of cardiac muscle.

The subject is asked to run on a treadmill. Speed and gradient is gradually increased till the subject can no longer continue the exercise due to exhaustion or reaches the predicted heart rate whichever occurs earlier. ECG is continuously recorded during the activity. Any demonstrable change in ECG with special reference to ST segment confirms the presence of ischemia.

Failure to achieve desired increase in BP is suggestive of ventricular decompensation secondary to extensive ischemia.

Ambulatory ECG (Holter Monitoring)

Holter monitoring is useful in detecting the episodes of ischemia or arrhythmia which occur occasionally.

ECG from one or more leads is recorded continuously by using small portable device. These recordings are later transmitted to the cardiac center for evaluation.

Types

Hypovolemic Shock

This occurs in cases of hemorrhage, trauma, burns, vomiting, and diarrhea. The condition is caused due to a reduction in blood volume. It is characterized by rapid thready pulse, hypotension, cold clammy skin, restlessness, rapid respiration, and excessive thirst. In hypovolemic shock, inadequate supply of blood to the tissues leads to an increase in anerobic glycolysis. It results in the production of large amounts of lactic acid. Lactic acidosis depresses the myocardium and responsiveness of the blood vessels to catecholamines.

Distributive Shock

It comprises **anaphylactic shock, septic shock,** and **neurogenic shock.** In this type of shock, blood volume is normal but the capacity of circulation is increased due to intense vasodilation. It is also termed **warm shock.**

Anaphylactic Shock   The hypersensitivity reaction releases histamine. Histamine causes vasodilation and increased permeability of blood vessels. There is loss of fluid resulting in decreased venous return and cardiac output. These changes produce shock.

Septic Shock   It is produced due to uncontrolled infection. The bacterial toxins released cause generalized vasodilation and increased permeability of blood vessels. This reduces the circulating blood volume resulting in shock.

Neurogenic Shock   It is produced due to sudden autonomic activity resulting in marked vasodilation. There is peripheral pooling of blood associated with fainting. It is also called vasovagal syncope. It lasts for a short duration and is reversible.

Other forms of syncope include the following:

- **Postural syncope:** Change in position results in fainting due to pooling of blood in dependent parts of the body.

- **Micturition syncope:** This is commonly seen in subjects with orthostatic hypotension. Fainting occurs during urination due to orthostasis and reflex bradycardia.

- **Carotid sinus syncope:** Pressure on the carotid sinus causes marked bradycardia and vasodilation resulting in syncopal attacks.

Cardiogenic Shock

It is seen in conditions of myocardial infarction, congestive cardiac failure, and arrhythmias. In this type of shock, heart fails to pump sufficient quantity of blood to maintain normal tissue perfusion. It is due to extensive infarction of the left ventricle or diseases that depress the ventricular function. This is also called **congested shock** as the lungs and viscera get congested due to ineffective pumping of heart.

Obstructive Shock

It is seen in conditions like cardiac tamponade, cardiac tumors, pulmonary embolism, and tension pneumothorax.

Compensatory Mechanisms

Compensatory mechanisms are aimed at restoring blood pressure. It comes into play within few seconds from the onset of shock.

Immediate Mechanism

1. Baroreceptor mechanism

2. Chemoreceptor mechanism

3. VMC ischemic response (*Refer to the section Regulation of Blood Pressure.*)

Long-Term Mechanism

Reverse Fluid Shift Mechanism   In normal circulation, the hydrostatic pressure (which depends on the blood pressure) at the arterial end of the capillary exceeds the tissue pressure and colloidal osmotic pressure. Hence, fluid comes out of the capillary. But it reenters at the venous end. When the SBP decreases as in the case of shock, the hydrostatic pressure is less than the other two pressures put together. This causes the entry of fluid into the blood vessel from extravascular space. These changes enhance the blood volume, venous return, and therefore increase the BP.

Water Conservation   ADH hormone is released in a state of shock. It helps in reabsorption of water from the kidney. In large doses ADH produces vasoconstriction and increases the peripheral resistance, helping to increase BP. Reduced blood flow to kidney causes the release of renin.

By renin–angiotensin–aldosterone mechanism sodium and water are retained. This increases the blood volume and hence increases BP.

Irreversible Shock

If prompt treatment is not given during the state of shock, it becomes irreversible. Death can be caused due to the following:

- Ischemic cardiac damage resulting in failure of the heart to pump blood.
- Accumulation of metabolic end products due to poor perfusion of the tissues causes acidosis. Acidosis results in peripheral vasodilation and peripheral pooling of blood. There is decreased venous return and reduced cardiac output producing irreversible cardiac damage.
- Hypoxia and hypercapnia due to poor perfusion of the tissues promote growth of microorganisms. These organisms produce toxins, which cause the paralysis of vascular smooth muscle and peripheral pooling of blood.
- Ischemia of the VMC results in its paralysis and failure of sympathetic system to restore the blood pressure.

Management of Shock

General principles in management of shock are

- restoration of fluid volume by blood or plasma transfusion,
- administration of plasma substitutes and plasma expanders,
- maintenance of oxygen concentration in the blood by administering oxygen,
- correction of acidosis,
- maintenance of functions of vital organs, and
- use of sympathomimetic drugs and steroids to restore blood pressure.

Regional Circulation

Coronary Circulation (Fig. 4.15)

The heart is supplied by right and left coronary arteries. Coronary arteries arise from sinuses at the root of the aorta.

The right coronary artery is dominant in 50% and left coronary artery in 20% of the individuals. In the remaining 30%, flow in right and left coronary artery is equal.

The capillary density of coronary arteries is very high when compared to other sites in the body.

The venous blood is drained into the right atrium through the coronary sinus and the anterior cardiac veins.

In addition, blood is drained directly into the chambers through

- thebesian veins,
- arteriosinusoidal vessels, and
- arterioluminal vessels.

Coronary arteries are end arteries with little anastomosis.

However, in patients with coronary artery disease, these blood vessels increase in number and size.

The normal coronary blood flow in human beings at rest is 250 mL/min (5% of the cardiac output).

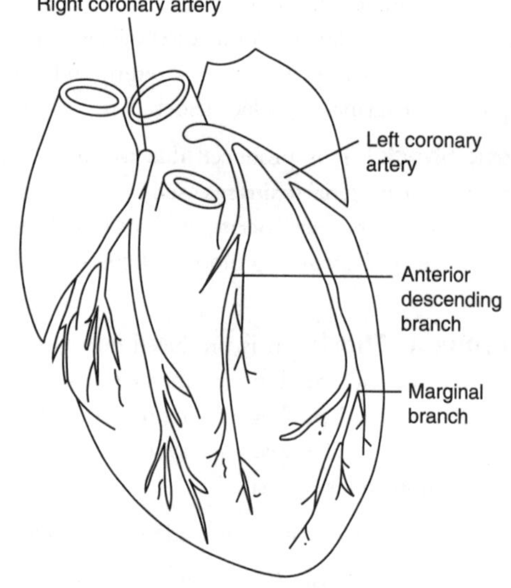

Fig. 4.15   Coronary arteries and their branches.

Evaluation of Myocardial Blood Flow

The coronary blood flow is evaluated by using radioactive tracers. Radionucleotide such as thallium-201 is introduced by intravenous injection. It is pumped into the cardiac muscle by the sodium–potassium ATPase. After a lapse of about

10–15 min, concentration of radioactive tracers is estimated by using radiation detectors placed over the chest. The distribution of thallium-201 is proportional to myocardial blood flow.

Uptake of radionucleotide is reduced in areas of ischemia.

Exertion-induced compromise in blood flow can be detected by measuring the uptake of radioactive isotope immediately after exercise and after few hours of rest.

Factors Influencing Coronary Circulation

- **Phases of cardiac cycle:** The blood vessels supplying the myocardium and endocardium pass through layers of the heart, arising perpendicular to the main artery. Hence, the blood vessels are compressed during the cardiac systole. The myocardium and endocardium do not get the blood supply during systole but get major part of the blood supply during diastole.

- **Chemical factors:** Metabolic activity results in the accumulation of end products like lactates and hydrogen ions. During anerobic metabolism there is formation of adenosine from ATP and prostaglandins in the cardiac tissue. These substances cause increased blood flow due to local vasodilation.

    The other factors known to produce local coronary vasodilation are

    (a)   oxygen lack,
    (b)   carbon dioxide excess,
    (c)   increased potassium ion concentration,
    (d)   adenine nucleotide accumulation, and
    (e)   intracoronary injection of cyanide.

    The coronary artery occlusion followed by release of occlusion increases the blood flow through it due to the release of adenosine. This is termed **reactive hyperemia.**

- **Autoregulation:** It is the ability of vital organs like heart, brain, and kidney to regulate its blood flow within narrow range of fluctuation. This operates between arterial blood pressures of 60 and 160 mm Hg.

- **Neural factor:** Stimulation of sympathetic nerves to the heart increases the heart rate and produces initial vasoconstriction. The accumulation of metabolic end products and adenosine finally

produces vasodilation by its local action.

Cerebral Circulation

In human beings two internal carotid and two vertebral arteries supply the brain.

The normal cerebral blood flow is 750 mL/min or 54 mL/100 g of the tissue.

Factors Influencing Cerebral Circulation

- **Autoregulation:** Brain maintains its blood flow in spite of variation in the arterial blood pressure.

- **Hypoxia:** Increases blood flow by vasodilation.

- **Oxygen excess:** High oxygen concentration produces vasoconstriction. This reduces the blood flow to the brain to prevent its damage.

- **Hypercapnia:** Increased carbon dioxide concentration in the blood causes cerebral vasodilation due to local effect enhancing the blood flow.

- **Intracranial pressure:** An increase in the intracranial pressure decreases cerebral blood flow. However if the intracranial pressure is reduced, the blood flow is restored.

- **Perfusion pressure:** The pressure difference between arterial and venous system to the brain plays an important role in the regulation of blood flow to the brain. Perfusion pressure helps to maintain a constant flow of blood.

- **Autonomic stimulation:** Sympathetic stimulation does not significantly alter the blood flow to the brain.

- **Anesthetics:** They reduce the flow of blood to the brain.

    Blood flow to the brain can be monitored by

- positron emission tomography and
- functional magnetic resonance imaging.

Cutaneous Circulation

It is circulation through the skin (Fig. 4.16)

Blood flow to the skin is about 400–450 mL/min. It can vary from 50 to 4500 mL/min.

Features

The cutaneous circulation plays an important role in the regulation of body temperature.

It acts as a reservoir for blood.

Blood flow to the skin is highly variable.

Applied Physiology

Angina Pectoris

It is a severe constricting pain in the chest radiating from precardium due to ischemia of cardiac muscles. In this condition, pain is produced due to hypoxia of myocardial tissue. An obstruction of about 75% to the coronary artery produces angina pectoris. Reduction in blood flow causes local accumulation of pain-producing factors.

Nitroglycerin (nitrates) is used in the management of pain during angina pectoris. Nitroglycerin generates nitric oxide (NO) and dilates the normal arteries.

Nitrates dilate the capacitance vessels and reduce the venous return. This reduces myocardial oxygen consumption due to decreased stroke volume.

NO production is defective in atherosclerotic vessels.

Myocardial Infarction

It is the death of the myocardial tissue. It is caused due to sudden stoppage of blood supply to an area of the myocardium. Blood flow to the myocardium is stopped due to

- formation of thrombus in already narrowed coronary blood vessel,
- spasm of coronary artery,
- platelet aggregation in severely sclerotic artery,
- rupture of atherosclerotic plaque, and
- hemorrhage into atherosclerotic plaque.

Management

Intracoronary clots are lysed by thrombolytic agents to restore the blood flow.

Streptokinase is a lytic agent obtained from the bacteria hemolytic streptococci. It converts plasminogen to plasmin in the clot.

Tissue-type plasminogen activator (t-PA) activates plasminogen bound to fibrin. It brings about fibrinolysis in the clots.

Thrombolytic agents are very effective if they are used within few hours after the onset of pain.

Angiography

This is a procedure to detect the presence of block in the blood vessels due to a clot. A radio-opaque dye is injected into the artery and demonstration of filling defect radiographically confirms the presence of a block.

Angioplasty

It is the procedure by which clot obstructing the coronary artery is removed by catheterization.

Stent

It is a mesh-like device placed in the coronary artery after the removal of the clot. This is done to prevent the reocclusion of the blood vessels due to its spasm.

Coronary Bypass

This is a surgical procedure in which proximal and distal parts of the coronary artery are connected bypassing the areas of obstruction due to a clot. A healthy blood vessel taken from different parts of the body is used in this procedure to restore the blood flow to the cardiac tissue.

Factors Influencing Cutaneous Circulation

- Sympathetic stimulation decreases blood flow to the skin.
- Increased body temperature causes vasodilation and hence increases blood flow.
- Epinephrine and norepinephrine cause vasoconstriction reducing the blood flow. Bradykinin and histamine cause vasodilation increasing the blood flow.

White Reaction

When the skin is stroked lightly the skin appears pale due to reduced blood flow. This response is due to the contraction of precapillary sphincter. It is called **white reaction.**

Triple Response

When the skin is stroked (scratched) firmly, it shows three reactions. They are as follows:

1. **Red reaction:** A red line appears when the stroke is made. This is due to relaxation of precapillary sphincter and engorgement of capillary under the influence of histamine. The line appears in about 10 s and becomes well developed in 1 min.
2. **Flare or flush:** When stroking is firm, an area of redness develops surrounding the site of stroking. This is caused due to arteriolar dilatation as a result of axon reflex. The area has increased temperature.
3. **Wheal:** In this stage fluid collects around the area of stroking resulting in edema. Fluid is a transudate produced due to increased hydrostatic pressure in the dilated capillaries. Triple response is largely due to local release of histamine.

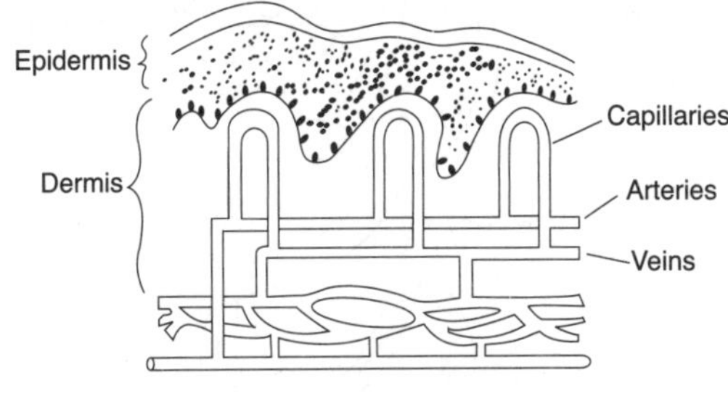

Fig. 4.16   Cutaneous circulation.

Fetal Circulation (Fig. 4.17)

The fetal oxygen and nutritional requirements during intrauterine period are obtained from maternal circulation through the placenta.

The placenta has the maternal portion and fetal portion.

The **maternal portion** consists of uterine spiral arteries which open into intervillous space. The **fetal portion** consists of umbilical arteries and umbilical vein. The umbilical vein carries blood from placenta. Later, it passes through the inferior vena cava and reaches the left ventricle through foramen ovale and left atrium. This blood bypasses the lungs.

Applied Physiology

Stroke

Stroke is a condition of paralysis produced due to lack of oxygen supply to the brain.

Neurons in the brain are sensitive to the supply of oxygen. Anoxia of 3–4 min results in death of these neurons. When blood supply to a part of brain is interrupted, it produces signs and symptoms of stroke.

The types of stroke are

- hemorrhagic stroke and
- ischemic stroke.

Hemorrhagic stroke occurs when the blood vessels to the brain rupture.

Ischemic stroke occurs when the flow of blood in the vessels is reduced or stopped by thrombus or atherosclerotic plaques. Thrombus may also be formed elsewhere and reach the brain as emboli.

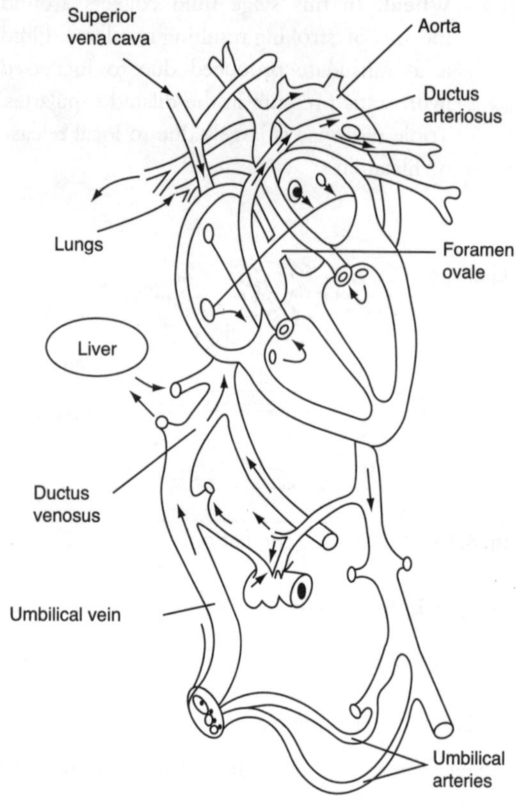

Fig. 4.17 Foetal circulation.

Blood from superior vena cava enters the right atrium and right ventricle. It later passes through pulmonary trunk and gets shunted via ductus arteriosus to aorta. From the aorta, blood goes to the placenta through umbilical arteries.

Changes at Birth

The placental circulation is cut off immediately after birth and peripheral resistance rises suddenly. Pressure in the aorta rises till it exceeds pressure in pulmonary artery. The infant gasps because of asphyxia and the lungs expand. Once the lungs expand, pulmonary vascular resistance falls to less than 20% of intrauterine levels and hence pulmonary blood flow increases markedly. Blood returning from the lungs raises the pressure in left atrium closing the foramen ovale. The ductus arteriosus constricts within few minutes after birth and finally it is shut off completely.

Capillary Circulation

The capillary is the connection between arterial and venous ends of the vascular tree.

The capillaries contain about 250 mL of blood (5% of circulating blood).

The capillary circulation helps in the exchange of gases, supply of nutrients, and removal of waste from the tissues.

The types of capillaries are

1. continuous capillary,
2. fenestrated capillary, and
3. sinusoidal capillary.

Continuous Capillaries (Nonfenestrated)

The majority of the capillaries are of this type. They have a single layer of continuous endothelial lining. They permit the exchange of fluid and water-soluble substances.

Fenestrated Capillaries

These capillaries are found in glomerulus of the kidney, intestinal villi, and endocrine glands. They have fenestrations or pores which allow rapid movement of molecules.

Sinusoidal Capillaries

They are found in liver, spleen, and bone marrow. They are lined by single layer of endothelial cells. There are large gaps in between the cells. They help in the passage of bigger molecules.

The filtration across the capillary wall depends on Starling's forces. These forces are acting in opposite directions. The resultant pressure influences the movement of fluid across the blood vessel.

- Capillary hydrostatic pressure
- Plasma colloid osmotic pressure
- Interstitial fluid hydrostatic pressure
- Interstitial fluid colloid osmotic pressure

At the arterial end of capillary, the net pressure is directed outward. Hence, fluid moves out of the capillary.

At the venous end, the resultant pressure is negative. Hence, fluid is drawn back into the capillary.

CHAPTER 5

Respiratory System

Respiration is a process of uptake of oxygen and removal of carbon dioxide from tissues of the body.

The cells in the body derive energy mainly by utilizing oxygen. Carbon dioxide (CO_2) is produced as a by-product. Carbon dioxide has to be eliminated from the cell.

Unicellular organisms exchange oxygen and CO_2 directly with the external environment. Multicellular organisms require a specialized system to exchange O_2 and CO_2 with the external environment. This complex function is performed by the respiratory system (Fig. 5.1).

Exchange of gases between the atmosphere and lungs is called **external respiration.**

Exchange of gases between blood and tissues is called **internal respiration.**

Respiration involves two processes:

1. **Inspiration:** During this phase air is taken into the lungs from the atmosphere.

2. **Expiration:** During this phase air is expelled out of the lungs.

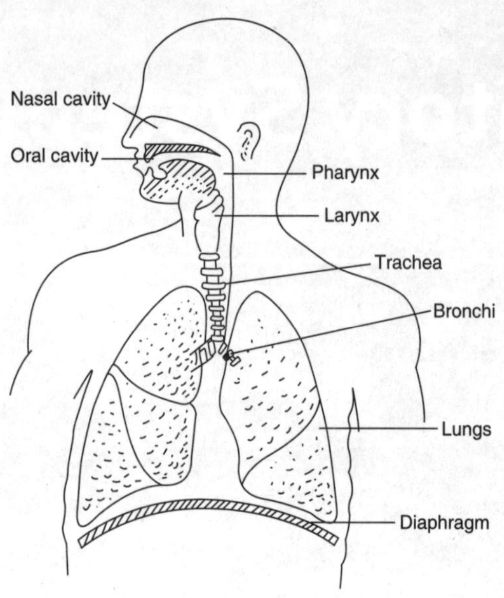

Fig. 5.1   Respiratory tract.

Normal respiratory rate is 12–18 cycles/min.

Functional Anatomy

The respiratory tract includes nasal cavities, paranasal sinuses, pharynx, larynx, trachea, bronchi, bronchioles, and alveoli.

Airways

The air passes from the nose to the nasal cavities and later into the pharynx. The pharynx is a common passage for air and food. It continues into larynx. The larynx contains vocal cords.

The larynx opens into a long tube called the **trachea**. The trachea divides into two bronchi. Each bronchus enters the lungs. Within the lungs, they branch further into bronchioles. The terminal parts of the bronchioles are termed **respiratory bronchioles**. The respiratory bronchioles end in the alveoli.

Upper Respiratory Tract

The part of the respiratory passage from the nostrils up to the vocal cords is called the upper respiratory tract.

Lower Respiratory Tract

The respiratory passage below the vocal cords is called the lower respiratory tract.

The lower respiratory tract begins with the trachea and divides into two bronchi, which subdivide repeatedly to form bronchioles, which end as the alveoli.

Respiratory tract divides 23 times (Fig. 5.2). First 16 generations form the **conducting zone**. Seventeenth to nineteenth generations form the **transition zone**. Twentieth to twenty-third generations form the **exchange zone**.

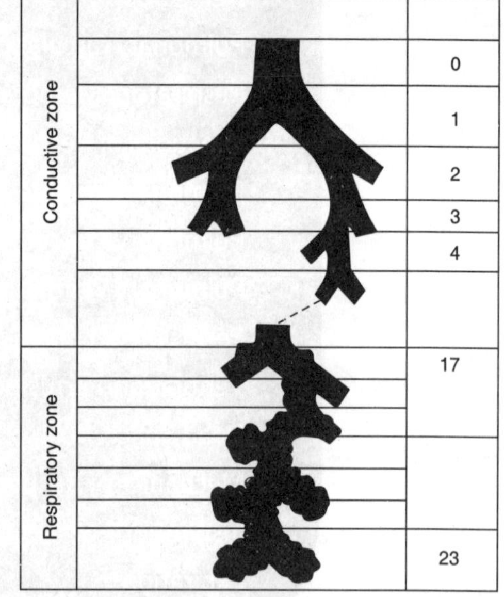

Fig. 5.2   Weibel model of respiratory tract.

Exchange of gases can take place from seventeenth to twenty-third generations.

Alveoli

The alveoli are the sites for gas exchange. These are tiny hollow sacs which continue with the lumen of the bronchioles.

The cells are flattened and form a single layer.

The alveoli contain two types of cells: (i) Type I and (ii) Type II.

Type I Cells   They are the main lining cells of the alveoli. Gas exchange occurs through these cells.

Type II Cells   They are specialized thicker cells that produce a substance called **surfactant**.

Other cells present are alveolar macrophages, mast cells, plasma cell, and APUD (amine precursor uptake decarboxycation) cells.

Histology

The respiratory tract is made up of three layers:

1.   outer fibrous layer,
2.   middle muscular layer, and
3.   inner epithelial layer.

Outer Fibrous Layer

It is made up of C-shaped cartilage in the trachea. As the respiratory tree divides, cartilage decreases and ultimately there is no cartilage in the terminal bronchiole and the alveoli.

Middle Muscular Layer

It is made up of smooth muscles. When these muscles contract, there is narrowing of bronchial lumen producing bronchoconstriction. Relaxation of muscles results in bronchodilatation.

Inner Epithelial Layer

It is formed by mucus membrane. It is made up of ciliated columnar cells in the upper respiratory tract. The cilia help to clear dust particles. The epithelium in the respiratory bronchiole is cuboidal and has no cilia.

This layer also contains glands that secrete mucus. Dust particles and particulate matter stick to the mucus. This is slowly moved upward toward the pharynx by the movement of cilia.

Nerve Supply

The respiratory tract is supplied by autonomic nervous system.

The sympathetic stimulation causes dilatation of bronchioles by relaxation of smooth muscles. This action is mediated through β_2 receptors.

The parasympathetic stimulation increases the bronchial secretion and causes narrowing of the respiratory passage (bronchoconstriction).

Pulmonary Circulation

The pulmonary circulation is between the right ventricle and the left atrium (Fig. 5.3). The pulmonary artery arises from the right ventricle and divides into right and left branches. These branches subdivide and form pulmonary capillaries. The pulmonary capillaries are lined by a single layer of epithelium and form a dense network around the alveoli.

The pulmonary arteries and their branches are thin walled and distensible. Therefore, pulmonary circulation is a low-pressure, low-resistance, and high-capacitance system.

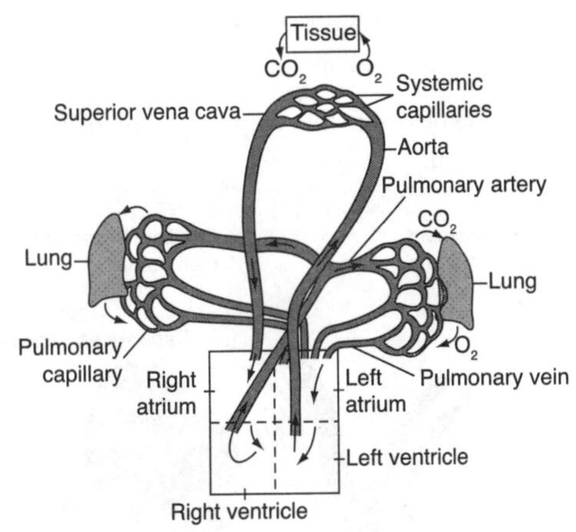

Fig. 5.3   Circulation in pulmonary system.

Pressures in Pulmonary System

The right ventricular pressure reaches a peak of 25 mm Hg during systole and falls to 0 mm Hg during diastole.

The pressure in the pulmonary artery during systole is 25 mm Hg and during diastole is 8 mm Hg.

The pulmonary capillary pressure is about 10 mm Hg.

The diameter of pulmonary capillary is about $10\,\mu m$ which is just enough for the RBC to pass through.

The RBC spends about three-fourth of a second in the pulmonary capillary network. The gas exchange between the alveolar air and the RBC occurs within this short period.

The gas exchange occurs between the alveolar air and the blood in the pulmonary capillaries through the **respiratory membrane**.

Respiratory Membrane

It is a thin membrane separating blood in the pulmonary capillaries and air in the alveoli (Fig. 5.4). Respiratory membrane consists of

- layer of surfactant lining the alveolus,
- alveolar epithelium,
- basement membrane of the alveolar epithelium,
- interstitial space between the alveolar epithelium and the capillary membrane,
- capillary basement membrane, and
- capillary endothelium.

The thickness of the respiratory membrane is around 0.6 μm.

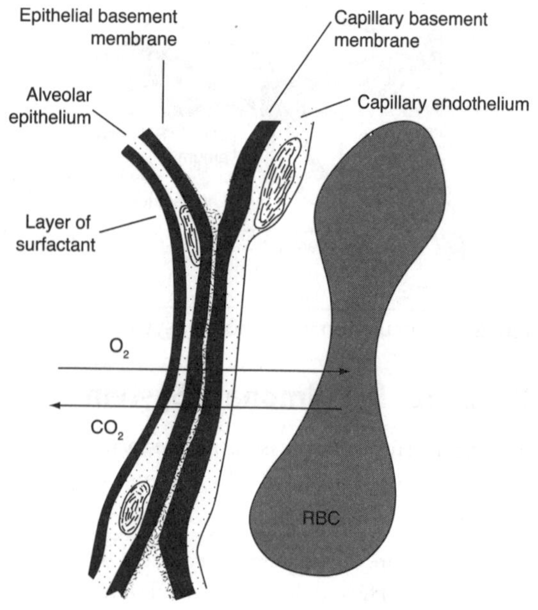

Fig. 5.4   Respiratory membrane.

The total surface area of the respiratory membrane is about 70 m² in normal adults.

Since about 150 mL of blood present in the pulmonary capillaries is spread over this large area, diffusion of gases is very rapid across the respiratory membrane.

Diffusion across Respiratory Membrane

The following factors affect this process:

- **Thickness of the membrane:** The rate of diffusion through the respiratory membrane is inversely proportional to the thickness of the membrane.
- **Surface area of the membrane:** The rate of diffusion is directly proportional to the surface area of the membrane.
- **Diffusion coefficient:** The rate of diffusion is directly proportional to the diffusion coefficient of the gas.
- **Pressure gradient across the respiratory membrane:** The rate of diffusion is directly proportional to the pressure difference between the partial pressures of gas in the alveoli and the pulmonary capillary.

Functions of Respiratory System

Nasal Cavity

- Filtration of dust particles
- Humidification
- Olfaction
- Modification of temperature of inspired air

Lungs

- **Uptake of O_2 from the atmosphere:** Oxygen is taken from the inspired air. It is transported through the blood to the tissues where it is utilized.
- **Expulsion of CO_2 from the body:** Carbon dioxide in the tissues is taken up by the blood and delivered to the lungs from where it is expelled.

Nonrespiratory Functions

- Defensive action—the mucosa of lungs produces secretory antibody IgA. Alveolar macrophages are phagocytic; i.e., they engulf foreign particles. Cilia present in the lungs trap microbes.
- Synthesis of surfactant, collagen, and elastic fibers.
- Fibrinolysis and removal of clots.

- Conversion of angiotensin I to angiotensin II by ACE (angiotensin converting enzyme).
- Temperature regulation—heat is lost from the body along with water during expiration.
- Acid–base balance—lungs regulate CO_2 content of blood and thereby help in acid–base balance.
- Excretory function—removal of volatile substances.
- Voice production—it helps in speech.

Pulmonary Volumes and Capacities

Lung Volumes

Lung volumes are the amount of air breathed by an individual under a specific condition. The lung volumes are as under.

Tidal Volume

Tidal volume (TV) is the volume of air inspired or expired during normal breathing at rest.

Normal value is 500 mL.

Inspiratory Reserve Volume

Inspiratory reserve volume (IRV) is the volume of air inspired with maximum effort over and above the normal tidal volume.

Normal value is 3000 mL.

Expiratory Reserve Volume

Expiratory reserve volume (ERV) is the volume of air expired forcefully after a normal expiration.

Normal value is 1100 mL.

Residual Volume

Residual volume (RV) is the volume of air remaining in the lungs after a forceful expiration.

Normal value is 1200 mL.

Lung Capacities

Inspiratory Capacity

Inspiratory capacity (IC) is the amount of air a person can inspire forcefully after a normal expiration:

$$IC = TV + IRV.$$

Normal value is 3500 mL.

Functional Residual Capacity

Functional residual capacity (FRC) is the amount of air that remains in the lungs at the end of normal expiration:

$$FRC = ERV + RV.$$

Normal value is 2300 mL.

Vital Capacity

Vital capacity (VC) is the maximum volume of air exhaled forcefully from the lungs after a maximum inspiration:

$$VC = TV + IRV + ERV.$$

Normal value is 4600 mL.

Total Lung Capacity

Total lung capacity (TLC) is the volume of air present in the lungs after maximum inspiration:

$$TLC = VC + RV.$$

Normal value is 5800–6000 mL.

Measurement of Lung Volumes and Capacities

Lung volumes and capacities are measured by an instrument called **spirometer**.

The graph obtained is called **spirogram** (Fig. 5.5).

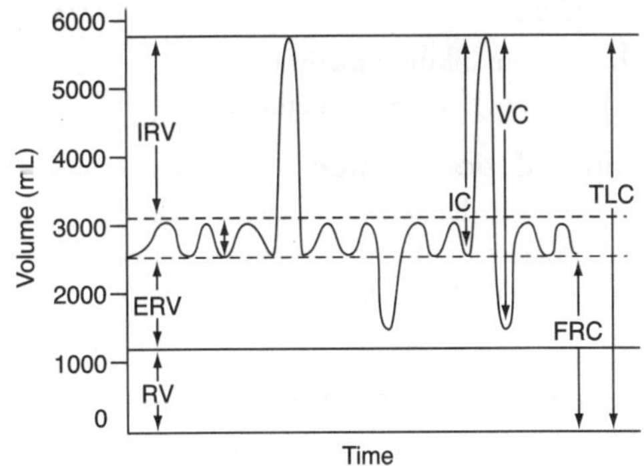

Fig. 5.5 Spirogram.

All the lung volumes and capacities are approximately 20–25% less in females as compared to males.

Spirometer (Fig. 5.6)

This apparatus consists of two concentric drums. The outer drum is filled with water. A lightweight drum (bell) is placed inverted between the two drums so that it dips into water. The top of the inverted drum is attached to a chain. This chain passes over a pulley and is connected to a counterweight and a writing pen. As the air in the bell is altered the pen moves up and down. The pen records the graph on a revolving drum which can be adjusted to rotate at a known speed.

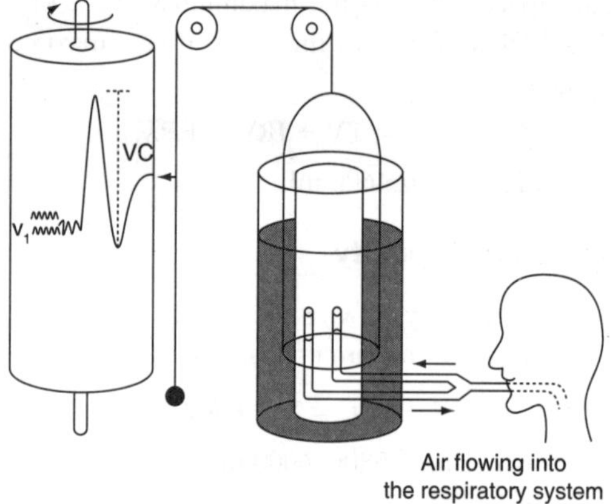

Fig. 5.6   Spirometer.

Simple spirometer can record all volumes and capacities except FRC, RV, and TLC.

FRC, RV, and TLC are determined by two methods:

1.   helium dilution method and
2.   nitrogen washout method.

Helium Dilution Method   Spirometer is filled with air mixed with helium of known concentration. The subject inhales air from the spirometer commencing from the end of normal expiration. FRC can be determined by the degree of dilution of helium.

Nitrogen Washout Method   The subject is asked to breathe normally. At the end of normal expiration, the subject inspires pure oxygen and later exhales into a Douglas bag. This procedure is repeated for 7 min till the nitrogen in the lungs is displaced by oxygen. FRC can be calculated by knowing the volume of air in the Douglas bag, N_2 concentration in the atmosphere, and the air sample in Douglas bag.

Once FRC is determined, RV and TLC can be calculated by

$$RV = FRC - ERV,$$
$$TLC = FRC + IC.$$

Pulmonary Function Tests

Pulmonary function tests (PFT) are a series of tests performed to assess the lung functions in an individual.

PFT include the following:

1.   **All lung volumes and capacities:** Discussed earlier.

2.   **Respiratory minute volume (RMV):** This is the volume of air that can be breathed in and out of the lungs every minute under resting condition. It is equal to the tidal volume times the respiratory rate:

     $$RMV = TV \times RR \text{ (respiratory rate)}.$$
     Normal value is 6 L/min.

     A person can sustain an RMV as low as 1.5 L/min or as high as 200 L/min for very short periods.

3.   **Maximum voluntary ventilation (MVV; maximum breathing capacity, MBC):** The maximum volume of air that can be breathed in and out of the lungs by maximum respiratory effort in 1 min is called MBC or MVV.

     Normal value is 125–170 L/min in males and 80–100 L/min in females.

     The subject is asked to breathe forcefully and rapidly into the spirometer for 15 s. The amount of air inspired and expired is measured. MVV is calculated by multiplying the measured volume by 4.

4.   **Timed vital capacity (FEV, forced expiratory volume):** It is the measurement of vital capacity in relation to time. FEV is the volume of air expired forcefully in unit time.
     - *FEV1:* Volume of air expired forcefully in 1 s. Normal value is 83%.
     - *FEV2:* Volume of air expired forcefully in 2 s. Normal value is 94%.

- *FEV3:* Volume of air expired forcefully in 3 s. Normal value is 97–100%.

FEV values are decreased significantly in obstructive airway diseases like asthma and emphysema.

In restrictive airway diseases, vital capacity is reduced but FEV can be normal.

FEV values are helpful to distinguish between obstructive and restrictive lung disorders.

5. **Peak expiratory flow rate (PEFR):** The maximum rate at which air can be exhaled forcefully after a deep inspiration is known as PEFR.

Normal value is 300–400 L/min.

PEFR is measured by using an instrument called Wright's peak flow meter. This is useful in assessing obstructive airway diseases like asthma, cystic fibrosis, and emphysema.

Pulmonary Ventilation

It is the process by which air enters the lungs or the air goes out of the lungs.

Alveolar Ventilation

It is the volume of air entering the alveoli in 1 min, which is used for the exchange of gases.

$$\text{Alveolar ventilation} = (\text{Tidal volume} - \text{Dead space}) \times 12$$
$$= (500 - 150) \times 12$$
$$= 350 \times 12$$
$$= 4200 \text{ mL/min.}$$

Alveolar ventilation determines the amount of oxygen and carbon dioxide in the alveoli. Alveolar ventilation decreases in rapid shallow breathing and increases in slow deep breathing.

Breathing Reserve Volume

This is the volume of air breathed in and out with maximum respiratory effort over and above the normal respiration.

It is the difference between the maximum voluntary ventilation and respiratory minute volume:

$$\text{Breathing reserve} = \text{MVV} - \text{RMV.}$$

Dyspneic Index

Dyspneic index (DI) is an index to evaluate if a person has dyspnea:

$$DI = \frac{MVV - RMV}{MVV} \times 100.$$

Value less than 70% indicates that the person is dyspneic.

Perfusion of Lungs

Perfusion is the volume of blood available for gas exchange which passes through pulmonary capillaries every minute.

Normal blood flow to the lungs is 5 L/min. The amount of blood present in the lungs is about 450 mL. The systolic pressure in the right ventricle is around 25 mm Hg and the diastolic pressure is 0 mm Hg. The pressure in the pulmonary system is low.

Hydrostatic pressure in the lungs determines the amount of blood flow to different zones of the lungs. The blood flow to the apex of the lungs is less than the blood flow to the base of the lungs. Ventilation is more to the base than to the apex. The blood flow is also greater at the base than at the apex. However, change in the blood flow from the apex to base is greater than change in ventilation. Therefore, ventilation perfusion ratio is more at the apex and low at the base of the lungs.

Ventilation–Perfusion Ratio

It is the ratio between the alveolar ventilation and the volume of blood perfusing the alveoli.

It is expressed as

$$\frac{\text{Alveolar ventilation}}{\text{Perfusion}} = \frac{V_A}{Q}.$$

Normal value is 0.8.

It is more at the apex (up to 3) than at the base (0.6) of lungs.

Ventilation-perfusion ratio is altered in respiratory diseases like emphysema and pulmonary embolism.

Dead Space

The part of the respiratory passage where there is no exchange of gases is called dead space. It corresponds to the conducting zone of respiratory passage.

Types

Dead space is of two types:

1. **Anatomical dead space (ADS):** It is that part of the respiratory passage which is not involved in the exchange of gases. This includes air in the nose, pharynx, larynx, trachea, and bronchi up to terminal bronchioles.

   The gas exchange does not occur in these areas because the walls of the respiratory passages are too thick for the gas exchange.

   Normal value is 150 mL.

   It is measured by single breath nitrogen analyzer method.

2. **Physiological dead space (PDS):** It includes anatomical dead space and the part of lungs where the exchange of gases does not take place.

   Physiological dead space
   = Anatomical dead space
   + Alveolar dead space.

   In healthy individuals, ADS = PDS.

   PDS is more significant than ADS. It is increased in case of arteriovenous shunts and pulmonary embolism.

Measurement

ADS is measured by analysis of single breath N_2 curve (Fowler's method). The subject is asked to inhale 100% pure O_2 and then exhale into a nitrogen meter. The initial air exhaled corresponds to the ADS. This air contains only oxygen and no nitrogen. Later when the alveolar air reaches the nitrogen meter, N_2 concentration increases steadily and reaches a plateau level.

The dead space volume will be equal to the volume of gas exchanged from the peak inspiration to midportion of phase II as shown in Fig. 5.7.

Mechanics of Respiration

Respiration is a process in which air moves into the lungs during inspiration and moves out of the lungs during expiration. Mechanics of respiration deals with various physical forces that are involved in the process of respiration.

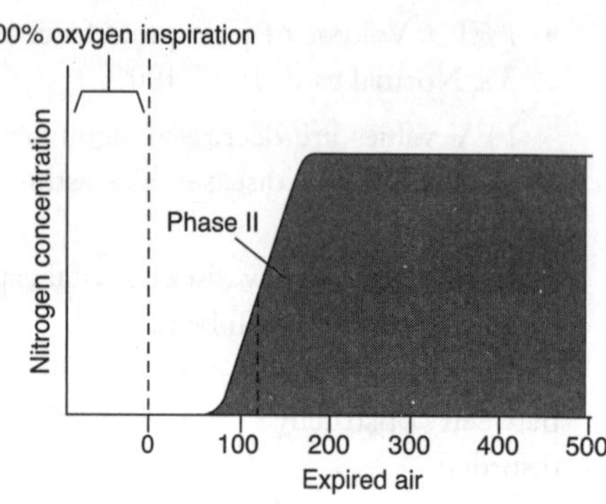

Fig. 5.7   Dead space.

Muscles of Respiration

These muscles are necessary for the process of inspiration and expiration.

Inspiratory Muscles

Diaphragm   This is a dome-shaped muscle with convexity upward. It separates the thorax and abdomen. It is supplied by the phrenic nerve.

It moves 1–1.5 cm during normal breathing. During deep breathing it moves by 10 cm.

Normal quiet breathing is due to the action of the diaphragm.

External Intercostals   These muscles are present between the ribs. The fibers are directed downward and medially.

Contraction of the external intercostal muscles causes

- increase in transverse diameter of rib cage and
- increase in the anteroposterior diameter of rib cage.

Expiratory Muscles

Muscles of Anterior Abdominal Wall   They include rectus abdominis, internal and external oblique, and transversus abdominis.

Contraction of muscles of anterior abdominal wall causes increased intra-abdominal pressure resulting in elevation of diaphragm.

Internal intercostals   They are present between the ribs. They pull the ribs downward, thereby reducing both the anteroposterior and transverse diameter of the thorax. This causes a reduction in the volume of the thoracic cage.

Internal intercostals are particularly important during coughing.

Accessory Muscles of Respiration

These muscles normally do not take part in inspiration but are active during forceful inspiration such as during exercise and conditions like asthma.

The accessory muscles are as under:

(a) **Scaleni:** Cause elevation of thoracic cage
(b) **Sternocleidomastoid (SCM):** Cause elevation of thoracic cage
(c) **Serratus anterior:** Help in fixing the thoracic cage so that ribs can move efficiently

Inspiration (Fig. 5.8a)

The discharge from inspiratory center through the phrenic nerve results in the descent of diaphragm and increase in the vertical diameter.

Contractions of the external intercostals increase the transverse diameter by bucket handle movement. The anteroposterior diameter is increased by the pump handle movement. This occurs by elevation of the anterior portion of the ribs. The second to fifth ribs assume horizontal position due to the contraction of external intercostal muscles. The sternum moves forward and upward.

Expansion of the thoracic cage creates negative pressure within the lungs.

Air enters the lungs from atmosphere to equalize the pressure.

During forced expiration neck muscles like sternocleidomastoid and scaleni are used. The exercise-induced increase in the respiratory effort involves all the accessory muscles of respiration.

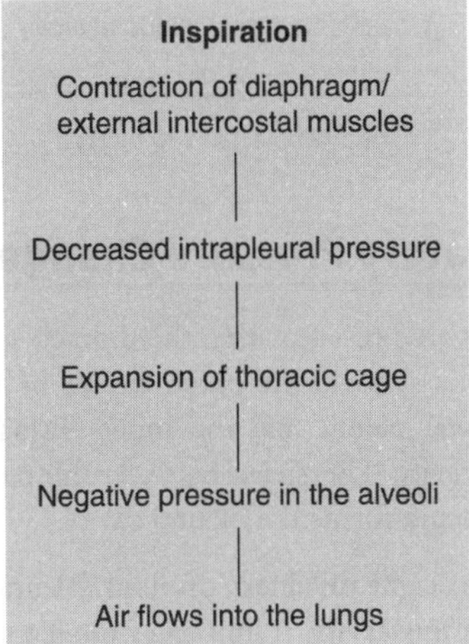

Expiration (Fig. 5.8b)

In quiet breathing, expiration is a passive process.

It is produced by relaxation of inspiratory muscles assisted by elastic recoil of the thoracic cage.

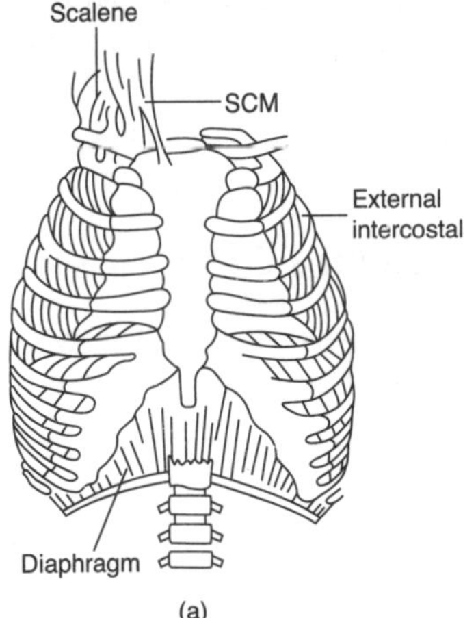

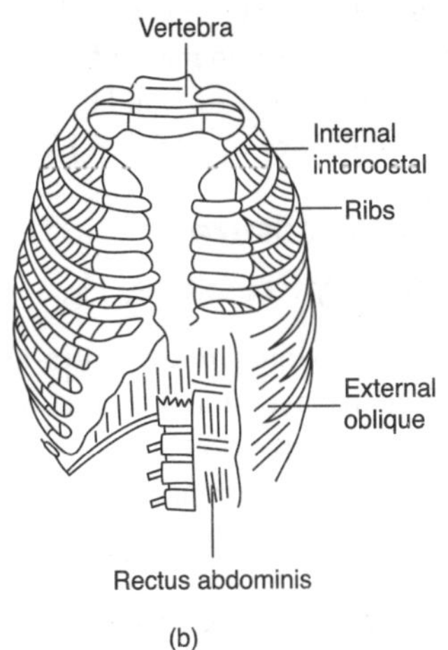

Fig. 5.8   (a) Inspiration and (b) expiration.

Expiratory muscles are active during forced expiration.

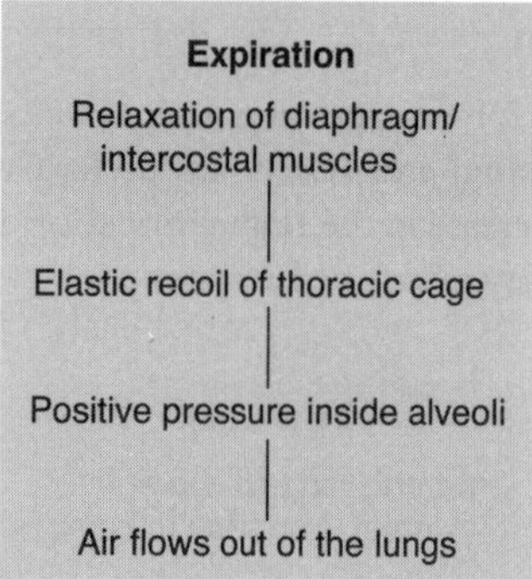

Respiratory Pressure Changes

The lungs are present within the thoracic cavity. The visceral pleura cover the outer surface of the lungs. The parietal pleura line the inner surface of the thoracic cavity. The space between the parietal and visceral pleura forms the pleural cavity.

Four to eight milliliters of fluid (pleural fluid) is present in this cavity. It lubricates movement of the lungs.

Intrapleural Pressure (Fig. 5.9a)

The pressure within the pleural cavity is termed **intrapleural pressure**. This pressure is normally negative. However, during forced expiration it can be positive. The normal intrapleural pressure varies between −2.5 and −6 mm Hg (−5 and −8 cm H_2O). At the beginning of inspiration it is −2.5 mm Hg and at the peak of inspiration it is −6 mm Hg. At the end of expiration it comes back to −2.5 mm Hg.

Intra-alveolar Pressure (Intrapulmonary Pressure; Fig. 5.9b)

The pressure within the lungs is termed **intra-alveolar pressure**. During inspiration it becomes negative (−1.5 mm Hg). During expiration it becomes positive (+1 mm Hg). At the end of inspiration and expiration the intra-alveolar pressure is zero.

Transpulmonary Pressure

The pressure difference between the intrapleural and intra-alveolar pressure is called **transpulmonary**

pressure. Transpulmonary pressure is a measure of the elastic forces in the lungs.

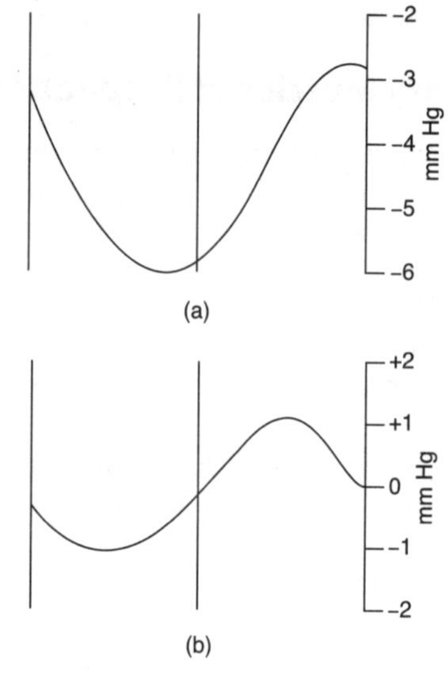

Fig. 5.9 (a) Intrapleural pressure and (b) intra-alveolar pressure.

Compliance

Compliance is stretchability of the lungs.

It is the extent to which lungs expand for each unit increase in the transpulmonary pressure. Normal compliance is 200 mL/cm H_2O. This means every time the transpulmonary pressure increases by 1 cm H_2O, the lungs expand by 200 mL. Compliance is due to elasticity of the lungs and the thoracic cage.

$$\text{Compliance} = \frac{\text{Change in volume}}{\text{Change in pressure}} = \frac{\Delta V}{\Delta P}.$$

Compliance Curve (Fig. 5.10)

The pleural pressure is plotted along X-axis and the lung volumes are plotted on Y-axis.

The transpulmonary pressure is changed in small steps. The record of lung volumes shows two curves—one inspiratory and another expiratory curve separately. These are called **compliance curves**. The inspiratory and expiratory curves do not overlap. The curves obtained are due to the elastic forces of the lungs.

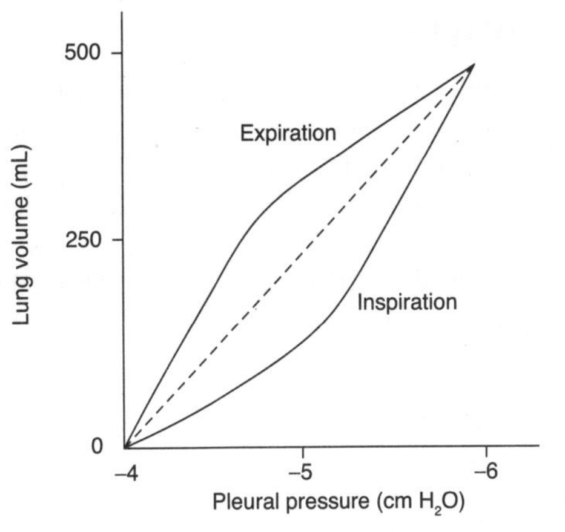

Fig. 5.10 Compliance curve.

Types

Specific Compliance

The compliance expressed as a function of FRC is termed specific compliance.

$$\text{Specific compliance} = \frac{\text{Compliance}}{\text{FRC}}.$$

This is a more specific measure of compliance especially in persons having only one lung and in children.

Dynamic Compliance

The compliance measured with respect to time is called dynamic compliance. The measurement of

Applied Physiology

Pleural Effusion (Fig. 5.11)

The accumulation of fluid in the pleural cavity is termed pleural effusion. The commonest cause of pleural effusion is TB. The accumulation of pus is called pyothorax, accumulation of fluid is hydrothorax, and accumulation of blood is hemothorax. This diminishes expansion of the lungs and leads to difficulty in breathing.

In pneumothorax (presence of air inside the pleural cavity), the normal negative intrapleural pressure is lost. It results in collapse of the lungs.

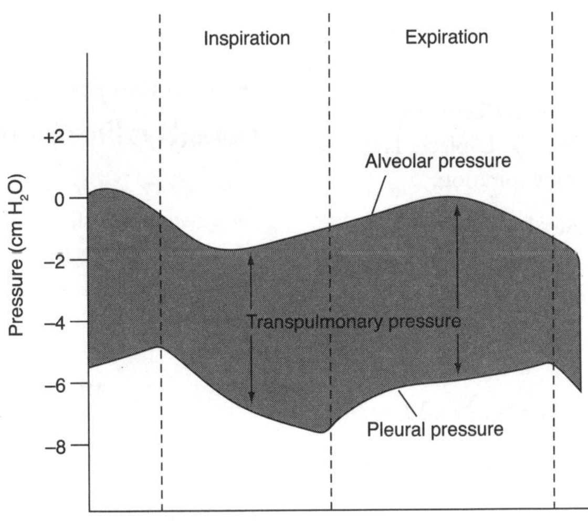

Fig. 5.11 Pressure changes during respiration.

dynamic compliance is useful in conditions like bronchial asthma wherein static compliance is normal but dynamic compliance is reduced.

Factors Affecting Lung Compliance

Lung compliance is mainly determined by the elastic forces:

- elastic forces of the lung tissue and
- elastic forces caused by surface tension within the alveoli.

Elastic forces of the lung tissue are due to elastic and collagen fibers. They contribute little to the elasticity.

Elastic forces produced by surface tension within the alveoli contribute about two-thirds of total elastic forces in the lungs.

Abnormal Lung Compliance

Decrease in lung compliance is seen in lung diseases which cause fibrosis of lungs, e.g., tuberculosis and silicosis.

Increase in lung compliance is seen in conditions like emphysema.

Surface Tension

It is the force caused due to intermolecular attraction between the molecules on the surface.

The surface tension has to be kept low in the alveoli. Otherwise according to Laplace law, the alveoli tend to collapse during expiration.

According to Laplace law, the force or pressure on the wall of a hollow structure is equal to twice the tension divided by the radius:

$$P = \frac{2T}{R},$$

where P is pressure, T surface tension, and R radius.

Whenever the radius is reduced without a reduction in tension, tension on the wall exceeds the distending pressure causing collapse of the alveoli. The surfactant reduces this surface tension and prevents collapse of alveoli whenever the radius is reduced.

Surfactant

Surfactant is a surface-active agent that reduces the surface tension when it is spread over a surface. It is secreted by Type II alveolar cells that occupy 10% of the surface area of the alveoli. These cells are granular and contain lipid inclusions. They secrete tubes of lipid called tubular myelin. This tubular myelin forms a thin film over the surface and helps to reduce the surface tension.

Composition

- Dipalmitoyl phosphatidylcholine
- Phosphatidyl glycine
- Other phospholipids

Functions

- Reduces surface tension of fluid lining the alveoli
- Prevents collapse of the alveoli
- Increases lung compliance and reduces the work of breathing
- Keeps the alveoli dry by preventing the tissue fluid formation

Production of surfactant starts by seventh month of intrauterine life. The thyroid hormone and glucocorticoids enhance the production of surfactant.

Infant Respiratory Distress Syndrome (Hyaline Membrane Disease)

Respiratory effort by baby at birth expands the alveoli. Surfactant prevents the collapse of alveoli. In premature babies production of surfactant is reduced. Small diameter of alveoli along with reduced surfactant increases the tendency for alveoli to collapse. This is called **infant respiratory distress syndrome**, or hyaline membrane disease. This condition can be fatal if proper treatment is not given.

Treatment

- Continuous positive pressure breathing
- Administration of bovine surfactant

Regulation of Respiration (Fig. 5.12)

Respiration involves the process of inspiration and expiration. It is controlled by

1. neural regulation and
2. chemical regulation.

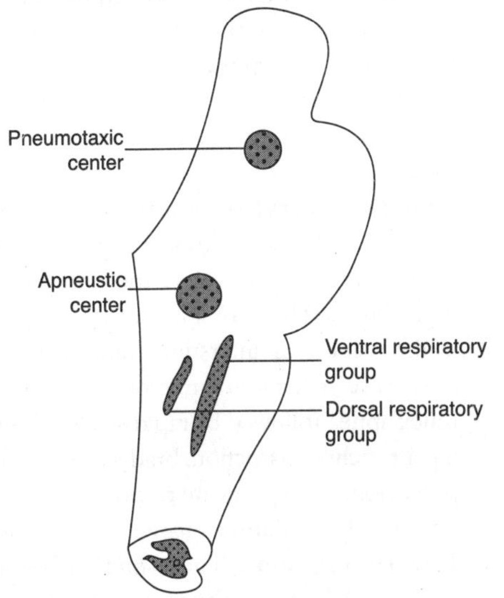

Fig. 5.12 Respiratory centers.

Neural Regulation

Neural regulation is by the involvement of

1. respiratory centers,
2. peripheral receptors, and
3. higher centers.

Respiratory Centers

The respiratory centers are a group of neurons present in the brainstem (Fig. 5.13). They are paired. These centers are as follows:

- dorsal respiratory group,
- ventral respiratory group,
- apneustic center,
- pneumotaxic center.

Dorsal Respiratory Group Dorsal respiratory group (DRG) is situated in the dorsal portion of the medulla around the nucleus of tractus solitarius.

The basic rhythm of respiration is generated and maintained by this group of neurons.

This group is responsible for the generation of inspiratory ramp. Inspiratory signals begin weakly and increase in a ramp manner (volley of impulses increasing in amplitude gradually). Later, they stop abruptly resulting in expiration.

Ramp signal steadily increases the volume of lungs during inspiration. DRG is autorhythmic (can generate its own signals). It can maintain respiration even when all the external signals are cut off.

Ventral Respiratory Group Ventral respiratory gr-oup (VRG) is present in the ventral aspect of the medulla. The neurons of this group remain inactive during normal respiration. When the respiratory drive becomes greater than normal, they participate in respiration.

Apneustic Center This is present in the lower pons. It gets feedback from the vagus and other respiratory centers. It acts with pneumotaxic center to control the depth of inspiration. Stimulation of apneustic center produces deep inspiration.

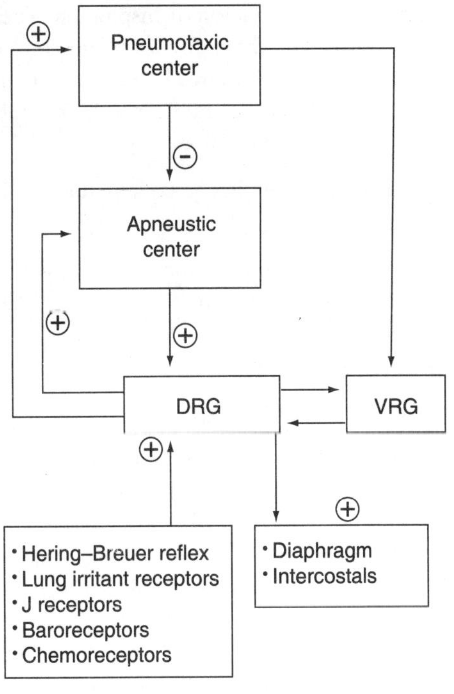

Fig. 5.13 Regulation of respiration.

Pneumotaxic Center This center is located in the upper part of the pons in the nucleus parabrachialis medialis. It controls the duration of inspiration by regulating the switch-off point of inspiratory ramp. Strong stimulation of the pneumotaxic center decreases the duration of inspiration and hence increases the rate of respiration. Damage to pneumotaxic center causes slower respiration and increases tidal volume.

Genesis of Respiratory Rhythm

The neurons of DRG generate rhythmic inspiratory signals. The signals are weak in the beginning, but rise rapidly to reach a peak in a **ramp** fashion and stop abruptly. After a brief period, the inspiratory neurons start discharging the impulses again. This cycle gets repeated. A negative feedback loop in the medulla regulates the cyclical discharges from the inspiratory neurons.

Pneumotaxic center also plays an important role in regulating the switch-off point of inspiratory ramp signals. It controls the duration of inspiration. Strong signals from pneumotaxic center reduce the duration of inspiration. There is an increase in the rate of respiration. In addition, signals from stretch receptors in the lungs control the duration of inspiration similar to pneumotaxic center.

Apneustic center has a limited role in the normal respiration.

The reflexes from within and outside the lungs influence respiration.

Peripheral Receptors

Intrinsic Reflexes of Lungs

1. **Hering–Breuer reflex:** Inflation of the lungs inhibits inspiration and initiates expiration. This is termed *Hering–Breuer inflation reflex*. Deflation of the lungs inhibits expiration and initiates inspiration. This is *Hering–Breuer deflation reflex*. This reflex is abolished by vagotomy. The reflex has limited role in quiet breathing in adults. The receptors for this reflex are located in airway smooth muscles, in the walls of the bronchioles, and the alveolar duct. Afferent impulses travel through the myelinated vagal fibers.

2. **Lung irritant receptors:** These receptors are located in between the epithelial lining of the airways. Myelinated vagal fibers carry afferent impulses. These receptors adapt rapidly. The receptors respond to chemical and mechanical irritants (inhalation of dust, irritant gases, cigarette smoke, and cold air). They also respond to sudden inflation and deflation of the lungs and pulmonary congestion. The response is hyperpnea, bronchoconstriction, and bradycardia. Unpleasant sensation produced in asthma is due to activation of this reflex.

3. **J (juxtacapillary) receptors:** The receptors are located close to pulmonary capillaries. The afferent impulses travel in the unmyelinated vagal fibers. They are stimulated by increase in the volume of interstitial fluid, pulmonary congestion, edema, and microemboli. There is reflex apnea followed by rapid shallow breathing, bronchoconstriction, bradycardia, and hypotension. J receptors are responsible for dyspnea produced during left-sided heart failure.

4. **Effect of vagotomy:** The respiration becomes slower and deeper (with prolonged inspiration) after bilateral vagotomy. This response is due to the abolition of Hering-Breuer inflation reflex. However, the pneumotaxic center maintains rhythmic breathing.

5. **Effect of vagal stimulation:** The stimulation of cut end of vagus produces varying results. The response depends on the type of fibers stimulated in the vagal trunk. The stimulation of the vagus can result in arrest of breathing or an increase in the rate and depth of respiration.

Extrinsic Reflexes of Lungs

1. Reflexes from baroreceptors—a sudden and significant increase in the arterial blood pressure stimulates the baroreceptors. There is reflex inhibition of respiration resulting in reduced rate and depth of breathing.

2. Reflexes from chemoreceptors—the chemoreceptors are sensitive to changes in partial pressure of oxygen and carbon dioxide. The reduction in PO_2 or an increase in PCO_2 stimulates the chemoreceptors. This increases the rate and depth of respiration.

3. There is reflex inhibition of respiration during the second stage of swallowing. This is termed **deglutition apnea**. It is a protective reflex to prevent the entry of food into the larynx. This reflex is produced by stimulation of the glossopharyngeal nerve.

4. The somatic pain sensation causes respiratory stimulation. It increases the rate and depth of respiration. The pain sensations arising from the internal organs and hollow viscus due to traction or distension inhibit the respiration.

5. The afferent proprioceptive impulses from the receptors from muscles and joints stimulate respiration. Hyperventilation observed during exercise is due to this reflex mechanism.

6. The stimulation of thermoreceptors in the skin by increased environmental temperature increases the rate and depth of respiration. This mechanism helps to regulate the body temperature in lower animals.

Influence of Higher Centers

The respiration is mainly an involuntary act. The respiratory muscles are skeletal muscles. Therefore, voluntary control of respiration is possible, but to a limited extent. Breathing can be voluntarily stopped for about a minute. Rate and depth of respiration can also be increased by voluntary effort for a short duration.

The voluntary breath holding builds up the carbon dioxide concentration. When it reaches a critical level, it stimulates the respiratory center to restart respiration. This is termed **breaking point**.

The cerebral cortex, limbic system, hypothalamus, and reticular activating system influence respiration.

The cerebral cortex helps to exercise voluntary control over respiration.

Emotional disturbances influence the rate and depth of respiration by acting through the limbic system.

Higher centers are not essential for the normal respiration. However, they have a modifying effect on the pattern of breathing.

Chemical Regulation

There are three factors responsible for the chemical regulation of respiration. They influence the rate and depth of respiration by acting through the chemoreceptor. There are two types of chemoreceptors, namely,

1. central chemoreceptors and
2. peripheral chemoreceptors.

Central Chemoreceptors

They are located in the medulla oblongata and are therefore also called medullary chemoreceptors. These receptors monitor the H^+ concentration of the CSF and the brain interstitial fluid.

Peripheral Chemoreceptors

They are present in the carotid and aortic bodies. These bodies contain two types of cells: Type I and Type II. Type I cells (glomus cells) are closely associated with endings of the afferent nerves. These cells are excited by hypoxia. Type II cells are glia-like cells. They are supportive in function.

The factors influencing respiration are

- PCO_2,
- H^+ ion concentration, and
- PO_2.

Role of Carbon Dioxide The respiratory changes depend on CO_2 concentration in the blood. Carbon dioxide acts by influencing the central and peripheral chemoreceptors. A mild-to-moderate increase in the concentration of CO_2 increases the rate and depth of respiration. A severe increase in the concentration of CO_2 leads to loss of consciousness and respiratory depression.

Mode of Action Carbon dioxide stimulates respiration by acting on the central chemoreceptor and reflexly through the peripheral chemoreceptor.

It crosses the blood–brain barrier and combines with water in the presence of an enzyme carbonic anhydrase to form carbonic acid. Carbonic acid being a weak acid dissociates into H^+ ions and HCO_3^- ions. H^+ formed stimulates the central chemoreceptor to increase the rate and depth of respiration. The central effect of CO_2 is more dominant when compared to its influence on the peripheral chemoreceptor.

Role of Hydrogen Ions An increase in the hydrogen ion concentration stimulates respiration and increases the rate and depth of respiration. A decrease in the hydrogen ion concentration decreases respiration and reduces the pulmonary ventilation. H^+ acts mainly through the peripheral chemoreceptors. Its influence on the central chemoreceptor is limited, as the hydrogen ion does not cross the blood–brain barrier. The respiratory response to H^+ ion concentration is to adjust the pulmonary ventilation to restore the pH of blood.

Role of Oxygen   The oxygen lack stimulates respiration, increasing the rate and depth of breathing. The stimulant effect is produced as a reflex by stimulation of the peripheral chemoreceptor located at the carotid body and the arch of aorta. The direct effect of oxygen lack is depressant on the respiratory center. However, the depressant effect is overcome by the stimulatory effect on the peripheral chemoreceptor.

A mild reduction in the oxygen concentration has little influence on the respiration. A moderate decrease in the oxygen concentration stimulates respiration, resulting in hyperventilation. A severe decrease in the oxygen concentration depresses respiration resulting in respiratory paralysis.

Principles of Gas Exchange

Atmospheric air contains gases like N_2, O_2, and CO_2. At sea level it contains 79% of N_2 and 21% of O_2. The total pressure of gases at sea level is 760 mm Hg. Partial pressure of a gas (P) is the pressure exerted by that gas in a mixture of gases. Partial pressure of oxygen is denoted as PO_2, nitrogen as PN_2, and carbon dioxide as PCO_2.

Transfer of gases from the alveoli to the pulmonary blood occurs by diffusion. Diffusion through tissue is described by Fick's law.

Fick's law states that the rate of transfer of a gas through a tissue is directly proportional to

- surface area,
- difference in partial pressure of the gases between two sides, and
- solubility of gas in the fluid.

It is inversely proportional to

- thickness of the tissue (distance) and
- molecular weight of the gas.

$$D \propto \frac{\Delta P \times A \times S}{d \times MW},$$

where ΔP is pressure difference between the two sides, A cross-sectional area of tissue, S solubility of the gas, d distance of diffusion, and MW molecular weight of the gas.

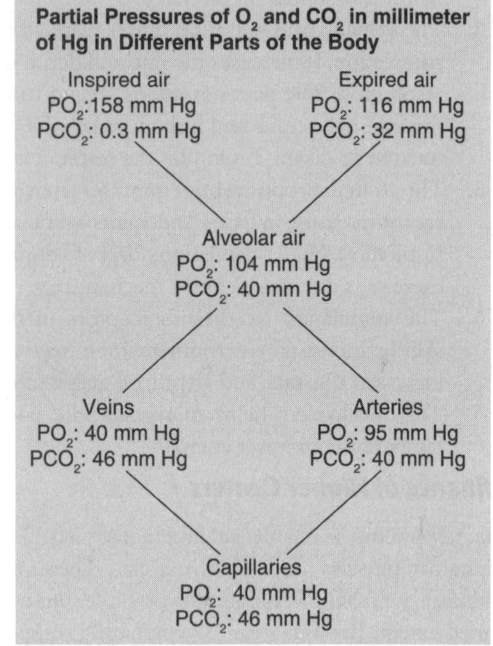

Alveolar air does not have the same concentration of gases as atmospheric air. This is because

- O_2 is constantly absorbed from alveolar air;
- CO_2 is diffusing from blood into the alveolar air;
- alveolar air is partially replaced by atmospheric air with each breath;
- water vapor is added to alveolar air.

Transport of Blood Gases

Tissues require oxygen for their metabolic activity. Atmospheric oxygen is taken up by the lungs. The oxygen is transported from the lungs to the tissues through blood. Tissues liberate carbon dioxide during metabolism. It is transported to the lungs through blood for expulsion to the atmosphere.

Oxygen Transport

O_2 is transported in the blood in two forms:

1. physical solution and
2. combination with hemoglobin.

Physical Solution

Oxygen in physical solution is the amount of oxygen carried in dissolved state in plasma.

Normal arterial blood with PO_2 of 100 mm Hg contains 0.3 mL of O_2/100 mL.

Only 3% of total O_2 transport occurs in the dissolved state.

Combination with Hemoglobin

About 97% of oxygen is transported from the lungs to the tissues in combination with hemoglobin.

Oxygen molecules combine loosely and reversibly with heme portion of Hb (oxygenation).

When PO_2 is high, O_2 binds with Hb, and when PO_2 is low, O_2 is released from hemoglobin. The combination of O_2 with Hb is better understood by studying the oxygen dissociation curve.

The curve is obtained by plotting the partial pressure of O_2 against percentage saturation of Hb. Curve shows a progressive increase in the percentage saturation of Hb as the PO_2 increases.

Arterial Blood	
PO_2	95 mm Hg
O_2 saturation	97%
Venous Blood	
PO_2	40 mm Hg
O_2 saturation	75%

O_2 dissociation curve is **sigmoid shaped** (Fig. 5.14). This sigmoid shape is physiologically significant.

The middle steep part of the curve shows that a small change in PO_2 leads to a significant change in percentage saturation of Hb. This helps in easy delivery of O_2 to the tissues and also uptake of O_2 in the lungs.

Top portion of this curve is flat. A considerable change in PO_2 results in a slight change of percentage saturation. Advantage is that a slight fall in alveolar PO_2 does not significantly alter the oxygenation of Hb.

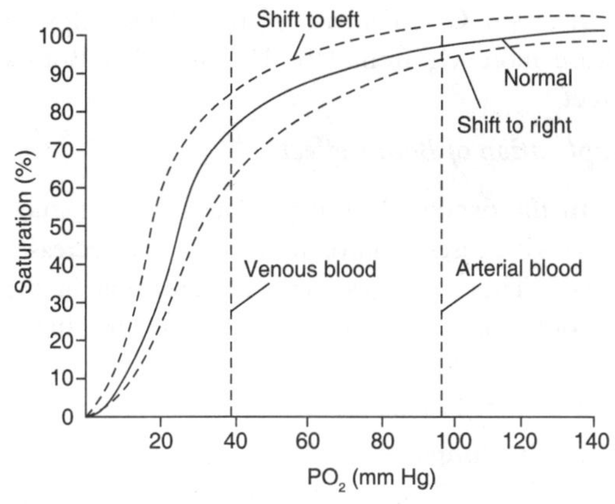

Fig. 5.14 O_2 dissociation curve.

P50   This is the partial pressure of O_2 at which Hb is 50% saturated.

P50 is an index of affinity of Hb with O_2. Higher the P50 value lower is the affinity.

Normal P50 is about 26 mm Hg.

Normal person has 15 g of Hb/100 mL of blood. Each gram of Hb can combine with 1.34 mL of O_2. Therefore, 100 mL of blood can carry 19.8 mL of O_2 when Hb is fully saturated.

Since Hb is usually saturated to about 95%, O_2 carrying capacity is 19 mL of O_2/100 mL of blood.

Venous blood contains 14 mL of O_2/100 mL of blood. Therefore, the net utilization of O_2 by tissues is around 5 mL/100 mL of blood.

Factors Affecting O_2 Dissociation Curve   If the affinity of Hb toward O_2 decreases, O_2 dissociation curve shifts to right.

Shift to the right occurs in conditions of

- ↑ PCO_2,
- ↑ H^+ ion concentration (decreased pH),
- ↑ temperature, and
- ↑ 2,3-DPG (diphosphoglycerate).

Effect of CO_2 and H^+ Ions

Bohr's Effect   It is the influence of CO_2 on the release and uptake of oxygen by hemoglobin.

Increased CO_2 content of the blood helps to release more O_2 from Hb. This is called **Bohr's effect**.

Application of Bohr's effect

- **In the tissues:** CO_2 is produced in the tissues. This increases H^+ ion concentration and decreases pH. These changes cause an alteration in the configuration of Hb molecule. Hence, its affinity to O_2 is reduced. Therefore, more amount of O_2 is delivered to the tissues.

- **In the lungs:** CO_2 diffuses from blood into the alveoli. This reduces CO_2 and H^+ ion concentration in blood. The affinity of Hb to O_2 is increased. Therefore, more oxygen binds to Hb.

Effect of DPG   2,3-DPG is formed inside the RBC during glucose metabolism. It has an affinity for Hb. It causes release of O_2 from Hb. Therefore, when 2,3-DPG is increased in RBC, more O_2 is released and delivered to the tissues. This is very helpful during chronic hypoxic conditions.

Effect of Exercise   Exercise causes shift of O_2 dissociation curve to the right. During exercise there is an increase in temperature and release of large quantities of CO_2 and acid metabolites. It enhances the release of O_2 to the muscle from Hb. Increased release of O_2 satisfies enhanced O_2 need of the muscle.

Diffusion of O_2 to Tissues

O_2 is continuously used by the tissues. Therefore the intracellular PO_2 remains lower than PO_2 in the blood. The normal intracellular PO_2 is 5–40 mm Hg. Therefore, O_2 diffuses easily from the blood into the tissues.

Cells require PO_2 between 1 and 3 mm Hg for their function. PO_2 of 23 mm Hg in tissues, therefore, provides a wide safety factor for its diffusion.

Carbon Dioxide Transport

The tissues during metabolic activity utilize oxygen and produce carbon dioxide. It is taken up from the tissues by blood in the capillaries. It is transported through the venous system and expelled from the lungs.

Carbon dioxide is transported by the blood in three forms:

1.   as bicarbonate,
2.   in combination with Hb and plasma proteins as carbamino compounds, and
3.   in physical solution.

As Bicarbonate Ions

This is the major mechanism of CO_2 transport. About 70% of CO_2 is transported in this form. RBC plays a major role in this mechanism. Carbon dioxide produced in the tissues diffuses into the plasma and from plasma into the RBC. Inside the RBC the dissolved CO_2 reacts with water to form carbonic acid. This occurs very rapidly due to the presence of enzyme carbonic anhydrase. Carbonic anhydrase enzyme accelerates the reaction 5000 times.

$$H_2O + CO_2 \rightleftharpoons H_2CO_3.$$

Subsequently, carbonic acid dissociates into H^+ ions and HCO_3^- ions. H^+ ions combine with Hb to form HHb in the red cells. Bicarbonate ions diffuse from red cells into plasma in exchange for chloride ions. This exchange is possible due to the presence of bicarbonate–chloride carrier protein present in the RBC membrane. The movement of chloride ions from plasma into RBC is termed **chloride shift** (Hamburger's phenomenon; Fig. 5.15). Chloride shift occurs at the tissues. Thus chloride content of RBC in venous blood is greater than in arterial blood.

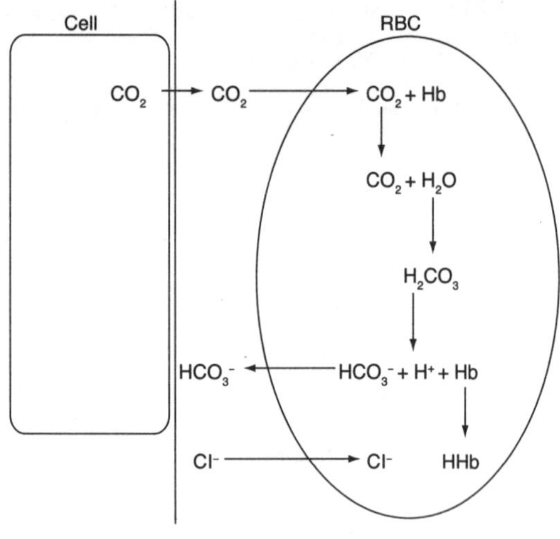

Fig. 5.15   Chloride shift.

When blood reaches the lungs, there is reversal of changes that occurred at the tissues. Hemoglobin is oxygenated releasing H^+ ions from hemoglobin. H^+ ion combines with HCO_3^- ion to form CO_2 and H_2O. CO_2 diffuses out of RBC into the alveoli. HCO_3^- ion is supplied from the plasma in exchange for the chloride ions. This is termed **reverse chloride shift** (Fig. 5.16).

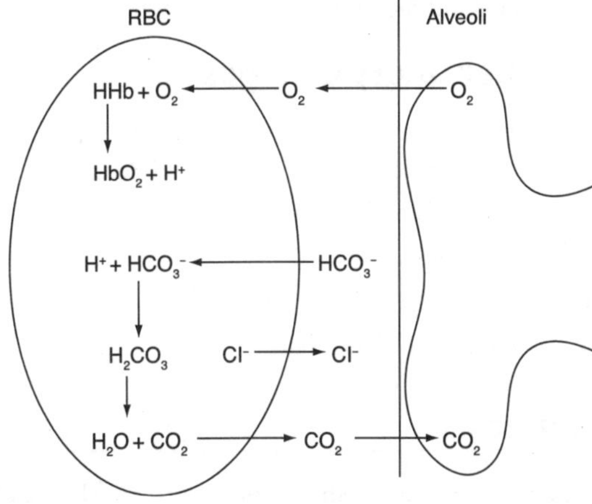

Fig. 5.16   Reverse chloride shift.

As Carbamino Compounds

CO_2 combines chemically with Hb and plasma proteins to form carbamino compounds. Since, Hb is the most abundant protein in blood, CO_2 combines mainly with Hb. It is carried as carbamino hemoglobin. About 20% of the total CO_2 transport occurs in this form.

In Dissolved Form

About 7% of the CO_2 is transported in dissolved state to the lungs.

PCO$_2$ of venous blood is 45 mm Hg. Hence, the dissolved CO_2 is 2.7 mL/dL.

PCO$_2$ of arterial blood is 40 mm Hg. Therefore, dissolved CO_2 is 2.4 mL/dL.

About 0.3 mL/dL of CO_2 is transported in dissolved state.

CO$_2$ Dissociation Curve (Fig. 517)   Relationship between PCO$_2$ and volume of CO_2 carried by blood is depicted by CO_2 dissociation curve.

CO_2 present in arterial blood is 48 mL/100 mL at PCO$_2$ of 40 mm Hg.

CO_2 present in venous blood is 52 mL/100 mL at PCO$_2$ of 45 mm Hg.

Haldane Effect   Influence of O_2 on the release and uptake of CO_2 by Hb is termed **Haldane effect**.

Combination of Hb with O_2 causes Hb to become a stronger acid. The highly acidic Hb has a lesser tendency to combine with CO_2. Therefore, CO_2 present in carbamino form is displaced from the blood.

Increased affinity of Hb with oxygen releases excess of H^+ ions. H^+ ions bind with HCO_3^- to form carbonic acid. This dissociates into CO_2 and water. CO_2 is released from the blood into alveoli.

$$HHb + O_2 \longrightarrow HbO_2 + H^+$$

$$H^+ + HCO_3^- \longrightarrow H_2CO_3$$

$$H_2CO_3 \longrightarrow CO_2 + H_2O$$

- **In tissue capillaries:** Haldane effect increases the uptake of CO_2 due to the removal of O_2 from Hb.

- **In the lungs:** Haldane effect causes increased release of CO_2 due to O_2 uptake by Hb. Volume of CO_2 eliminated is doubled by Haldane effect.

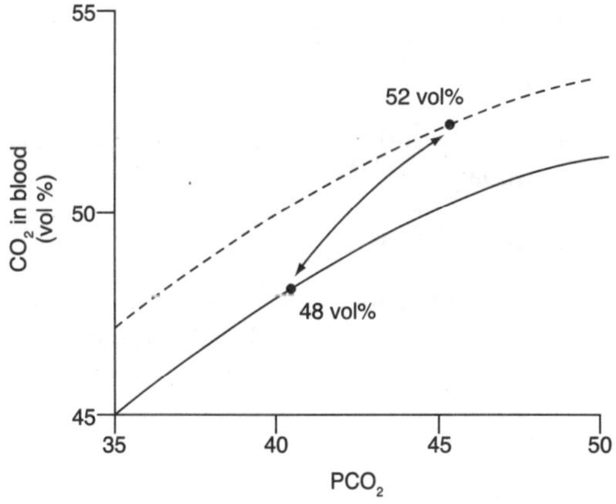

Fig. 5.17   CO$_2$ dissociation curve.

Hypoxia

Hypoxia is a condition characterized by deficiency of O_2 at tissue level.

Types

Types of hypoxia are

1. hypoxic hypoxia,
2. anemic hypoxia,
3. stagnant hypoxia, and
4. histotoxic hypoxia.

Hypoxic Hypoxia

In this type of hypoxia PO_2 decreases in the blood. O_2 saturation of Hb is reduced. However, the Hb content is normal.

It occurs at

- high altitude,
- ill-ventilated rooms,
- in conditions like pneumonia,
- respiratory paralysis,
- arteriovenous shunts, and
- collapse of lungs.

Anemic Hypoxia

Hemoglobin content is reduced but PO_2 is normal. There is a decrease in O_2 carrying capacity of blood.

It is seen in severe anemia and carbon monoxide poisoning.

Stagnant Hypoxia

This is seen when the blood flow through a tissue is sluggish.

It occurs in cardiac failure, circulatory shock, and hemorrhage.

Histotoxic Hypoxia

The tissues are unable to use oxygen present in the blood due to damage of cytochrome oxidase enzyme system.

It is seen in cyanide poisoning.

Symptoms

Hypoxia initially causes

- impaired judgment,
- drowsiness and excitement,
- disorientation,
- loss of time sense, and
- headache.

Other symptoms include anorexia, nausea, vomiting, and tachycardia.

Hypoxia affects the brain. A sudden drop in PO_2 to 20 mm Hg causes unconsciousness in 10–15 s and death in about 4–5 min.

Compensatory Changes

- Hyperventilation (increased rate and depth of respiration)
- Increased blood pressure and cardiac output
- Polycythemia
- Increased 2,3-DPG in RBC
- Excretion of alkaline urine

Cyanosis

Cyanosis is the bluish discoloration of skin and mucus membrane.

It is observed in lips, nail bed, earlobes, and cheeks.

It occurs when the amount of reduced Hb in blood is more than 5 g/dL.

It is of two types:

1. central and
2. peripheral.

Central cyanosis occurs in hypoxic hypoxia, e.g., right to left shunts (mixing of oxygenated and deoxygenated blood).

Peripheral cyanosis occurs due to reduced peripheral circulation, e.g., exposure to severe cold and frostbite.

Asphyxia

Asphyxia is a condition characterized by decreased O_2 and increased CO_2 in the body.

It is of two types:

1. generalized asphyxia and
2. local asphyxia.

Generalized asphyxia is produced by occlusion of airway, e.g., strangulation and drowning.

Local asphyxia is produced due to obstruction of blood supply to a particular region, e.g., accidental ligature of blood vessel during surgery.

Dyspnea

Abnormal awareness of breathing is termed dyspnea. This condition is characterized by distress and discomfort during breathing. A person generally feels dyspneic if his/her breathing reserve falls below 70% of normal.

Its causes are bronchial asthma, severe anemia, and cardiac failure.

Orthopnea

Dyspnea in lying-down position is orthopnea.

Periodic Breathing

When a normal person hyperventilates for a few minutes, there is a period of apnea alternating with shallow breathing following hyperventilation. This is termed periodic breathing. Periodic breathing is due to lack of stimulation of respiratory center by CO_2.

Cheyne-Stokes Breathing

Cheyne-Stokes breathing occurs in patients with congestive cardiac failure, uremia, brain diseases, and during deep sleep.

Breathing is characterized by alternate apnea and hyperventilation.

It is due to the sluggish chemical regulation of respiration.

Biot's Breathing

In this condition there is alternate eupnea (normal breathing) and apnea.

This is seen in meningitis and severe brain damage.

Kussmaul's Breathing

This occurs in metabolic acidosis like diabetic ketoacidosis or renal failure. There is rapid and deep breathing due to respiratory stimulation by increased hydrogen ion concentration.

Apnea

Apnea is temporary cessation of respiration.

Types

Types of apnea are as under:

1. sleep apnea,
2. deglutition apnea,
3. voluntary apnea,
4. hyperventilation apnea, and
5. sudden infant death syndrome.

Sleep Apnea

This is a temporary cessation of breathing during sleep. It occurs due to failure of respiratory centers to discharge impulses or due to airway obstruction. Sleep apnea is common during REM sleep since muscles are hypotonic. This condition can occur in any age group.

If sleep apnea becomes severe, there are recurrent periods of hypoxia and hypercapnia, which leads to polycythemia, right-sided heart failure, and pulmonary hypertension.

Deglutition Apnea

It is a temporary stoppage of respiration during swallowing. This prevents the entry of food into the respiratory passage.

Voluntary Apnea

It is the temporary cessation of respiration by voluntary effort. Higher centers override the respiratory control by medullary and pontine centers.

Hyperventilation Apnea

It is a phase of apnea following hyperventilation due to the removal of CO_2. There is lack of stimulation of respiration due to excessive CO_2 washout.

Sudden Infant Death Syndrome

Death of an apparently healthy infant in the crib (cot) for no detectable reason is termed sudden infant death syndrome (SIDS). It is common in premature infants due to repeated apneic spells.

Coughing

Coughing is a respiratory act wherein forced expiration occurs after a deep inspiration. This is produced due to stimulation of irritant receptors in air passages. It helps to keep the airways clear.

- First, there is deep inspiration.
- Closure of glottis and building up of intrapleural pressure.
- Sudden opening of glottis.
- Air rushes out at the rate of 600 miles/h.

Sneezing is a similar respiratory effort which occurs with a continuously open glottis.

Hiccup

Spasmodic contraction of diaphragm and other inspiratory muscles during inspiration produces hiccup. Sound is produced due to a sudden closure of glottis.

High-Altitude Sickness

Acute Mountain Sickness

It is a condition that develops in a person who rapidly ascends to high altitudes. It is caused due to decreased alveolar PO_2. This occurs due to fall in barometric pressure at high altitude and also partial pressure of O_2.

Symptoms

- Headache, dizziness, palpitation, insomnia, nausea, vomiting, breathlessness, and hyperventilation.
- Severe conditions result in cerebral edema, convulsions, and unconsciousness.

- The symptoms start at heights above 12,000 ft. They begin 8–12 h after arrival at high altitude and last for 4–8 days.

Treatment

- Descent to lower altitude.
- Acetazolamide (diuretic).
- Oxygen therapy.

Chronic Mountain Sickness

This is seen in persons staying at high altitudes for longer durations.

Features

- Easy fatigability
- Polycythemia
- Pulmonary hypertension

Acclimatization

It is the ability of the body to adjust to an altered environmental condition.

Changes Occurring During Acclimatization

- Hyperventilation
- Polycythemia (physiological)
- ↑ Diffusion capacity of lungs
- ↑ Vascularity of tissues
- ↑ Ability of cells to use oxygen despite low PO_2
- ↑ Cardiac output
- Excretion of alkaline urine. This helps to combat respiratory alkalosis caused by excessive removal of CO_2

Acclimatization in natives of high altitudes occurs during infancy itself.

They are short statured; chest becomes broader (barrel shaped); and there is hypertrophy of right heart. They have polycythemia.

Dysbarism (Decompression Sickness, Caisson's Disease)

It is a condition occurring in persons who move to low-barometric-pressure region from a region of high barometric pressure.

This occurs in deep sea divers staying underwater for prolonged periods. Rapid ascent from underwater causes decompression sickness.

Under high barometric pressure, gases especially N_2 are dissolved in blood. When such persons are suddenly exposed to lower barometric pressure, the gases tend to escape. N_2 bubbles are formed in blood and there is pain due to local ischemia.

Symptoms

- Bends in the knee
- Chokes in the lungs
- Strokes in the brain

Treatment

- Slow ascent
- Stay in decompression chambers where rapid recompression followed by slow decompression is done

Eupnea: It is normal respiration.

Dyspnea: It is the abnormal awareness of one's own breathing (labored breathing).

Orthopnea: It is dyspnea in lying-down position.

Tachypnea: Tachypnea is increased rate of respiration.

Hyperventilation: This is a condition wherein both rate and depth of respiration are increased.

Hypoventilation: This is a condition where alveolar ventilation is less than normal.

Applied Physiology

Artificial Respiration

Artificial respiration is a process of restoring the respiratory activity which has stopped suddenly. Respiratory arrest can occur as a result of drowning, poisoning, suffocation, electrocution, myocardial infarction, or cerebrovascular accidents.

This can lead to death unless the oxygen supply to vital organs is restored within 2–3 min.

Therefore, it is important to restart respiration artificially as a life-saving measure.

Methods

- Manual methods

  Mouth-to-mouth breathing

  Schafer's method

  Holger Neilson's method

- Mechanical methods

Manual Methods

- **Mouth-to-mouth breathing**

  Subject is placed in supine position; airway is cleared, neck extended, nose closed.

  Resuscitator blows air twice the tidal volume into the subject's mouth.

  Procedure is repeated 12 times a minute.

- **Schafer's method**

  Subject is placed in prone position and the head is turned to one side.

  Operator kneels down and presses the loin for 2–3 s and then releases the pressure.

  On application of pressure there is expiration and release of pressure causes inspiration.

- **Holger Neilson's method**

  Subject is placed in prone position and arms are kept in folded position in front of the head.

  Operator kneels down near the head of patient, places his hand on the back, and compresses the chest. This effort forces the air out of the lungs.

  After 3 s the operator lifts the arms of the subject to produce inspiration.

  Inspiration occurs due to elastic recoil of the lungs.

Mechanical Methods   These are used to treat chronic respiratory insufficiency due to inadequate ventilation.

- **Drinker's method:** In this method, subject is placed in airtight metal or plastic container and the head is kept outside. Now portable respirators are available that cover only the chest. Negative pressure is created around the chest at regular intervals with the help of a motor. The chest wall is moved in a way that resembles normal breathing. Air moves in and out of the lungs with the movement of chest.

- **Positive pressure breathing:** In this method, inspiration is produced by forcing air into the lungs by application of positive pressure. Release of pressure results in expiration.

- **Intermittent positive pressure ventilation (IPPV):** This is a technique used in most of the respirators. Positive pressure is applied intermittently to introduce air into respiratory passage.

Oxygen Therapy

Oxygen therapy is required in conditions of respiratory failure due to lung diseases or poisoning.

Oxygen is administered through nasal catheters. Usually pure oxygen is not administered; it is mixed with air. Masks are used for giving oxygen in higher concentrations.

Oxygen therapy is useful in

1. Atmospheric hypoxia–O_2 therapy can correct depressed O_2 levels in inspired air. It provides 100% effective therapy.
2. Hypoventilation hypoxia as seen in neuromuscular disorders.
3. Hypoxia caused by impaired alveolar membrane diffusion.

Oxygen therapy is **not useful** in hypoxia caused by anemia, abnormal transport of oxygen, circulatory deficiency, and physiological shunt.

Hyperbaric Oxygen Therapy

Hundred percent oxygen is administered at 2–3 atmosphere pressure. This is helpful in the treatment of carbon monoxide poisoning, radiation-induced tissue injury, gas gangrene, severe blood loss anemia, and diabetic leg ulcers. It is also used in the treatment of decompression sickness and air embolism.

Oxygen Toxicity

Inhalation of 100% oxygen causes toxicity due to the production of superoxides. Infants administered with oxygen continuously develop lung cysts and densities.

Withdrawal of O_2 therapy produces corneal opacities due to vascularization (retrolental fibroplasia).

6 Gastrointestinal System

The gastrointestinal (GI) system is the route through which the nutritive substances, vitamins, minerals, and fluids enter the body. The food consumed cannot be utilized by the body directly. It is broken down into simpler substances like glucose, amino acids, and fatty acids. The process of conversion of complex substances into simple chemical substances that can be absorbed is termed **digestion**.

The GI tract (Fig. 6.1) consists of the following parts:

Mouth → Pharynx → Esophagus → Stomach → Duodenum → Jejunum → Ileum → Caecum → Ascending colon → Transverse colon → Descending colon → Sigmoid colon → Rectum → Anal canal.

It also includes salivary glands, liver, gallbladder, and pancreas.

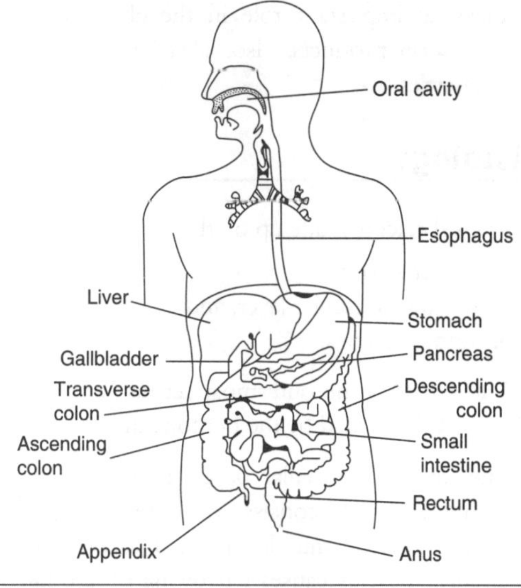

Fig. 6.1 Gastrointestinal tract.

Functions

The GI system has the following functions:

- **Secretion of digestive juices:** Hydrochloric acid (HCl) is secreted by the stomach, bile is secreted by the liver, and various digestive juices are secreted by the salivary glands, pancreas, and intestinal epithelial cells.
- **Digestion of food:** The churning and mixing action of the GI tract causes breakdown of the large food particles into smaller size; thereafter, the enzymes secreted in the digestive juices cause the breakdown of various components of the food into smaller molecules.
- **Absorption of digested food products, water, and electrolytes:** The digested food particles are absorbed from the lumen of the small intestine (SI) into the blood.
- **Movement of food from the mouth toward the anus:** While the processes of digestion, secretion, and absorption are going on in the GI tract, the smooth muscles mix the contents in the lumen of the GI tract with various juices and enzymes and move them from the mouth toward the anus.
- **Protection of gut against harmful and toxic substances in the food:** The HCl secreted in the stomach causes destruction of harmful bacteria and toxins.
- **Elimination of waste products:** The GI tract plays an important role in the elimination of solid waste products. Also, saliva has antibacterial properties.

Histology

The GI tract is made up of three layers (Fig. 6.2):

1. outer serosa,
2. middle muscular layer, and
3. inner mucosa.

The serosa is the outermost serous layer of the GI tract. It is formed by the peritoneum.

The middle muscular layer is made up of smooth muscles. It consists of outer longitudinal and inner circular muscle layers. The contraction of circular muscles causes narrowing of the lumen and contraction of longitudinal muscles causes

shortening of the gut. The muscle fibers are electrically connected with one another through a large number of gap junctions. The bundle fuses with one another at many points and therefore the muscle layer functions as syncytium.

The inner mucosa has the submucus layer which is composed of areolar tissue, blood vessels, lymphatics, and nerves. It is lined by a single layer of columnar cells called the **mucosa**. It also has a thin layer of muscle called the **muscularis mucosae**.

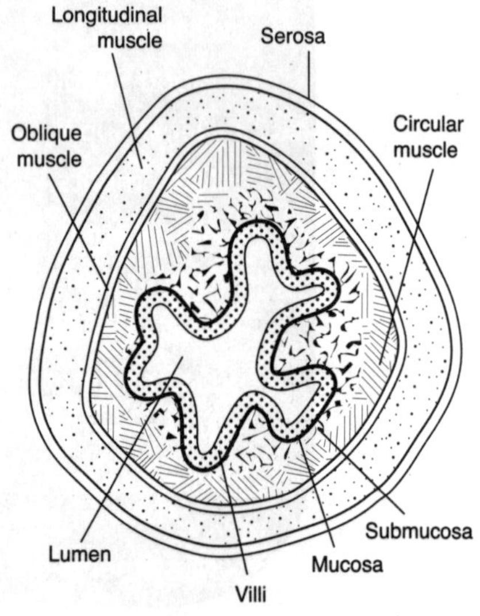

Fig. 6.2   Layers of GI tract.

Blood Supply

The blood supply to the GI tract is from the following branches of the aorta:

- celiac plexus and
- superior and inferior mesenteric arteries.

The blood leaving the GI tract is drained by the portal vein to the liver.

The GI tract receives nearly 30% of the cardiac output. The GI circulation to the abdomen is termed the **splanchnic circulation**. The splanchnic circulation supplies the stomach, pancreas, SI, colon, liver, spleen, omentum, and mesenteric tissues. The splanchnic circulation is arranged both in parallel and in series.

Nerve Supply

The GI tract is supplied by an intrinsic as well as an extrinsic nerve supply.

Intrinsic Nerve Supply

The intrinsic nerve supply is by the enteric nervous system.

Extrinsic Nerve Supply

The extrinsic nerve supply is by afferent and efferent nerves from both the sympathetic and parasympathetic nervous systems.

Enteric Nervous System

There are two major networks in the GI tract:

1. **Myenteric plexus of Auerbach:** This is present between the outer longitudinal and inner circular layer of muscles.
2. **Submucus plexus of Meissner:** This is present between the circular muscle layer and the mucosa.

The enteric nervous system is connected to the central nervous system (CNS) by the sympathetic and parasympathetic fibers, but they can function independently without these connections.

Extrinsic Innervation

The extrinsic innervation consists of the following components:

1. **Afferent nerves:** These nerves transmit information from the GI tract to the CNS. They pass through the spinal cord and vagus nerve.
2. **Efferent nerves:** These are of two types:
   (a) *Parasympathetic:* The parasympathetic supply to the GI tract is mainly through the vagus nerve. The parasympathetic stimulation increases secretion and motility.
   (b) *Sympathetic:* The sympathetic nerve supply to the GI tract arises from the fifth thoracic segment to second lumbar segment of the spinal cord. It inhibits the GI smooth muscles except the sphincters. It reduces GI motility and secretions.

Influence of Higher Center   Autonomic output is modified by influences from higher centers particularly from the limbic system and cerebral cortex.

Electrical Activity of GI Smooth Muscle

The GI smooth muscle shows two types of electrical waves:

1. slow waves and
2. spikes.

Slow Waves

The spontaneous rhythmic fluctuations in the membrane potential (between −65 and −45 mV) are termed the **basal electrical rhythm** (BER). These fluctuations produce slow waves.

The BER is initiated by the stellate muscle cells. These cells are termed the **pacemaker cells**. The slow waves are not action potentials but are slow undulating changes in the resting membrane potential. Their intensity ranges from 5 and 15 mV. The frequency ranges from 3 to 12/min.

In the stomach their frequency is about 4/min. In the duodenum it rises to 12/min and falls to around 8/min in the terminal ileum.

The slow waves arise due to slow undulation of the sodium–potassium pump. These slow waves do not cause muscle contraction, but control the appearance of intermittent spike potentials.

Spike Potentials

They are true action potentials. They occur when potential rises above −40 mV. Their frequency increases if the spike potential value increases. Spike potentials last for a duration of about 10–20 ms.

These spike potentials occur due to the entry of large amounts of calcium ions along with small amounts of sodium ions.

Spike potentials do not propagate for more than a few millimeters in the intestinal muscles.

Acetylcholine increases the number of spikes and epinephrine decreases the number of spikes.

Migrating Motor Complex

The migrating motor complex (MMC) occurs between the periods of digestion. Each cycle of MMC begins with a slow period (Phase I), continues with a period of irregular electrical and mechanical (Phase II) activity, and ends with a burst of regular activity. They occur at intervals of approximately 90 min. They migrate at a rate of about 5 cm/min.

Function

The MMC clears the contents of the GI lumen to prepare for the next meal.

Movements

Food taken from the mouth has to be moved in a regular fashion along the length of the GI tract. This movement depends mainly on the activity of the GI smooth muscles.

The movements are regulated by the autonomic nervous system. The parasympathetic stimulation causes release of acetylcholine, which increases the movement. The sympathetic stimulation causes release of norepinephrine, which inhibits movements.

The GI hormones like gastrin stimulate movements, while secretin and gastric inhibitory polypeptide (GIP) inhibit movements.

Two basic types of movements occur in GI tract:

1. propulsive movements and
2. mixing movements.

Propulsive Movements

These movements propel the food along the GI tract. The basic propulsive movement is **peristalsis**.

Peristalsis

Peristalsis is a reflex response that begins when the GI wall is stretched by the food present in the lumen. It occurs throughout the GI tract from the esophagus to the rectum. Peristalsis occurs at the rate of 2–25 cm/min.

It consists of a ring of contraction in one segment and receptive relaxation in the immediate distal segment. Apart from the GI tract, peristalsis occurs in the bile ducts and ureters.

The stimulus for peristalsis is distention of the gut. Distention stimulates the gut wall and a contractile ring appears which initiates peristalsis.

Peristalsis is brought about by the myenteric plexus. It occurs only in one direction, i.e., from the esophagus toward the rectum.

The occurrence of peristalsis and its movement toward the anus is termed the **law of the gut**.

Mixing Movements

The mixing movements are caused by either the peristaltic contractions or the local constrictions of small segment of the GI tract. These constrictions last for a few seconds and new contractions occur at other points of the gut.

Mastication (Chewing)

Mastication is a process by which food taken in the mouth is crushed into small particles by grinding action of the teeth. The anterior teeth (incisors and canines) provide cutting action and the posterior teeth (premolars and molars) provide the grinding action. The muscles of mastication are innervated by various branches of the trigeminal nerve.

The process of mastication is controlled by the nuclei in the brainstem.

Chewing Reflex

The presence of food in the mouth causes reflex inhibition of the muscles of mastication, causing lower jaw to drop. This activates a stretch reflex of muscles resulting in its contraction. The jaw is raised to cause apposition of the teeth and compression of the bolus. The compression of the bolus inhibits contraction of the jaw muscles and the process is repeated.

Functions of Mastication

- It increases the surface area of the food by breaking it into small particles for better digestion.
- The grinding action prevents excoriation of the GI tract and increases the rate of emptying of food from the stomach.

Deglutition (Swallowing)

Deglutition is the process of transfer of food from the mouth to the stomach. Deglutition is a reflex response.

Phases

The phases of deglutition are (Fig. 6.3)

- buccal phase,
- pharyngeal phase, and
- esophageal phase.

Buccal Phase

The food present in the mouth is converted to a bolus by the process of mastication and mixing with saliva. Later, the food is pushed backward by pressure of the tongue against the palate.

Pharyngeal Phase

As the food enters the pharynx, a series of changes occur to allow the food to pass through the pharynx.

- The soft palate is raised to close the posterior nares so that the food does not enter the nasal cavity.
- The palatopharyngeal folds are pulled medially to form a sagittal slit which allows the masticated food to pass through it.
- The vocal cords come close to each other. The hyoid bone and larynx are pulled upward and anteriorly by the neck muscles causing the epiglottis to swing back over the laryngeal opening. This prevents the entry of food into the trachea.
- The opening of the esophagus stretches and the upper esophageal sphincter relaxes, allowing the food to pass down into the esophagus. Normally this sphincter is strongly contracted so that air does not enter the esophagus during respiration.
- At the same time, the superior constrictor muscle of the pharynx contracts, giving rise to a rapid peristaltic wave which passes down into the esophagus.

The entire process occurs in 1–2 s. During this period, respiratory centers of the medulla are inhibited causing interruption of respiration (deglutition apnea).

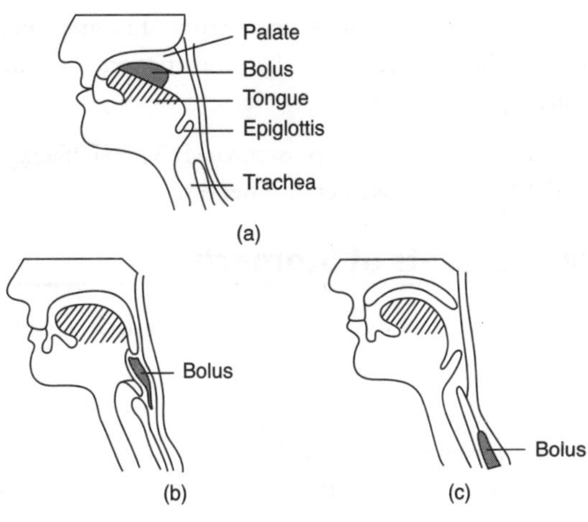

Fig. 6.3   Phases of deglutition: (a) buccal phase, (b) pharyngeal phase, and (c) esophageal phase.

Esophageal Phase

The esophagus conducts the food from the pharynx to the stomach. It exhibits two types of peristaltic movements: (i) primary peristalsis and (ii) secondary peristalsis.

Primary Peristalsis   This is continuation of peristalsis from the pharynx; it causes movement of food in 8–10 s.

Secondary Peristalsis   It causes the movement of food not propelled by primary peristalsis.

As the food reaches the lower esophageal sphincter, there is relaxation of the stomach and sphincter to receive the food. This is termed **receptive relaxation**.

The esophageal phase ends with the entry of food into the stomach.

Control

The presence of food in the mouth causes stimulation of the tractus solitarius of the medulla through V (trigeminal), IX (glossopharyngeal), and X (vagus) cranial nerves. The afferent impulses from these nerves are integrated at the nucleus of tractus solitarius and the nucleus ambiguus present in the medulla.

Deglutition Center

The deglutition center is present in the reticular areas of the upper medulla and lower pons. It consists of the nucleus of tractus solitarius and nucleus ambiguus.

The motor impulses arise from this area and bring about swallowing by constriction of the pharyngeal muscles.

The efferent fibers pass through V, VII (facial), and XII (hypoglossal) cranial nerves.

Movements of Stomach

The movements observed in the stomach are of three types:

1. movements in empty stomach,
2. receptive relaxation, and
3. digestive peristalsis.

Movements in Empty Stomach

The various movements of the empty stomach are as under:

- **Type I movements:** They are mild movements occurring at the rate of 3/min. These are discrete movements.

- **Type II movements:** They are stronger movements, called hunger contractions. They are rhythmic, tetanic peristaltic contractions lasting for 2–3 min. They are more intense in healthy adults. The hunger contractions are increased by low blood sugar levels.

- **Type III movements:** They occur in conditions of extreme hunger, termed hunger pangs. They begin 12–24 h after the last meal and reach greatest intensity in 3–4 days. They gradually weaken in the succeeding days. It produces pain in pit of the stomach.

Receptive Relaxation

Receptive relaxation occurs after a meal. There is active relaxation of the stomach which causes increase in the volume of the stomach. It is caused by the vagovagal reflex originating in the pharynx and esophagus. The neurotransmitters involved are vasoactive intestinal polypeptide (VIP), nucleotides, and dopamine.

Digestive Peristalsis

The digestive peristalsis begins as soon as the food enters the stomach (Fig. 6.4). It starts in the form of small indentation on the wall and encircles the middle part of the stomach in the form of a ring. Later, it proceeds toward the pylorus.

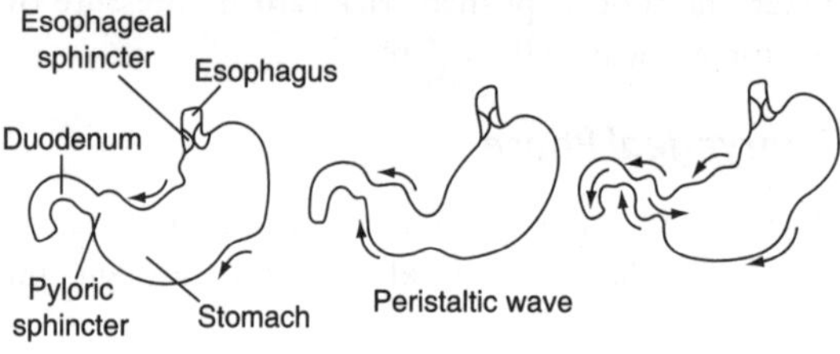

Fig. 6.4 Movements of stomach: digestive peristalsis.

The contractions are initially weak, but gradually increase in strength. Each time the peristaltic waves pass down the wall of the gastric antrum it digs deeply into the food contents in the antrum. As each peristaltic wave reaches the pyloric region, the pyloric muscles contract and the contents are pushed upward. These two mechanisms help in mixing the food particles and secretions.

Applied Physiology

Bulbar Paralysis (Bulbar Polio)

It is caused due to infection by the poliovirus. In this condition, food regurgitates through the nose.

Paralysis of Laryngeal Muscles

In this condition, food enters the respiratory tract causing suffocation and death.

Achalasia Cardia

In this condition, the lower esophageal sphincter fails to relax during swallowing. There is excessive dilatation of the esophagus.

Gastric Emptying

This is a process by which the stomach empties its contents into the duodenum. Normally, the pylorus remains closed, partially allowing only fluids to pass through it. Whenever food is present in the stomach as chyme, the contractions become intense and cause gastric emptying. It occurs till the stomach is totally emptied and this pumping action is called the **pyloric pump**.

Pyloric Pump

The presence of food in the stomach causes contractions of the stomach to become intense. These contractions are strong ring-like constrictions that begin in the region of the midstomach and then progress distally. These strong contractions push the contents toward the duodenum.

As the stomach becomes empty, these constrictions begin further up on the body of the stomach and push the contents toward the duodenum.

Each peristaltic wave pushes several milliliters of chyme into the duodenum every time.

The degree of constrictions of pylorus can be controlled by various nervous and hormonal factors. These factors regulate emptying of the stomach contents into the duodenum.

Factors Regulating Gastric Emptying

The gastric emptying is promoted by secretion of gastrin, food volume, and increase in parasympathetic stimulation.

The secretion of cholecystokinin (CCK) secretin, increased acidity in the intestine, products of fat and protein digestion, and hypertonicity of the food inhibits gastric emptying.

Movements of Small Intestine

Movements of the SI are required for proper mixing of chyme with the digestive juices for propulsion of food and absorption of digested materials.

The various movements of small intestine are

- mixing movements,

- propulsive movements, and
- antiperistalsis.

Mixing Movements

Mixing movements of the SI cause proper mixing of food with digestive juices secreted into the lumen of SI.

These movements include the following.

Segmentation Contraction (Fig. 6.5)

When a portion of the SI gets distended with the entry of chyme, stretch of the intestinal wall elicits localized constrictions spaced at intervals along the intestine. As one set of segmentation contraction relaxes, a new set begins between the previous contractions. These segmentation contractions chop the chyme eight to twelve times a minute.

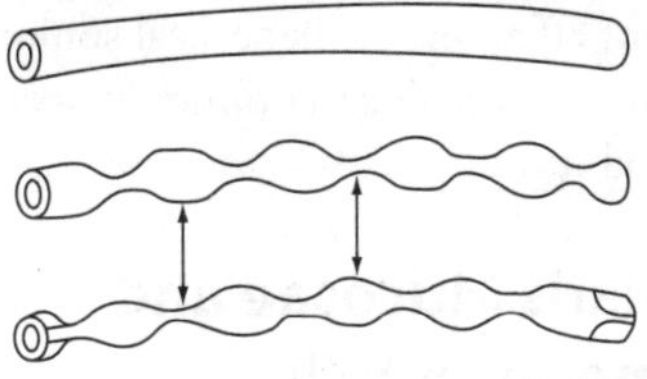

Fig. 6.5   Segmentation contraction of intestine.

Pendular Movements

This type of movement helps in mixing of intestinal contents. A long segment of intestine moves over its contents to and fro like a pendulum and hence it is called pendular movement.

Propulsive Movements

Peristalsis

The chyme is propelled through the SI by peristaltic waves. Normally, 3–5 h are required for the passage of chyme through the SI.

Peristaltic Rush

This occurs due to intense irritation of the intestinal mucosa. It causes powerful and rapid peristalsis as in severe cases of intestinal infections resulting in diarrhea.

Antiperistalsis

It is the peristaltic movement in the opposite direction (anal to oral direction).

It occurs normally in the region of duodenum. It results in vomiting.

Ileocaecal Valve

The ileocaecal valve is located at the junction of ileum and caecum. The main function of this valve is to prevent the movement of fecal contents from the colon back to the SI. The lips of the ileocaecal valve protrude when the caecum gets filled.

The wall of the ileum for a short distance preceding the ileocaecal valve has a thickened muscular coat called the **ileocaecal sphincter**. This normally remains mildly constricted. The gastroileal reflex and the hormone gastrin have a relaxant effect on the ileocaecal sphincter. The abdominal tuberculosis commonly occurs at the ileocaecal region.

Muscularis Mucosae and Movements of Villi

The muscularis mucosae can cause short or long folds to appear in the intestinal mucosa. This increases the surface area exposed to chyme, thereby increasing the rate of absorption.

The contractions of the villi, i.e., repeated shortening and elongation of the villi, milk the villi facilitating free flow of the lymph.

Movements of Colon

The movements of colon are sluggish in nature. These movements are necessary for mixing, propulsion, and absorption.

Mixing Movements (Haustrations)

Large circular constrictions appear in the large intestine narrowing the lumen of the colon, sometimes leading to complete occlusion. At the same time, the longitudinal muscles of the colon contract. The combined contractions of the longitudinal and circular smooth muscles cause the unstimulated portion of the large intestine to bulge outward like a sac called **haustration**. Thus, the fecal matter is gradually exposed to the surface of the large intestine and a major part of the fluid is absorbed.

Propulsive Movements (Mass Movements)

These movements occur only a few times each day.

First, a constrictive ring appears at the distended or irritated point in the colon, usually in the transverse colon. Then about 20 cm of the colon distal to the constriction contracts almost as a single unit, forcing the fecal matter to move down the colon.

When the fecal matter enters the rectum, the subject gets the urge to defecate.

Functions of Colon

The colon helps in

- absorption of water and electrolytes from the chyme and

- storage of fecal matter until it is excreted.

The proximal half of the colon is concerned with the absorption and distal half with the storage of fecal matter.

Defecation

The rectum is empty most of the time. When a mass movement forces the feces into the rectum, desire for defecation is initiated. Defecation occurs if the conditions are favorable.

The dribbling of fecal matter is prevented by the tonic contraction of the following:

1. **Internal anal sphincter:** Composed of smooth muscles
2. **External anal sphincter:** Composed of striated muscles

The internal sphincter is supplied by the autonomic nervous system; the external anal sphincter is supplied by the pudendal nerve. The external anal sphincter is under voluntary control.

Defecation Reflex

The defecation reflex occurs in the following steps:

- The entry of feces into the rectum causes its distension.
- The afferent signals are initiated in the myenteric plexus. It results in the formation of peristaltic waves in the descending colon, sigmoid colon, and rectum.
- The movement of feces toward the anal canal relaxes the internal sphincter.
- Defecation occurs if the external anal sphincter is also relaxed.

The contraction of the abdominal muscles helps in the process of defecation.

If the circumstances are not favorable, defecation is inhibited by voluntary contraction of the external anal sphincter. Soon, the internal anal sphincter and the rectum also relax. The reflex disappears but reappears a few minutes later.

Salivary Secretion

Salivary Glands (Fig. 6.6)

There are three pairs of salivary glands:

1. **Parotid glands:** Serous secretion
2. **Submandibular glands:** Serous and mucus secretion
3. **Sublingual gland:** Mucus secretion

The parotid gland opens on the inner surface of the cheek opposite the second molar tooth, by the **duct of Stenson**.

The submandibular gland opens by the **Whartons duct** in the floor of the mouth by the side of the frenulum of the tongue.

The sublingual gland opens by several fine ducts in the floor of the mouth on either side of the frenulum of the tongue. These are called the **ducts of Rivinus**.

Saliva

Composition

Total volume	1200–1500 mL/24 h
Appearance	Slightly cloudy
Reaction	Slightly acidic
Specific gravity	1.002–1.012

Contents

Water	99.5%
Solids	0.5%

Cellular Constituents (0.3%) It contains yeast cells, bacteria, and desquamated epithelial cells.

Inorganic Salts (0.2%) NaCl, KCl, and $CaCO_3$.

Organic Constituents

- Enzymes—ptyalin (salivary amylase), lipase, and carbonic anhydrase
- Mucin
- Soluble specific blood group substances
- Urea, amino acids, cholesterol, and vitamins

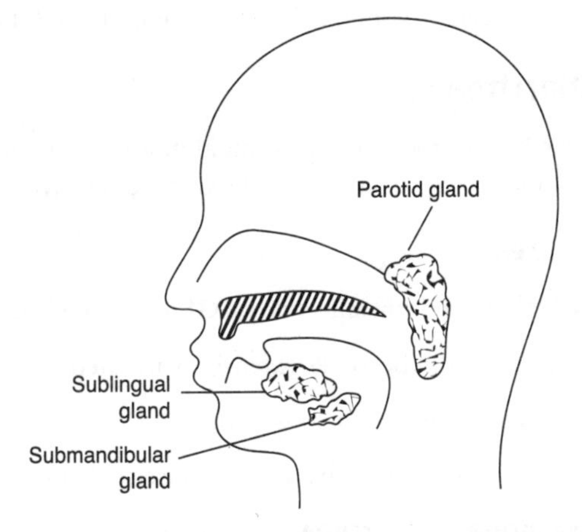

Fig. 6.6 Salivary glands.

Functions

The various functions of saliva are summarized as follows:

1. **Mechanical functions**
   - Keeps the mouth moist and helps in speech (articulation).
   - Acts as a lubricant for the formation of the bolus of food.
   - Dilutes hot and irritant substances, thereby preventing injury to the mucus membrane.
   - Washes down the food debris and prevents bacterial growth.

Applied Physiology

Vomiting

Vomiting is a process by which the upper GI tract empties its contents when it is excessively irritated or overdistended. The process of vomiting occurs by antiperistalsis.

The impulses are transmitted by both sympathetic and parasympathetic nerves to the vomiting center. The efferent impulses from vomiting center reach the upper GI tract to induce vomiting.

Vomiting Center

The vomiting center is present bilaterally in the medulla. It lies near the tractus solitarius at the level of the dorsal motor nucleus of the vagus.

Chemoreceptor Trigger Zone

This is a small area located bilaterally on the floor of the fourth ventricle near the area postrema. Drugs like morphine and apomorphine can stimulate the chemoreceptor trigger zone (CTZ) to initiate vomiting. Motion sickness causes vomiting by stimulation of the CTZ.

Diarrhea

Diarrhea is produced due to rapid movement of the fecal matter through the intestine. This is accompanied by loss of large quantities of fluid and electrolytes from the body.

Causes

Enteritis   It is the infection of GI tract caused either by a virus or by bacteria.

The mucosa becomes extensively irritated and secretion becomes greatly enhanced.

There is passage of loose stools.

Toxins secreted by pathogens cause secretion of large quantities of fluid and electroloytes.

Psychogenic Diarrhea   It is caused by excessive stimulation of parasympathetic nervous system, which increases both motility and secretion of mucus in the distal colon. This results in the passage of frequent loose stools.

Ulcerative Colitis   This is a disease in which extensive areas of the large intestine become inflamed and ulcerated. The motility of the ulcerated colon increases significantly. As a result, the patient has repeated loose motions.

Megacolon

Megacolon is a congenital condition characterized by the absence of intrinsic nerve plexus (Auerbach plexus). It results in the accumulation of fecal matter, resulting in distension of sigmoid (a segment of colon) with improper defecation.

Intestinal Bacterial Flora

Intestinal bacteria supply vitamin K and vitamin B complex. They have an important role in preventing infection. Destruction of intestinal flora can result in loose stools, commonly seen following the administration of broad-spectrum antibiotics.

2. **Digestive functions**
    - The following enzymes are secreted in the saliva and act as follows:

      Ptyalin splits cooked starch into maltose.

      Maltase converts maltose to glucose.

3. **Excretory functions**
    - Excretes urea, drugs, heavy metals, and thiocyanates.

4. **Taste**
    - Helps in sensation of taste.

5. **Water balance**
    - Helps in water balance. Saliva keeps the mouth moist. When body water is lost, saliva is reduced and sensation of thirst is felt.

6. **Heat loss**
    - Helps in heat loss from the body.

7. **Buffering action**
    - Bicarbonate in saliva acts as buffers.

8. **Bacteriolytic action**
    - Lysozyme, the enzyme present in the saliva, dissolves the cell wall of many bacteria and destroys them.

Mechanism of Secretion

The salivary secretion occurs in two stages: the first stage involves changes in the acini and the second stage involves secretion from the ducts.

The acini secrete ptyalin and mucin.

As the secretion passes through the ducts, Na^+ is reabsorbed and K^+ is secreted.

Cl^- is passively absorbed. HCO_3^- is secreted by the ductal epithelium into the lumen.

Regulation

The salivary secretion is predominantly under the neural control from the superior and inferior salivary nuclei present in the brainstem.

Salivary secretion increases by

- parasympathetic stimulation,
- smelling or eating favorite foods, and
- presence of irritating food in the stomach.

  Salivary secretion decreases by

- atropine and other cholinergic blockers.

Stimulation of sympathetic nerve causes secretion of small amounts of saliva rich in organic constituents.

Stomach (Fig. 6.7)

It is a J-shaped hollow structure. Its average capacity is 1.2–1.7 L.

It is divided into three parts: fundus, body, and pylorus.

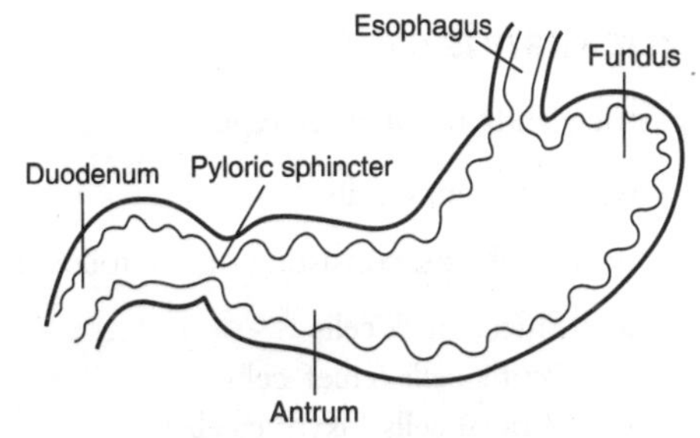

Fig. 6.7   Stomach.

Applied Physiology

Mumps

It is a viral infection affecting the parotid gland.

Xerostomia

It is a condition due to reduced salivary secretion resulting in dryness of mouth.

Unlike other parts of the GI tract, muscular layer of the stomach contains outer longitudinal, middle circular, and inner oblique layers.

Inlet of the stomach is guarded by esophageal sphincter and the outlet by pyloric sphincter.

Gastric mucosa is thick, thrown into folds called rugae, and has a number of gastric glands.

Functions

The functions of the stomach are as follows:

- Helps in storage of food. The food is stored in the stomach for 3–4 h and slowly emptied into the duodenum.

- Helps in proper mixing of food and converts it into semisolid substance called chyme.

- Helps in digestion of food by secretion of gastric juice.

- HCl secreted by the stomach destroys microorganisms and other harmful substances present in the food.

- Secretes intrinsic factor which helps in the absorption of vitamin B_{12}.

Gastric Glands (Fig. 6.8)

The gastric glands are of three types:

1. Mucus-secreting cells

2. Oxyntic glands, consisting of the following:

    (a) Mucus neck cells
    (b) Peptic cells (chief cells)
    (c) Parietal cells (oxyntic cells)

3. Pyloric glands, consisting of the following:

    (a) Mucus cells
    (b) G cells
    (c) Enterochromaffin cells

Mucus Cells

They are columnar in shape. They absorb carbohydrates from the bloodstream and convert them into mucin. Mucin when hydrated forms mucus.

Functions of Mucus

- Forms a protective barrier against acid and prevents peptic damage.

- Lubricates the food particles as they pass through the gut.

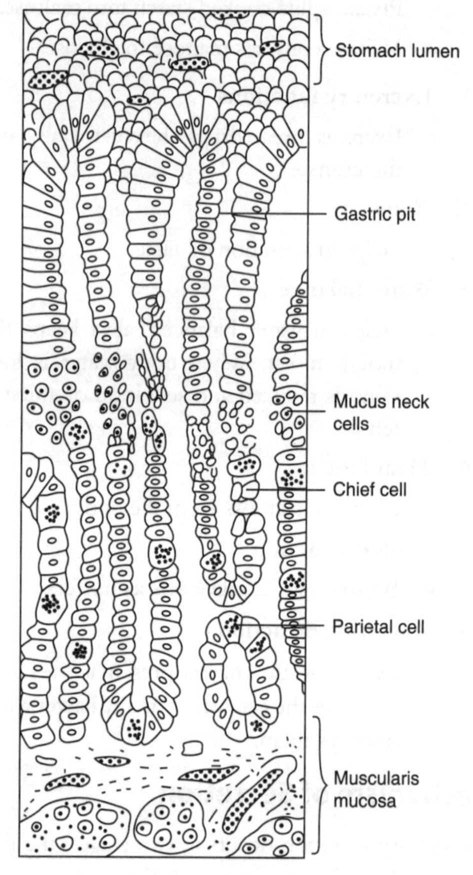

Fig. 6.8   Gastric glands.

Oxyntic Glands

Peptic Cells (Chief Cells)   They are primarily found at the base of the oxyntic glands in the body of the stomach.

They produce pepsinogen. Pepsinogen is an inactive form which gets converted to active form pepsin when it comes in contact with the HCl.

Parietal Cells (Fig. 6.9)   The parietal cells secrete HCl and intrinsic factor.

HCl Secretion (Fig. 6.10)   The parietal cells contain many large branching intracellular canaliculi. HCl is formed in these canaliculi and secreted when these cells are stimulated.

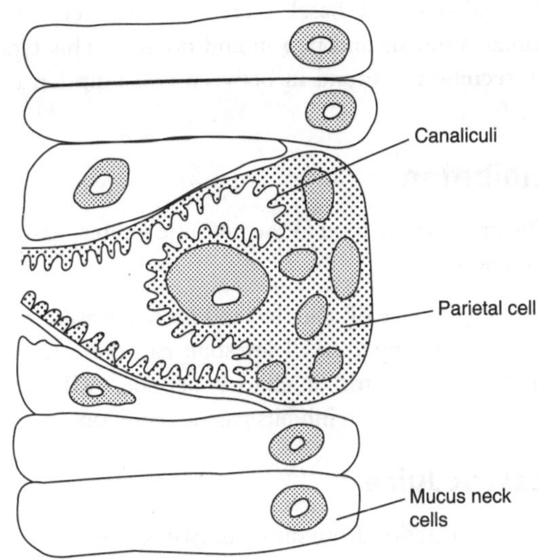

Fig. 6.9   Parietal cell.

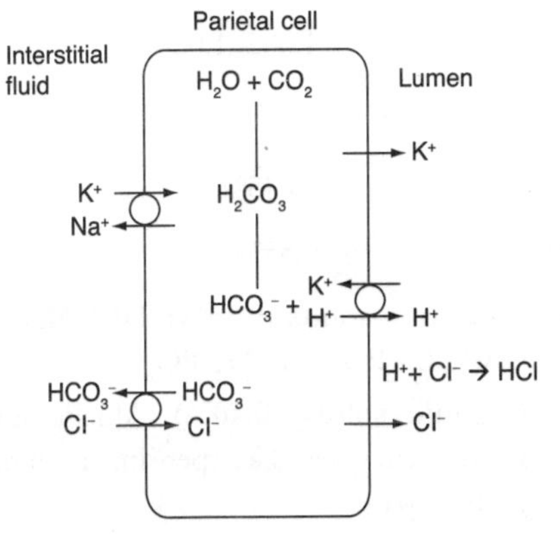

Fig. 6.10   HCl secretion.

Steps in HCl synthesis:

1. Water present inside the parietal cell is ionized into hydrogen ions and hydroxyl ions. Hydrogen ions are actively secreted into the canaliculi.

$$H_2O \longrightarrow H^+ \text{ and } OH^-.$$

2. CO_2 combines with H_2O in the presence of carbonic anhydrase to form carbonic acid.

$$CO_2 + H_2O \longrightarrow H_2CO_3.$$

3. Carbonic acid dissociates to form hydrogen ions and bicarbonate ions.

$$H_2CO_3 \longrightarrow H^+ + HCO_3^-.$$

4. Chloride enters the parietal cell in exchange for bicarbonate ions. This chloride is secreted into canaliculi.

5. H^+ ion is pumped into canaliculi. It combines with Cl^- to form HCl.

Intrinsic Factor   The intrinsic factor is a glycoprotein with a molecular weight of 45,000.

It is synthesized and secreted by the parietal cells. It is required for the absorption of vitamin B_{12}. Deficiency of vitamin B_{12} causes failure of maturation of red blood cells. This leads to a condition called megaloblastic anemia.

Pyloric Glands

They are present in the pyloric antrum. They contain mucus-secreting cells and G cells.

G-Cells   They secrete the hormone **gastrin**.

Gastrin   It is a large polypeptide secreted in two forms. The large form is called G_{34}. It contains 34 amino acids.

The smaller form is called G_{17}. It contains 17 amino acids.

Gastrin is absorbed into blood and carried to the oxyntic glands in the body of the stomach. It stimulates the parietal cells strongly and the peptic cells to a lesser extent.

Its functions include the following:

- It enhances gastric secretion.
- Gastrin secretion is increased by the food rich in proteins.

Gastric Secretion

The secretion of gastric juice occurs continuously. However, the volume of secretion is variable.

Phases

Gastric secretion occurs in the following phases:

- cephalic phase,
- gastric phase,

- intestinal phase, and
- interdigestive phase.

Cephalic Phase

Gastric secretion in this phase occurs even before the food enters the stomach.It is due to sight, smell, thought, or taste of the food.

The signals originate in the cerebral cortex and reach the stomach through the vagus.

It accounts for 20% of the total gastric secretion.

Gastric secretion is due to both conditioned and unconditioned reflexes.

The conditioned reflexes are sight, smell, and thought of food.

The unconditioned reflex are food in the mouth, chewing, and swallowing.

The secretion of gastric juice starts in about 5 min and continues for 20–30 min.

Gastric Phase

Once the food enters the stomach, it excites the long vagovagal reflex and the local myenteric reflex causing secretion of the gastric juice. The secretion continues as long as the food remains in the stomach. This phase accounts for 70% of the total gastric secretion.

The main hormone involved in this phase is **gastrin**.

Bombesin, histamine, Ca^{++} ions, and products of protein digestion increase the gastric secretion.

Cortisol, parathormone, and insulin increase gastric secretion.

CCK-PZ, secretin, VIP, and somatostatin reduce the gastric secretion

Intestinal Phase

The presence of food in the upper portion of the SI causes the stomach to produce small amounts of gastric juice.

The hormones responsible are gastrin and bombesin.

Interdigestive Phase

It is also called basal secretion. The secretion contains mucus and pepsin and no acid. This type of secretion is found in between consumption of the food.

Inhibition

The presence of food in the intestine inhibits gastric secretion.

The presence of acid, fat, and protein breakdown products in upper small intestine causes secretion of secretin, gastric inhibitory peptide, VIP, and somatostatin, which inhibits gastric secretion.

Gastric Juice

It is the secretion from different gastric glands.

Composition

Volume   1200–1500 mL/day

pH   0.9–1.5

Specific gravity 1.002–1.004

Contents

Water   99.45%

Solids   0.55%.

- **Inorganic solids (0.15%):** HCl, NaCl, KCl, $CaCl_2$, Ca_2PO_4, and Mg_2PO_4
- **Organic solids (0.40%):** Mucin, intrinsic factor, enzymes like pepsin, rennin, and gastric lipase

Functions

The enzyme pepsin digests proteins up to the stage of peptones.

Rennin coagulates caseinogen of milk. (It is present in infants.)

Gastric lipase digests fat.

HCl acts as an antiseptic and causes hydrolysis of foodstuff. It converts pepsinogen to pepsin.

Toxins, heavy metals, and certain alkaloids are excreted through the gastric juice.

Experiments to Study Gastric Secretion

1. **Sham feeding (false feeding; Fig. 6. 11a):** The esophagus of a dog is exposed in the neck, divided in the middle. Both the cut ends are kept open to the exterior. A canula is introduced into the stomach to drain the gastric juice. The food given to the animal comes out through the cut end of the esophagus without reaching the stomach. There will be gastric secretion even without food reaching the stomach. This experiment is helpful to prove the cephalic phase of gastric secretion.

2. **Pavlov's pouch (Fig. 6.11b):** It is a small diverticulum prepared from the body of the stomach, representing about one-eighth of the whole stomach. A pouch is prepared in such a way that one end is shut off from the main cavity of the stomach by two layers of mucus membrane, while the other end communicates with the exterior through an opening in the abdominal wall. Vagus nerve supply is kept intact for the pouch.

   Its advantage is that uncontaminated gastric juice can be collected.

3. **Heidenhain's pouch:** This is a denervated pouch made of the gastric mucus membrane. Secretion from this pouch occurs only under the influence of bloodborne chemicals. This experiment helps to study the hormonal control of gastric secretion.

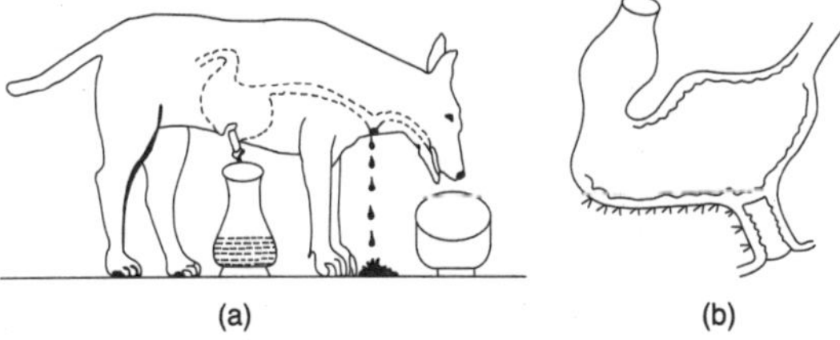

Fig. 6.11 (a) Sham feeding and (b) Pavlov's pouch.

Gastric Function Tests

HCl Secretion

Gastric juice is collected by a Ryle's tube introduced through the nose.

Basal Acid Output

It is the acid output in the interdigestive phase. Normal value is 0.5–2 mEq/h. Basal acid output is increased in duodenal ulcer and Zollinger–Ellison syndrome.

Peak Acid Output

It is measured from the gastric juice collected after the stimulation of gastric glands by the food or other agents. Normal value is 40–60 mEq/h. It is measured by

(a) histamine test,

(b) pentagastrin test, and

(c) insulin test.

Fractional Test Meal

Fractional test meal gives an indication about the acid output and also other functions of the stomach.

Barium Meal X-Ray

Barium meal X-ray is helpful in evaluating the movements of the stomach and gastric emptying. It is also helpful in the diagnosis of peptic ulcer.

Endoscopy

Endoscopy is helpful in diagnosing various conditions like gastritis, peptic ulcer, and study of gastric emptying.

Biopsy

Biopsy is helpful in diagnosing gastric malignancy and atrophic gastritis.

Liver and Bile

The liver is the largest gland in the body (Fig. 6.12). It is present in the right upper part of the abdominal cavity. It weighs around 1.5 kg.

The liver is both an exocrine and endocrine gland since part of its secretions directly drains into the blood and remaining is drained through the ducts.

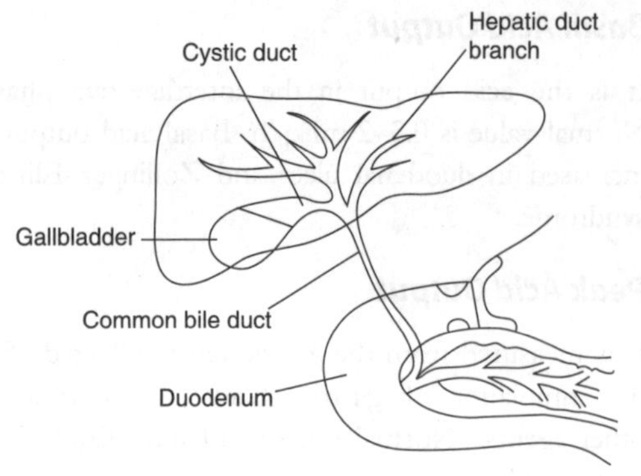

Fig. 6.12   Liver with gallbladder.

The liver is made up of cells termed **hepatocytes**. In between the layers of hepatocytes are the sinusoids.

- **Secretions from the hepatocytes drain through:** Intralobular bile duct → Right and left hepatic duct → Hepatic duct → Cystic duct → Common bile duct → Enters duodenum.

- **Blood flow through the liver:** Branch of portal vein and hepatic artery → Sinusoids → Central vein → Hepatic vein → Inferior vena cava (Fig. 6.13).

- **Portal triad:** This is made up of a branch of portal vein, branch of hepatic artery, and tributary of bile duct.

Functions of Liver

The functions of liver are as follows:

- **Formation and secretion of bile:** The bile is continuously produced in the liver cells. About 500 mL of bile is produced each day.

- **Metabolism of nutrients and vitamins:** The liver is essential for the metabolism of glucose, amino acids, lipids, and vitamins.

Applied Physiology

Gastritis

It is the inflammation of gastric mucosa, caused by nonsteroidal anti-inflammatory drugs, alcohol, and smoking.

Achlorhydria

This is a condition wherein the stomach fails to secrete HCl as in **atrophic gastritis**.

It is associated with pernicious anemia due to reduced secretion of intrinsic factor and hence absorption of vitamin B_{12}.

Peptic Ulcer

This is an excoriated area of mucosa caused by the digestive action of gastric juice.

Peptic ulcer is caused by an imbalance between the rate of secretion of gastric juice and the degree of protection offered by gastroduodenal mucosal barrier.

Helicobacter pylori infection is said to be the cause for peptic ulcer.

Anti-inflammatory drugs, alcohol, and smoking also cause gastric ulcers.

Management

Gastritis and peptic ulcer are treated with antacids, H_2 receptor antagonists (ranitidine), and proton–pump inhibitor (omeprazole).

Combinations of antibacterials are used to treat *H. pylori* infection in patients not responding to conventional treatment.

- **Inactivation of various substances:** Various toxins and hormones are inactivated in the liver.
- **Synthesis of plasma proteins:** Albumin, globulins, and clotting factors are synthesized in the liver.
- **Immunity:** Kupffer cells present in the liver are protective in function.
- **Hemopoiesis:** The liver is a major site of hemopoiesis during the first few weeks of intrauterine life.
- **Storage:** It stores vitamins A, D, B_{12} iron, and glycogen in significant quantities.

Bile

The bile is secreted by cells of the liver into the bile duct. Later, it drains into the duodenum. The bile is actually a product of secretion as well as excretion.

Composition

Total quantity	500–1000 mL/day
Specific gravity	1.010–1.011
Color	Yellowish green
Taste	Bitter
Reaction	Alkaline
pH	7–7.6
Solids	2–11%

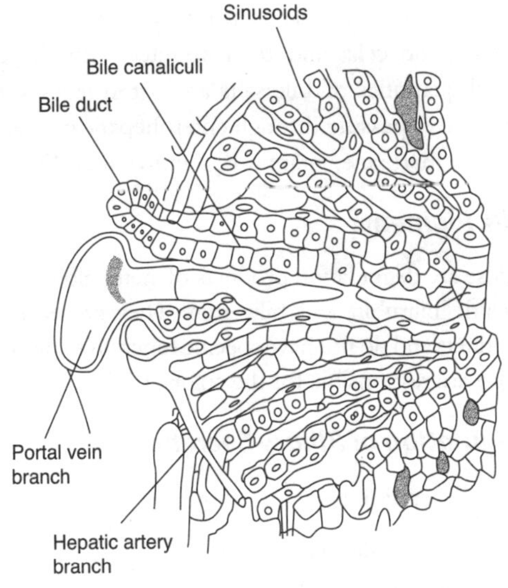

Fig. 6.13 Hepatic lobule.

Contents

- **Inorganic salts:** Chlorides, carbonates, phosphates of sodium, potassium, and calcium
- **Cholesterol and lecithin**
- **Bile salts:** Sodium taurocholate and sodium glycocholate
- **Bile pigments:** Bilirubin and biliverdin

Functions

1. **Digestion**

   The bile helps in digestion and emulsification of fats by the following:

   - *Reducing the surface tension:* Fats are converted to emulsion.
   - *Activating lipases:* Bile salts act as specific activator for different lipases.
   - *Solvent action:* Bile acts as a solvent.

2. **Absorption**
   - The bile is necessary for fat absorption by hydrotropic action.
   - Insoluble fatty acids and cholesterol are made readily soluble in the watery contents of intestinal canal.
   - Absorption of iron, calcium, and fat-soluble vitamins is facilitated by bile.

3. **Excretion**
   - Metals, toxins, bile pigments, and cholesterol are excreted through bile.

4. **Laxative action**
   - The bile salts stimulate peristalsis and act as laxative.

5. **Choleretic action**
   - The bile acts as its own stimulant for further secretion. This is brought about by bile salts present in the bile.

6. **pH**
   - The bile helps to *maintain a suitable pH* of duodenum.

7. **Emulsification**
   - Lecithin and cholesterol present in the bile act as an *adjuvant* to bile salts during the process of *fat emulsification.*

8. **Cholagogue action**

- The bile salts present in bile cause contraction of gallbladder and result in expulsion of bile.

Secretion

The bile is secreted in two stages by the liver. The initial portion containing bile acids and cholesterol is secreted by the liver cells.

Sodium, bicarbonate, and water are added as it passes through the canaliculi.

Bilirubin, the metabolic end product of Hb breakdown, is actively secreted into the bile canaliculi. Cholesterol and lecithin are also secreted into the bile canaliculi.

Storage and Concentration

The bile is secreted by the liver and stored in the gallbladder. It is normally concentrated five times. Capacity of gallbladder is 30–60 mL.

Emptying of Gallbladder

When food starts getting digested, the gallbladder begins to empty its contents by rhythmic contractions. Main stimulus for the contraction of gallbladder is the hormone **cholecystokinin**.

Gallbladder

This is a sac present underneath the liver. The capacity of the gallbladder is around 50 mL. It is connected to the common hepatic duct through the cystic duct.

Function

- Stores bile.
- Concentrates bile.

Shortly after the consumption of food, the smooth muscles of the gallbladder contract rhythmically and empty gradually. The stimulus for its contraction is mainly hormonal. CCK is the most important hormone causing contraction of the gallbladder.

Bile Salts

Bile salts are sodium and potassium tauro and glycocholates. These are salts of bile acids.

Three to four grams of bile salts are present in the body. Bile salts recycle six to eight times per day.

Functions

- They have detergent action on fat. This decreases the surface tension of particles and allows breakdown of fat globules into smaller particles. This is called emulsifying or detergent function of bile salts.
- They help in the absorption of fatty acids, monoglycerides, cholesterol, and other lipids from the intestinal tract.
- They stimulate the peristaltic action of intestine and thereby have laxative effect.
- They prevent the formation of gallstones by keeping cholesterol and lecithin in solution.
- Choleretic action—bile salts stimulate the secretion of bile.

Bile salts form minute complexes with lipids and these complexes are called **micelles**.

Lipids collect in the form of micelles. The micelles play an important role in keeping lipids in solution and transporting them to the brush border of the intestinal epithelial cells, where they are absorbed.

Enterohepatic Circulation   About 94% of bile salts secreted are reabsorbed in the SI. They enter the portal circulation and pass back to the liver.

These salts are taken up totally by the liver into the hepatic cells and then secreted into the bile. Small quantities of bile salts are lost in feces. Other substances passing through enterohepatic circulation include thyroxine, vitamin B_{12}, and vitamin D.

Bile Pigments

These are degradation products of hemoglobin. They include bilirubin and biliverdin. They are excretion products and do not have specific function to perform. They are responsible for the color of bile.

Regulation of Biliary Secretion

Biliary secretion is increased by

- vagal stimulation,
- cholecystokinin, and
- secretin.

When the food enters the mouth, sphincter of Oddi relaxes. Fatty acids and amino acids in the duodenum cause the release of CCK. CCK causes the gallbladder contraction. Stimulation of vagus and hormone secretin increases the water and HCO3 the content of the bile.

Choleretics Choleretics are the substances that increase the secretion of bile. Bile salts themselves act as choleretics.

Cholagogues These are substances that cause contraction of the gallbladder, e.g., cholecystokinin.

Composition of Bile

	Liver Bile	Gallbladder
Water	97%	91%
Bile salts	1.1 g/dL	6 g/dL
Bilirubin	0.04 g/dL	0.3 g/dL
pH	7.8–8.6	7.0–7.4
Cholesterol	0.1 g/dL	0.3–0.9 g/dL
Na^+	145 mEq/L	130 mEq/L
Cl^-	100 mEq/L	25 mEq/L

Jaundice

Jaundice is yellowish discoloration of the skin and mucus membrane. It is caused due to excessive deposition of bile pigments.

Clinically, jaundice occurs when plasma bilirubin exceeds 2 mg%.

Pathological Jaundice

There are three types of jaundice:

1. prehepatic,
2. hepatic, and
3. posthepatic (obstructive).

Prehepatic Jaundice

This is caused due to excessive breakdown of RBCs. Therefore, it is also called **hemolytic jaundice**. The liver cannot conjugate bilirubin and therefore concentration of unconjugated bilirubin increases in the blood.

Hepatic Jaundice

This is caused due to infection or toxic damage to the liver. There is increase in both unconjugated and conjugated bilirubin in the blood.

Applied Physiology

Gallstones (Cholelithiasis)

This is a condition in which stones are formed in gallbladder. Its incidence increases with age.

Gallstones are of two types:

1. calcium bilirubinate stones, and
2. cholesterol stones.

Cholecystitis

It is inflammation of the gallbladder. It is more common in fatty, fertile females in their forties.

Cholecystography

This is an investigation in which radio-opaque substances are administered either orally or intravenously. This is excreted by the liver and gets concentrated in the bile. X-rays are taken after few hours to visualize the gallbladder.

Cholecystectomy

Removal of gallbladder is termed cholecystectomy.

Obstructive Jaundice

This is caused due to obstruction of bile ducts either by tumors or by stones. In this condition, conjugated bilirubin increases in the blood.

Physiological Jaundice

It occurs in newborn babies on the second or third day after birth and disappears before 10 days.

Cause

Physiological jaundice is caused by rapid hemolysis leading to increased bilirubin production and reduced conjugation due to deficiency of enzyme glucurony transferase. This condition is self-limiting and requires no treatment. However, globulin production is normal.

Van den Bergh Test

This test helps to identify the type of jaundice. The serum of patient is mixed with a diazo reagent. If red color develops immediately it is called **direct positive**. It happens if conjugated bilirubin is present.

In **indirect positive** test, patient's serum is first treated with alcohol and later mixed with diazo reagent. This causes development of red color. It is seen if unconjugated bilirubin is present.

If both conjugated and unconjugated bilirubin are present, the reaction is termed **biphasic reaction**.

In hemolytic jaundice, the unconjugated bilirubin is increased. The Van den Bergh reaction is indirect positive. Urobilinogen levels are increased.

In obstructive jaundice, bilirubin is conjugated type. The Van den Bergh reaction is direct positive. The serum alkaline phosphatase levels are increased. Bile salts are present in urine.

Liver Function Tests

1. **Serum bilirubin:** Normal plasma bilirubin is 0.2–0.8 mg%. Plasma bilirubin is increased in jaundice.
2. **Estimation of plasma proteins:** Normal albumin/globulin ratio (1.7:1) is reversed in liver diseases. Albumin production in the liver is reduced due to the disease process.
3. **Serum fibrinogen and prothrombin levels:** Levels of these two substances are decreased in liver diseases.
4. **Serum enzyme estimation:** SGOT (serum glutamic-oxalo acetic transaminase) and SGPT (serum glutamic-pyruvic transaminase) increase in liver disorders. Serum alkaline phosphatase is markedly increased in biliary obstruction.
5. **Hippuric acid excretion and bromsulphalein excretion test:** These tests are done to assess the detoxifying capacity of liver by measuring their excretion rate from liver.
6. **Ultrasound scan of liver:** It helps in the detection of abscess, cyst, or any malignant growth. It also gives information about the size of the liver.
7. **CAT scan:** It helps in detecting any malignancy in the liver.
8. **Liver biopsy:** Ultrasound scan of liver, CAT scan, and liver biopsy give an indication about the structural and functional changes in the liver.

Pancreatic Secretion

The pancreas is both an exocrine and endocrine gland (Fig. 6.14). The endocrine secretion is from the islet of Langerhans. The exocrine secretion is necessary for digesting carbohydrates, proteins, and fats, and neutralizing the acidity of the duodenal contents.

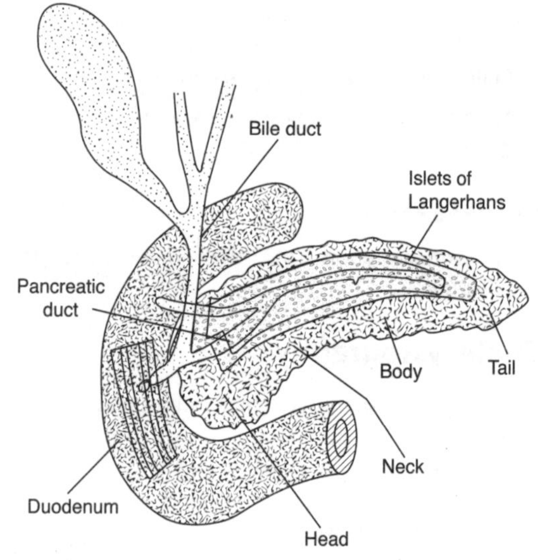

Fig. 6.14   Structure of pancreas.

Anatomy

The exocrine pancreatic gland is a compound alveolar gland resembling the salivary gland.

The secretory units are called **acini**. The acini secrete enzymes of pancreatic juice.

The secretions pass through

Intercalated duct → Interlobular duct → Extralobular duct → Larger duct → Main collecting duct (duct of Wirsung).

The pancreatic duct joins the common bile duct to form the ampulla of Vater, which drains into the duodenum.

Nerve Supply

The pancreas has the following nerve supply.

Sympathetic Supply

Celiac plexus → Superior mesenteric plexus.

Sympathetic stimulation inhibits the pancreatic secretion.

Parasympathetic Supply

It is through the vagus. The stimulation of the vagus increases the pancreatic secretion.

Composition

It is alkaline in nature. pH is 8–8.3. Quantity is 1500 mL/day.

Contents

98% water and 2% solids

Solids–Organic and inorganic

1. **Organic (0.8%)**
   - *Protein-digesting enzymes*
     Trypsinogen
     Chymotrypsinogen
     Nuclease
     Procarboxypeptidase
     Proelastase
   - *Fat-digesting enzymes*
     Phospholipase
     Lipase
   - *Carbohydrate-digesting enzymes*
     Amylase
2. **Inorganic (1.2%)**
   - *Cations:* Na^+, K^+, Ca^{2+}, Mg^{2+}, and Zn^{2+}
   - *Anions:* HCO_3^-, Cl^-, PO_4^{3-}, and SO_4^{3-}

Mechanism of Secretion

The enzymes are secreted by the acinar cells. They are stored as zymogen granules in the acinar cells. The stimulation of these cells leads to exocytosis of the zymogen granules and release of enzymes.

The fluid and electrolytes of the pancreatic juice are secreted by centroacinar cells and intercalated and interlobular ducts.

HCO_3^- ions are secreted in plenty.

Regulation of Pancreatic Secretion

The pancreatic secretion is regulated in relation to the food intake. Both hormonal and neural factors are involved in its regulation.

The parasympathetic stimulation increases the pancreatic secretion by releasing acetylcholine. Secretin and CCK increase the secretion of pancreatic juice.

There are three phases of the pancreatic secretion:

1. cephalic phase,
2. gastric phase, and
3. intestinal phase.

Cephalic Phase

In this phase, sight, smell, and taste of food stimulates the brain to send efferent impulses through the vagus to the pancreas. This causes secretion of enzymes. Acidic contents from the stomach on reaching the intestine cause secretion of bicarbonate-rich pancreatic juice.

Gastric Phase

The presence of food in the stomach induces the vagovagal reflex leading to pancreatic secretion. Hormone secretin stimulates the pancreatic secretion.

Intestinal Phase

This is the most important phase. It is mainly regulated by the hormones **secretin** and **cholecystokinin**.

Acid in the intestine stimulates the bicarbonate-rich pancreatic secretion by the action of secretin. Products of lipid and protein digestion, i.e., peptides and amino acids, stimulate cholecystokinin secretion. Cholecystokinin stimulates the formation of enzyme-rich pancreatic juice. This in turn enhances the secretion of digestive products by a positive feedback mechanism.

Functions

- **Digestion of proteins:** Trypsin, chymotrypsin, and carboxypeptidase hydrolyse proteins to amino acids.

    Proteolytic enzymes are present in the inactive form as trypsinogen, chymotrypsinogen, and procarboxypeptidase. They are activated on being secreted into the intestinal lumen.

    $$\text{Trypsinogen} \xrightarrow{\text{Enterokinase}} \text{Trypsin.}$$

    $$\text{Chymotrypsiongen} \xrightarrow{\text{Trypsin}} \text{Chymotrypsin.}$$

    $$\text{Procarboxypeptidase} \xrightarrow{\text{Trypsin}} \text{Carboxypeptidase.}$$

    Inside the pancreas, the action of proteolytic enzymes is inhibited by the presence of trypsin inhibitor in pancreatic juice. Trypsin inhibitor does not prevent the action of proteolytic enzymes in intestine since they are activated by enterokinase.

- **Digestion of carbohydrates:** Pancreatic amylase splits starch to maltose and α-dextrins.

    $$\text{Starch} \xrightarrow{\text{Amylase}} \text{Maltose} + \alpha\text{-Dextrin.}$$

- **Digestion of fats:** Pancreatic lipase splits fats into fatty acids and monoglycerides.

    Other enzymes present are colipase, phospholipase, and bile salt-activated lipase.

    $$\text{Fats} \xrightarrow{\text{Lipase}} \text{Fatty acids.}$$

- **Neutralization of acidic food:** This is brought about by HCO_3^- secreted in pancreatic juice.

    Maintenance of alkaline pH is necessary for the activity of digestive enzymes.

Secretions of Small Intestine

Small intestine does not secrete enzymes.

The digestive enzymes are intracellular and come into action only after desquamation.

Secretion of SI is called **succus entericus.**

Applied Physiology

Steatorrhea

Deficiency of pancreatic enzymes leads to indigestion of fats. This produces fatty, foul-smelling feces, steatorrhea. This can occur in pancreatitis, blockage of pancreatic duct by gallstones, or pancreatic malignancy.

Acute Pancreatitis

This is a serious disease, often fatal, caused by acute inflammation of the gland.

In this condition, pancreatic enzymes are activated within the pancreas. This damages the pancreas and the contents are released into the abdomen causing acute peritonitis.

Chronic Pancreatitis

It is a chronic condition caused by the consumption of alcohol and presence of gallstones.

Succus Entericus

Composition

Total quantity   1–2 L/day
Specific gravity   1.010
pH   6.3–9
Water   98.5%
Solids   1.5%

- **Inorganic (0.8%)**
  Salts of Na, K, Ca, and Mg

- **Organic (0.7%)**
  Enteropeptidase: Activates trypsinogen to trypsin
  Proteolytic enzymes: Erepsin, nuclease, nucleotidase, and arginase
  Carbohydrate splitting: Amylase, sucrase, maltase, and lactase
  Fat splitting: Lipase

Intestinal Villi (Fig. 6.15)

These are finger-like projections present in the mucus membrane of the SI.

Villi are composed of two types of cells:

1. goblet cells that secrete mucus and
2. a large number of enterocytes, which help in absorption.

Crypts of Lieberkuhn

They are small pits located on the entire surface of the SI. These crypts are formed in between the intestinal villi.

Secretion of Mucus

Mucus is produced by Brunner's glands located in the first few centimeters of the duodenum.

Mucus protects the duodenal wall from digestion by gastric juice.

Large amounts of mucus are secreted due to tactile stimulation of the mucosa, vagal stimulation, and secretion of hormones like secretin.

Secretion of Water

The enterocytes secrete large amounts of water and electrolytes along with end products of digestion.

Secretion of watery fluid is due to

- active secretion of chloride ions into the crypts,
- active secretion of bicarbonate ions,
- chloride ions drag sodium ions through the membrane, and
- all these ions together cause osmotic movement of water.

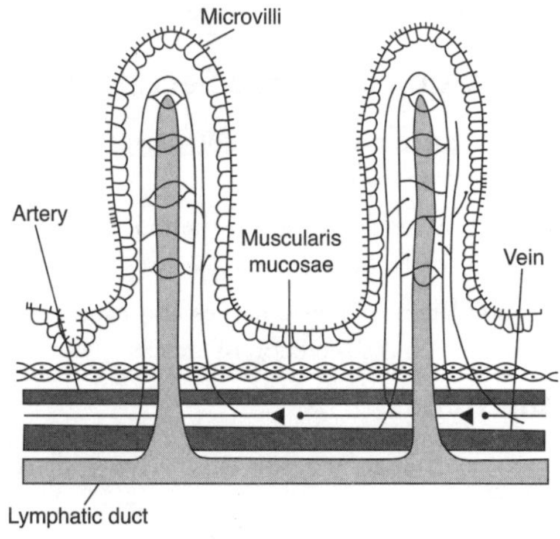

Fig. 6.15   Intestinal villi.

Enzymes of Small Intestine

Enzymes in the intestinal juice help in the conversion of partially digested food particle to simpler chemicals suitable for absorption.

Peptidase splits small peptides into amino acids:

$$\text{Peptides} \longrightarrow \text{Amino acids}.$$

Sucrase, maltase, isomaltase, and lactase split disaccharides into monosaccharides:

$$\text{Disaccharides} \longrightarrow \text{Monosaccharides}.$$

Intestinal lipase splits neutral fats into glycerol and fatty acids:

$$\text{Fats} \longrightarrow \text{Glycerol + Fatty acid}.$$

Enzymes cause hydrolysis of the food at the outer surface of the microvilli. The digested products are later absorbed through the intestinal mucosa into the blood.

Regulation of Intestinal Secretion

- **Local stimulus:** Chyme in the intestine increases the secretion of intestinal juice.

- **Hormonal regulation:** Secretin and cholecystokinin increase secretion.

Secretions of Large Intestine

The mucosa of large intestine has many crypts of Lieberkuhn but no villi.

The epithelial cells do not contain enzymes; instead, they have cells that secrete only mucus.

Regulation of Mucus Secretion

- Direct tactile stimulation of mucus cells on the surface of the mucosa
- Local nervous reflexes to the mucus cells in the crypts of Lieberkuhn
- Stimulation of pelvic nerves also causes marked increase in the secretion of mucus

Functions

- Mucus in large intestine protects its wall against excoriation
- Provides the adherent medium for holding fecal matter together
- Protects the intestinal wall from bacterial activity

GI Hormones

The GI hormones play a major role in the regulation of GI secretion and motility.

The GI hormones are classified into two groups:

1. **Gastrin family:** Gastrin and cholecystokinin
2. **Secretin family:** Secretin, glucagon, glicentin, VIP, and GIP

The cells secreting these hormones are called **enteroendocrine cells**.

Gastrin

Gastrin is produced by G cells present in the pyloric glands. These glands are present in the antral wall of the gastric mucosa.

It is found in the pancreatic islets in fetal life. Gastrin-secreting tumors, gastrinomas, occur in the pancreas.

Gastrin is a polypeptide hormone found in various forms.

G17 is the principal form of hormone connected with the gastric acid secretion.

Gastrins are inactivated primarily in the kidney and small intestine.

Functions

- Stimulates gastric acid and pepsin secretion.
- Stimulates mucosal growth of stomach, small intestine, and large intestine.
- Enhances gastric motility.
- Stimulates insulin secretion after protein intake.
- Causes contraction of gastroesophageal sphincter.

Regulation of Gastrin Secretion

Products of protein digestion, vagal stimulation, acetylcholine, Ca^{++} ions, and bombesin stimulate gastrin secretion.

Acidity in stomach, somatostatin, VIP, GIP, secretin, and glucagon inhibit gastrin secretion.

Cholecystokinin Pancreozymin (CCK–PZ)

This is a single hormone secreted by I cells of the upper small intestine.

It is a polypeptide hormone found in various forms.

The half-life of circulating CCK is about 5 min.

Functions

- Causes contraction of gallbladder and expulsion of bile.
- Causes secretion of pancreatic juice rich in enzymes.
- Increases the action of secretin in producing alkaline juice.
- Inhibits gastric emptying.
- Enhances the motility of small intestine and colon.
- Increases the secretion of enterokinase.
- Stimulates the secretion of calcitonin and glucagon.

In the brain, it may be involved in the regulation of food intake and appears to be related to the production of anxiety and analgesia.

Regulation of CCK-PZ Secretion

CCK secretion is increased by contact of intestinal mucosa with the products of digestion, particularly peptides and amino acids.

Secretin

This was the first hormone to be discovered in 1902 by Bayliss and Starling. Starling coined the word hormone.

Secretin is produced by S cells located in the mucosa of upper small intestine.

The half-life of secretin is 5 min.

Functions

- Increases the secretion of bicarbonate by the duct cells of pancreas and biliary tract.
- Causes secretion of a watery and alkaline pancreatic juice.
- Potentiates the action of CCK to produce enzyme-rich pancreatic secretion.
- Decreases gastric acid secretion and may cause contraction of pyloric sphincter.

Regulation

Products of protein digestion and acid bathing the mucosa of upper small intestine increase the secretion of secretin.

Bile salts in the intestine also stimulate secretin production.

Somatostatin

This is growth hormone–inhibiting hormone, isolated originally from the hypothalamus. It is secreted into circulation by D cells in the pancreatic islets and by similar D cells in the gastrointestinal mucosa.

It exists in two forms: somatostatin-14 and somatostatin-28.

Somatostatin inhibits the secretion of gastrin, VIP, GIP, secretin, and motilin.

It also inhibits the exocrine secretion of pancreas, gastric acid secretion, GI motility, contraction of gallbladder, absorption of glucose, amino acids, and triglycerides.

Its secretion is stimulated by the acid in the lumen.

GIP

This is a polypeptide containing 43 amino acid residues. It is produced by cells in the mucosa of duodenum and jejunum.

In large quantities, it inhibits gastric motility and secretion. GIP stimulates insulin secretion.

VIP

This is a polypeptide containing 28 amino acid residues. It is found in the nerves of GI tract. VIP is also found in blood.

- Stimulates intestinal secretion of electrolytes and water.
- Relaxes intestinal smooth muscle including sphincters.
- Causes dilatation of peripheral blood vessels.
- Inhibits gastric acid secretion.

  Other GI hormones are

- glucagon,
- guanylin,
- ghrelin,
- motilin,
- neurotensin,
- gastrin-releasing peptide, and
- substance P.

Digestion

Digestion is the chemical breakdown of food by the enzymes of the GI tract. The food that we consume contains carbohydrates, fats, proteins, vitamins, and minerals. These substances cannot be absorbed in their natural form and therefore have to be broken down into smaller particles.

Digestion and absorption of all major food substances take place in small intestine.

Digestion of Carbohydrates

Diet contains carbohydrates in disaccharide (sucrose and lactose), polysaccharide (starch), and monosaccharide (glucose and fructose) forms.

Diet also contains large amounts of cellulose. However, there are no enzymes in the human GI tract capable of hydrolyzing cellulose.

In the Mouth

The saliva contains an enzyme ptyalin (salivary amylase). This enzyme hydrolyses starch into maltose and other glucose polymers. Since the food stays for a very short period in mouth, only 5% of the starch is hydrolyzed before the food is swallowed. The action of salivary amylase continues in the stomach.

In the Stomach

Acidic gastric juice inhibits the action of salivary amylase, but before this action, about 30–40% of the starch is hydrolyzed.

In the Small Intestine

Pancreatic secretion contains pancreatic amylase. This enzyme digests starch into maltose completely in 15–30 min after the chyme enters the duodenum. The enterocytes lining the villi of SI contain lactase, sucrase, maltase, and α-dextrinase. These enzymes split disaccharides into their constituent monosaccharides:

$$\text{Lactose} \longrightarrow \text{Glucose} + \text{Galactose}$$
$$\text{Maltose} \longrightarrow \text{Glucose} + \text{Glucose}$$
$$\text{Sucrose} \longrightarrow \text{Fructose} + \text{Glucose}.$$

These final products of digestion are water soluble. They are immediately absorbed into portal circulation.

Digestion of Proteins

In the Stomach

Digestion of proteins begins in stomach. Pepsin secreted in the gastric juice is responsible for protein digestion. It is most active at a pH of 2–3. Pepsin is produced as inactive pepsinogen. It is later activated to pepsin by HCl. Ten to twenty percent of the protein digestion is by pepsin. Pepsin causes hydrolysis of bonds between amino acids. Pepsin converts protein to proteoses, peptones, and a few amino acids.

In the Small Intestine

Majority of protein digestion occurs in SI. Pancreatic proteolytic enzymes like trypsin, chymotrypsin, carboxypeptidase, and elastase cause digestion of proteins.

Trypsin and chymotrypsin convert protein molecules to small polypeptides. Carboxy peptidase cleaves individual amino acids from these polypeptides.

In the intestinal lumen, peptidase present in the brush border of enterocytes splits larger polypeptides into tripeptides, dipeptides, and aminoacids. These substances are transported through the microvilli into enterocyte.

Inside the enterocyte, dipeptides and tripeptides are broken down to amino acids. These amino acids are later absorbed into the bloodstream.

Digestion of Fats

In the Mouth

A small quantity of lingual lipase is secreted in the mouth. The amount of fat digested by this enzyme is very small (<10%). Majority of fat digestion takes place in the intestine.

In the Small Intestine

The first step in the digestion of fats is breakdown of fat globules into smaller particles. This process is termed **emulsification**. It is achieved partly by movements of stomach and by bile in the duodenum. Bile salts and lecithin are extremely important in emulsification of fat.

Pancreatic lipase present in the pancreatic juice splits triglycerides into free fatty acids and monoglycerides. Enteric lipase present in the enterocytes also helps in the digestion of triglycerides.

Accumulation of monoglycerides and free fatty acids causes interaction of bile salts to form micelles.

Micelles are small spherical globules 3–6 nm in diameter containing 20–40 bile salt molecules. Micelles transport monoglycerides and free fatty acids to the brush border of intestinal epithelium for absorption.

Absorption

The GI tract absorbs around 8–9 L of fluid every day (1.5 L of ingested fluid and 7 L of GI secretions).

Absorption mainly occurs in the SI.

The absorptive surface of SI is increased about three times by formation of folds termed **valvulae conniventes**.

The entire surface of SI contains millions of small projections called **villi**. These villi project about 1 mm from the surface of mucosa. Presence of villi increases the area about 10 times. Cells lining the villi are enterocytes. These cells have a brush border consisting of about 1000 microvilli. These microvilli increase the intestinal surface area by another 20 times.

The combination of valvulae conniventes, villi, and microvilli increases the surface area about 1000 times.

Absorption through the GI tract occurs by diffusion, active transport, and solvent drag.

Absorption of Carbohydrates

Carbohydrates are absorbed in the form of monosaccharides, especially glucose.

Transport of glucose is by cotransport with sodium. Sodium-dependent glucose transporter (SGLT) is the cotransporter responsible for this transport. Glucose moves with sodium into the intestinal cell. Sodium is then transported to the lateral intercellular spaces. Glucose is transported by GLUT-2 into the interstitium and later into the capillaries.

Galactose is transported by a similar mechanism. Fructose is transported by facilitated diffusion through intestinal epithelium by GLUT-5 and GLUT-2.

Absorption of Proteins

Proteins are absorbed in intestine as dipeptides, tripeptides, and amino acids.

Amino acids and peptides are transported by seven different types of transport systems. Five of these systems require Na ions. Transport of amino acids is by cotransport with Na^+. In two systems transport is independent of Na^+.

Absorption of Fats

Fats are absorbed in the form of free fatty acids and monoglycerides. Transport of fatty acids and monoglycerides in SI occurs by diffusion across the membrane of microvilli into the intestinal cell. From the intestinal cell, small fatty acids directly enter the portal blood and larger fatty acids are reesterified to triglycerides. Triglycerides are coated with protein, cholesterol, and phospholipids to form chylomicrons. These chylomicrons leave the enterocyte and enter the lymphatics.

Absorption of Water

Every day about 9 L of water is presented to the gut. Ninety-eight percent of the water is reabsorbed and only about 200 mL passes out of the gut in the stools.

Absorption of water starts from the stomach. Maximum water is absorbed from SI. Large intestine also absorbs significant amounts of water.

Absorption of Electrolytes

Sodium is absorbed from the lumen through diffusion and active transport. Chloride enters the enterocytes by diffusion. Chloride is secreted into the lumen of intestine.

HCO_3 is absorbed indirectly. It is secreted into the intestine in exchange for chloride ions. Calcium ions are actively absorbed from the duodenum.

Absorption of Vitamins

Water-soluble vitamins are rapidly absorbed from the intestinal lumen. Absorption of fat-soluble vitamins depends on fat absorption.

Metabolic activities of the body result in the formation of waste products. These are excreted through the kidneys, lungs, skin, and digestive tract.

The kidneys are essential for life. There are two kidneys present retroperitoneally in posterior part of the abdominal cavity, one on either side of the vertebral column. The consumption of water and electrolytes is greater than the quantity required by the body. The kidneys excrete this excess intake. Thus, they maintain fluid and electrolyte balance. They produce urine containing metabolic waste products, inactivated hormones, and their metabolic derivatives. They also produce hormones like erythropoietin, active metabolites of vitamin D, renin, and prostaglandins.

Each kidney weighs about 150 g. The kidneys are bean shaped (Fig. 7.1). The medial side of each kidney is indented and is called the **hilum**. Blood vessels, nerves, and ureter enter or leave the kidney through the hilum.

A cut section of the kidney shows the outer cortex and the inner medulla. The medulla has a number of cone-shaped structures called **renal pyramids**. The central portion of the kidney is called the **pelvis**.

The pelvis narrows down to continue as a tube-like structure called the **ureter**. The ureter leaves the kidney from the medial side and continues as a tube to open into the urinary bladder. The urinary bladder communicates with the exterior through the urethra.

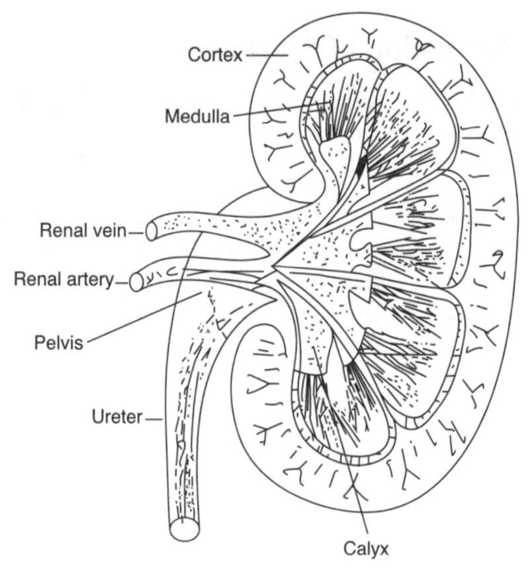

Fig. 7.1　Section of kidney.

Functions of the Kidney

Excretory Functions

The excretory functions of the kidney are

- formation of urine,
- excretion of waste products of metabolism, and
- maintenance of water balance.

Nonexcretory Functions

The nonexcretory functions of the kidney are

- regulation of acid–base balance,
- secretion of renin and erythropoietin,
- formation of active form of vitamin D, and
- secretion of prostaglandins.

Nephron

Nephron is the functional unit of the kidney (Fig. 7.2). There are about 1 million nephrons in each kidney. About 80–85% of the nephrons are located in the cortex, and they are called **cortical nephrons**. The remaining 15% are located more toward the medulla and are designated as **juxtamedullary nephrons**. Blood flow to the nephron is through the afferent arteriole that opens into the glomerular capillary bed. Blood from the glomerular capillary drains into the efferent arteriole. The efferent arterioles redivide to form the peritubular capillary or vasa recta.

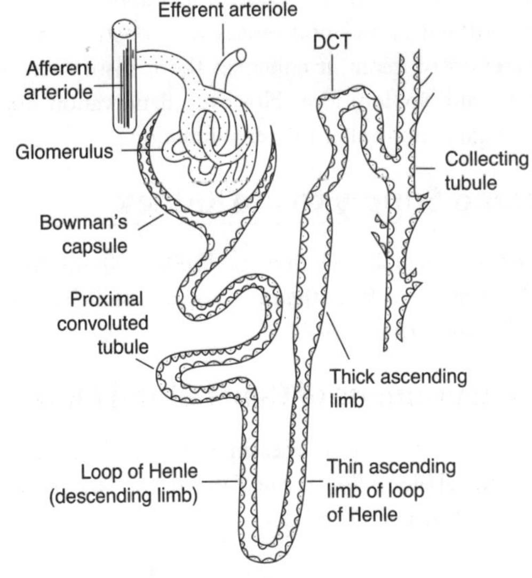

Fig. 7.2   Structure of nephron.

Cortical Nephron

The cortical nephrons are superficial nephrons having a short loop of Henle reaching only to the outer medullary zone. The loop of Henle is surrounded by the peritubular capillaries.

Juxtamedullary Nephron

The juxtamedullary nephrons are present in the medullary portion of the kidney. They have a long loop of Henle surrounded by vasa recta. Renal blood flow and glomerular filtration rate is greater in these nephrons. They have a greater capacity to absorb water and salt than the cortical nephrons. The juxtamedullary nephrons play a major role in concentrating the urine.

Parts of Nephron

Malphigian Corpuscle

Malphigian corpuscle is a flattened spheroidal structure consisting of glomerulus and Bowman's capsule. It helps in filtration, which is the first step in the formation of urine. Malphigian corpuscle is also called renal corpuscle.

Glomerulus

The glomerulus is formed by a tuft of capillaries arising from the afferent arteriole. The glomerular capillaries join to form the efferent arteriole. The glomerulus contains fenestrated capillaries supported by a basement membrane. Basement membrane is composed of loose fibrillar glycoprotein with negative charge.

The glomerular capillaries form the first capillary bed. The hydrostatic pressure in this capillary bed is determined by the resistance offered by the afferent and efferent arterioles to the flow of blood. This process regulates the capillary pressure for glomerular filtration.

The foot processes (pedicels) of the specialized epithelial cells (podocytes) are in contact with the other surface of the basement membrane.

The slit pores present between the foot processes of podocytes provide pathway for the flow of plasma into Bowman's space.

The interstitial mesangial cells support the glomerular capillary and basement membrane.

The mesangial cells affect the glomerular blood flow and thereby regulate the glomerular filtration.

Bowman's Capsule

Bowman's capsule is the blind end of the nephron, which is funnel shaped. It encloses the glomerulus. It has an inner visceral layer covering the glomerulus and an outer parietal layer. The parietal layer is made up of simple squamous epithelial cells.

Proximal Convoluted Tubule

Proximal convoluted tubule (PCT) is the continuation of Bowman's capsule measuring about 15 mm. It is made up of a proximal convoluted portion called **pars convoluta** and a straight part called **pars recta**. The pars recta forms the first part of the descending limb of the loop of Henle.

PCT is lined by a single layer of epithelial cells that are columnar in pars convoluta and cuboidal in pars recta. The luminal surfaces of the lining cells have microvilli that give it a brush-border appearance. The microvilli increase the surface area of the cells. The cytoplasm of the cells is granular and the nucleus is situated toward the base. Functionally useful substances are absorbed from this part of the nephron.

Loop of Henle

It is a continuation of the PCT. It is short in cortical nephrons and long in juxtamedullary nephrons.

The loop of Henle has the following parts:

- descending loop,
- hair pin bend, and
- ascending loop.

The descending loop is thin walled and permeable to water. It is the continuation of pars recta of the PCT. The thin descending limb of the loop of Henle after a variable length turns back to form the thin ascending limb. The thin descending and short ascending loops are lined by the squamous epithelium.

The thick ascending loop is the continuation of the thin ascending loop of Henle. The thick ascending loop is thick walled and impermeable to water. It ends at the macula densa. It is lined by

columnar epithelium with few microvilli without brush border. The nucleus is closer to the lumen and the cell contains numerous mitochondria.

Distal Convoluted Tubule

Distal convoluted tubule (DCT) is the distal coiled part of the nephron measuring about 5 mm. It is lined by cuboidal cells. The cells lining the DCT resemble the cells of the thick ascending limb with few microvilli and mitochondria.

Collecting Duct

The DCT continues as the collecting duct. The DCT and collecting duct are made up of P cells (principal cells) and I cells (intercalated cells). These cells contain an enzyme called carbonic anhydrase. In addition, the collecting duct has simple columnar cells. The collecting ducts receive the filtrate from the DCT and open into the renal pelvis. Two hormones, namely, ADH and aldosterone act on this part of the nephron.

Nerve Supply to the Kidney

The kidney is supplied by the sympathetic fibers from T_{11} to L_1 segments of the spinal cord through the celiac ganglion. The parasympathetic nerve supply is from the vagus nerve. The pain-mediating fibers pass through the sympathetic trunk. The nerve fibers accompany the blood vessels. They supply the blood vessels and juxtaglomerular apparatus. The sympathetic stimulation causes vasoconstriction and secretion of renin; it enhances the reabsorption of water and sodium ions. However, denervation does not significantly alter the renal function.

Blood Supply to the Kidney

Normal renal blood flow is 1100–1200 mL/min. Blood supply is from the renal artery, a branch of the abdominal aorta.

Measurement of Renal Blood Flow

Renal plasma flow is measured by PAH clearance test. Renal blood flow is calculated using renal plasma flow and hematocrit value.

$$\text{Renal blood flow} = \text{RPF} \times \frac{100}{100 - \text{Hematocrit}}.$$

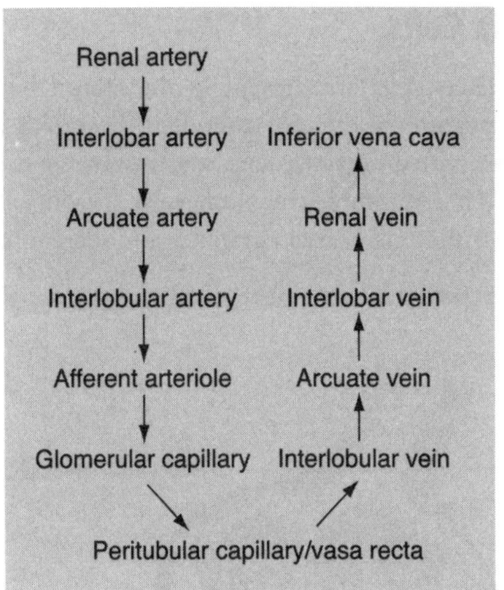

Regulation of Blood Flow

The nerves supplying the renal blood vessels do not significantly influence the blood supply to the kidneys. The sympathetic vasoconstrictor activity is minimal at rest. However, it increases with change of posture, pain, emotion, and exercise. Hence, the renal blood flow decreases.

The reduction of renal blood flow with erect posture and exercise is exaggerated in patients with cardiac failure.

Severe reduction of arterial blood pressure as in shock depresses the renal blood flow; this may precipitate renal failure.

Chronic diseases that destroy the nephrons also reduce the renal blood flow.

The kidney maintains its own blood supply by the mechanism of autoregulation.

Autoregulation

Autoregulation is the ability of the kidney to maintain a constant flow of blood despite a variation in the systemic arterial blood pressure from 60 to 160 mm Hg. It occurs in denervated and isolated kidneys. Vital organs like the brain and heart also have autoregulation.

Theories

Myogenic Theory   This theory is based on intrinsic contractile response of the smooth muscle to stretch. The smooth muscles contract in response to increase of tension on the walls of the blood vessel. Increase

in blood pressure enhances the flow of blood to an organ. Sudden rush of blood into a segment of blood vessel causes it to stretch. The stretching of the smooth muscle in the wall of the blood vessel results in its reflex contraction. Contraction of the muscle produces vasoconstriction and hence a reduction in the blood flow to the organ. Vasoconstriction increases resistance to the flow of blood.

The fall in blood pressure reduces the flow of blood into the blood vessel. The lack of stretching relaxes smooth muscle in the wall of the blood vessel. The blood vessel dilates, reducing resistance to the flow of blood. The blood flow improves through that blood vessel.

Interstitial Tissue Pressure Theory   This theory states that increased blood pressure will cause an increase in the flow of blood. As a result, more fluid comes out of the blood vessel and accumulates in the area surrounding the blood vessel. Progressive increase in the volume of accumulated fluid will exert pressure on the blood vessel making it narrow. This mechanical obstruction to the flow of blood will regulate the entry of blood to the organ.

Metabolite Theory   According to this theory, reduced blood flow to a vital organ due to decreased arterial pressure results in hypercapnia associated with hypoxia; this will lead to accumulation of metabolic end products locally. These end products of metabolism like lactic acid and pyruvic acid will produce local vasodilatation and restore the flow of blood.

Conversely, an increase in blood flow washes away the accumulated metabolites. The blood vessels constrict, restricting the flow of blood through the blood vessel.

Cell Separation Theory   When blood is flowing through the blood vessels, the blood cells are arranged centrally and plasma is arranged in the periphery surrounding the blood cells. If the branch arises perpendicular to the main artery, fluid portion of the blood separates out easily and flows into the branch leaving behind the cellular portion in the main artery. An increase in cellular component associated with a reduction in fluid portion will increase the viscosity of blood. This delays further entry of the blood into that segment of the vessel.

Special Features of Renal Circulation

- The kidneys receive a large quantity of blood in relation to their size. They recieve more than 25% of the cardiac output.

- The renal artery arises as direct branch of the aorta. Hence, it is a high-pressure system.

- The renal blood vessels form a portal system. They have two capillary networks.

- The kidneys have a system of autoregulation.

- The glomerular capillaries are a high-pressure bed and peritubular capillaries form a low-pressure bed.

Juxtaglomerular Apparatus

The juxtaglomerular apparatus (JGA; Fig. 7.3) is a specialized structure with vascular and tubular components. The ascending limb of the loop of Henle (beginning of DCT) passes close to its own glomerulus and comes in contact with the afferent and efferent arterioles. The modified cells of the afferent arteriole and the DCT along with the interstitial cells form the **juxtaglomerular apparatus**.

The JGA consists of

- macula densa,
- juxtaglomerular cells, and
- interstitial cells of Lacis.

Macula Densa

These are the modified cells of the DCT present close to the afferent arteriole. The cells of the tubule become narrower and taller. The cells of macula densa send cytoplasmic projections to the juxtaglomerular cells. The cells of macula densa contain a number of secretory granules which sense ionic changes in the filtrate.

Juxtaglomerular Cells

The cells of tunica media of afferent arteriole undergo modification to form the juxtaglomerular cells. The cells thicken containing a large number of granules. The granules are made up of precursors of renin. The juxtaglomerular cells secrete renin.

Lacis Cells

The Lacis cells are present in the region between the afferent and efferent arterioles; these cells are in contact with the macula densa and the juxtaglomerular cells. They resemble the glomerular mesangial cells. Few of the cells contain granules and secrete renin.

Sympathetic nerve fibers richly supply the JGA.

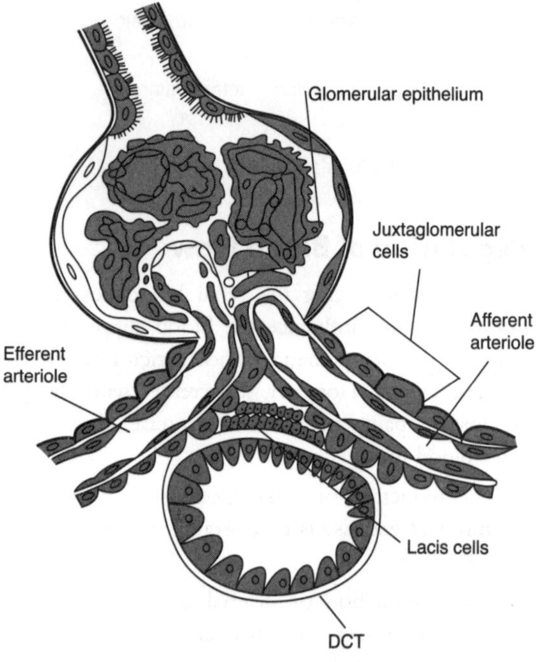

Fig. 7.3   Juxtaglomerular apparatus.

Functions of JGA

1. The JGA secretes renin in response to a drop in blood pressure and thus helps to regulate the blood pressure. The juxtaglomerular cells produce a glycoprotein hormone renin. Renin is a proteolytic enzyme that acts on the renin substrate present in the plasma (angiotensinogen). It converts angiotensinogen to a decapeptide angiotensin I. Angiotensin I gets converted to angiotensin II in lungs by angiotensin converting enzyme (ACE). Angiotensin II is a vasoconstrictor. It also stimulates the release of aldosterone. The juxtaglomerular cells detect changes in the blood volume from the degree of stretch of the walls of afferent arteriole.

2. The macula densa detects changes in the ionic concentration of the filtrate.

3. The JGA controls glomerular blood flow and glomerular filtration rate.

Formation of Urine

About 1.5–2 L of urine is formed per day by both the kidneys. Approximately 180 L of filtrate is formed per day. Almost 99% of the filtrate is reabsorbed as it passes through the nephron.

Urine is formed by the processes of

- glomerular filtration (ultrafiltration),
- tubular reabsorption, and
- tubular secretion.

Glomerular Filtration

Glomerular filtration is a passive process of formation of protein-free filtrate containing water and solutes.

Filtration takes place in the glomerulus and Bowman's capsule. It is influenced by various forces acting in opposite directions.

- Hydrostatic pressure is the pressure exerted by fluid on the walls of the blood vessel. It depends on the systemic arterial blood pressure and helps to push fluid out of the glomerular capillaries.

- Outward movement of the fluid is opposed by colloidal osmotic pressure exerted by the plasma proteins. The osmotic pressure retains the fluid within the blood vessel. It is the force that draws fluid due to the presence of plasma protein, especially albumin and colloids.

- The pressure exerted by Bowman's capsule resists the movement of fluid from the blood vessel to the exterior.

In a normal individual, hydrostatic pressure is about 45 mm Hg, colloidal osmotic pressure is 25 mm Hg, and Bowman's capsular pressure is 10 mm Hg. As the hydrostatic pressure is more than the other two pressures combined, fluid is pushed out of the blood vessel with an effective filtration pressure of 10 mm Hg.

Effective filtration pressure

= Hydrostatic pressure – (Colloidal osmotic pressure + Bowman's capsular pressure)

= 45 – (25 + 10)

= 10 mm Hg.

During the process of filtration, a protein-free filtrate is formed in the PCT. Hence, it is termed **ultrafiltration**.

Filtration occurs through the filtration membrane.

Layers of Filtration Membrane

- Endothelium of the glomerular capillary
- Basement membrane of the capillary endothelium
- Interstitial layer
- Epithelial lining of Bowman's capsule
- Basement membrane of the epithelial lining

Although the membrane is made up of many layers, filtration occurs because the capillary endothelium has pores termed **fenestrae**.

The basement membrane is made of meshwork of collagen fibers that have large spaces.

The epithelial cells (podocytes) have foot processes having gaps called **slit pores**.

Glomerular Filtration Rate

Glomerular filtration rate (GFR) is the rate at which filtrate is formed in all the nephrons in a minute.

GFR is 125 mL/min, and amounts to 180 L/day. It is estimated by inulin clearance.

Factors Influencing Glomerular Filtration

- **Capillary hydrostatic pressure:** Filtration is favored by the capillary hydrostatic pressure. An increase in the capillary hydrostatic pressure enhances the effective filtration pressure and hence the filtration.

  Constriction of the afferent arteriole reduces glomerular filtration.

  A marked decrease in blood pressure as in hemorrhage or shock reduces glomerular filtration.

- **Colloidal osmotic pressure:** It is the pressure exerted by plasma proteins and colloids in the blood. Effective filtration at the glomerulus is opposed by colloidal osmotic pressure.

  Dilution of blood or hypoproteinemia reduces

colloidal osmotic pressure. There is an increase in effective filtration pressure and GFR.

- **Bowman's capsular pressure:** It is the hydrostatic pressure exerted by the fluid present in Bowman's space. This will also oppose filtration of fluid at the glomerulus.
- **Thickness of filtration membrane:** The rate of filtration varies inversely to the thickness of the filtration membrane. Greater the thickness of membrane, lesser is the filtration.
- **Surface area of filtration membrane:** The rate of filtration depends on the surface area of the membrane. An increase in the surface area enhances the filtration. A reduction in the size of the glomerular capillary bed due to renal diseases or partial nephrectomy reduces glomerular filtration.
- **Size of the afferent and efferent arterioles:** The relative sizes of the afferent and efferent arterioles determine the glomerular capillary hydrostatic pressure. Normally, the efferent arteriole is narrower and longer as compared to the afferent arteriole. This anatomical character offers greater resistance to outward flow of blood from the glomerular capillaries. Hence, the hydrostatic pressure generated at glomerular capillary is increased. Constriction of the efferent arteriole associated with dilatation of the afferent arteriole can further enhance the glomerular capillary hydrostatic pressure.

Barriers for Filtration

There are two major barriers for the process of filtration:

1. mechanical or structural barrier and
2. electrical barrier.

Mechanical Barrier The glomerular basement membrane is the main mechanical barrier. The pores in the epithelial lining of the capsule and the endothelium of the blood vessel restrict the movement of large-sized particles.

Electrical Barrier Bowman's capsular cells and basement membrane have negative charge. They repel negatively charged particles in blood. Albumin is a large negatively charged protein repelled by this barrier. Hence, minimum amount of albumin enters the filtrate.

Due to these two barriers, molecules measuring more than 4 nm do not enter the filtrate.

Abolition of negative charge occurs in a number of renal diseases and advanced stage of diabetic nephropathy. Large amounts of protein (mainly albumin) get filtered resulting in proteinuria.

Measurement of GFR

Inulin clearance is used to measure GFR.

The substance used for the measurement of GFR should have the following properties:

- It should be filtered freely.
- It should be neither secreted nor absorbed.
- It should be nontoxic.
- It should not alter the function of kidneys.
- It should not be metabolized in the body.
- There should be an accurate and easy method to estimate it.

Principle

Amount of inulin filtered

$$= \text{Amount of inulin excreted}$$
$$= P \times \text{GFR}$$
$$= U \times V,$$

where P is the concentration of inulin in plasma, GFR glomerular filtration rate, U the concentration of inulin in urine, and V the volume of urine produced in unit time.

GFR is calculated using the formula

$$\text{GFR} = \frac{U \times V}{P}.$$

Creatinine clearance is also used to estimate GFR. Creatinine is produced in the body. It is neither secreted nor absorbed by the nephrons.

$$\text{Filtered load} = \text{GFR} \times \text{Plasma concentration of the solute.}$$

Variations in GFR

Glomerular filtration rate is reduced due to

- fall of blood pressure below 60 mm Hg as in circulatory shock,

- erect posture,
- emotion,
- pain,
- exercise,
- cold,
- loss of blood, and
- pathological processes that destroy the nephron.

GFR is increased when the extracellular fluid and blood volume are increased. It happens during the administration of saline. Infusion of saline dilutes the plasma proteins and decreases the colloidal osmotic pressure.

Filtration Fraction

It is the ratio between glomerular filtration rate and renal plasma flow. Normal value is about 20%.

Filtered Load

It is the amount of any solute filtered per minute.

Renal (Plasma) Clearance

Renal clearance of any substance is the volume of plasma from which that substance is completely removed by both kidneys in unit time. (It is the volume of plasma cleared off the substance in unit time.)

$$\text{Clearance of a substance} = \frac{\text{Mass of the substance excreted in unit time}}{\text{Plasma concentration of the substance}}.$$

Urea Clearance

It is the volume of plasma from which urea is removed in 1 min. Depending on the urine the output, it can be

1. **Maximal urea clearance:** Urine output is more than 2 mL/min. It is calculated by using the formula

$$\text{Maximal urea clearance} = \frac{U \times V}{P}.$$

Normal maximum urea clearance is 75 mL/min.

2. **Standard urea clearance:** Urine output is less than or equal to 2 mL/min.

$$\text{Standard urea clearance} = \frac{U \times \sqrt{V}}{P}.$$

Normal standard urea clearance is 54 mL/min.

Inulin Clearance and GFR   Inulin clearance is used to measure GFR. Inulin is introduced through intravenous route and the plasma level is maintained by continuous infusion. When the inulin attains equilibrium concentration with the body fluids, urine specimen and plasma samples are collected. The urine collected over a specified time and the plasma samples are analyzed for inulin concentration. Inulin clearance gives an estimate of GFR.

Creatinine Clearance as a Measure of GFR   Creatinine is produced by the metabolism of muscle creatine and creatine phosphate. Urinary creatinine is derived from endogenous creatinine. It is not absorbed in the renal tubule. However a small quantity of creatinine is secreted in the tubule. Hence, creatinine clearance is marginally higher than inulin clearance. Creatinine clearance is routinely used for the evaluation of GFR as it is produced in the body and its estimation is easy.

Para-amino Hippuric Acid Clearance   Para-amino hippuric acid (PAH) clearance is used to measure the renal plasma flow. It is freely filtered and completely excreted in the tubules. A known amount of PAH is infused intravenously; its concentration in plasma and urine is measured. About 90% of PAH is cleared. Clearance of PAH is calculated, which gives effective renal plasma flow. The extraction ratio for PAH is 90% or 0.9. The actual renal plasma flow is calculated:

$$\text{Actual renal plasma flow} = \frac{\text{Effective renal plasma flow}}{\text{Extraction ratio}}.$$

Based on the actual renal plasma flow and the hematocrit value, renal blood flow is calculated.

Normal renal plasma flow is about 600–650 mL/min. Normal renal blood flow is about 1100–1200 mL/min.

Tubular Reabsorption

The filtrate contains physiologically useful substances, namely, glucose, sodium, amino acids, chloride, bicarbonates, phosphates, potassium, and water, which are absorbed in different parts of the nephron.

Sodium

- Sodium is actively pumped out into the lateral intercellular space (space between the two adjacent cells lining the lumen of the nephron). This creates a concentration gradient between the lumen and the cell. Therefore, sodium ions move into the cell from the lumen.
- Sodium is transported along with glucose by cotransport.
- Sodium is also absorbed by countertransport. For every sodium ion absorbed one hydrogen ion is transferred to the lumen of nephron.
- Absorption is also influenced by chloride. Movement of chloride creates more positivity inside the lumen. This repels the positively charged sodium ions which move from the lumen into the cell.

Aldosterone, hormone of the adrenal cortex, increases sodium reabsorption from the DCT.

Potassium

A major part of the filtered potassium is absorbed in the PCT. Potassium is reabsorbed passively in PCT following the absorption of NaCl and other solutes along with water.

Calcium

Calcium ions bound to plasma proteins are not filtered by the kidneys. Ionized calcium is filtered. About 60% of the filtered calcium is absorbed in the PCT. The remaining part is absorbed in the ascending limb of the loop of Henle, DCT, and collecting duct. Less than 5% of filtered load of calcium is excreted. Parathormone stimulates calcium reabsorption from the distal tubule.

Magnesium

The kidneys filter ionic magnesium. Approximately 25% of filtered load is reabsorbed in PCT, 65% in thick ascending limb of the loop of Henle, and about 5% in the DCT. Parathormone, glucagon, calcitonin, and ADH stimulate magnesium absorption in the thick ascending limb.

Glucose

All the glucose that is filtered gets reabsorbed by cotransport or secondary active transport with sodium ions. Energy for transport is provided by the sodium–potassium ATPase pump.

Renal Threshold for Glucose   It is the concentration of glucose in the blood above which it starts appearing in the urine. It is 180 mg/dL of blood.

Tubular Maximum for Glucose   It is the maximum capacity of the nephrons to reabsorb glucose from the filtrate in an ideal condition.

It ranges from 325 to 375 mg/min.

Although the maximum capacity of reabsorption of glucose is reported to be 325–375 mg/dL, actual reabsorption is far below the expected level. This deviation of actual absorption compared to maximum capacity is called **splay**.

The variation is seen because
- all the nephrons do not have the same capacity of reabsorption as the ideal nephron;
- all the nephrons are not active and absorbing to their maximum at any given point of time.

Water

The PCT is highly permeable to water. About 85% of water filtered is reabsorbed passively. It depends on the reabsorption of other osmotically active substances. As the water absorption is obliged to absorption of other substances, it is called **obligatory water reabsorption**.

Applied Physiology

Renal Glycosuria

It is inability of the kidney to reabsorb glucose in spite of a normal blood glucose level. This is because of reduced tubular maximum for glucose.

A major portion of the remaining 15% of water is reabsorbed in the DCT and collecting duct under the influence of ADH (antidiuretic hormone or vasopressin). This process is called **facultative reabsorption of water**. Water channel proteins, termed aquaporins, help in the process of water reabsorption.

As the filtrate passes through the descending limb of the loop of Henle, water gets reabsorbed and filtrate gets concentrated. In the ascending limb of the loop of Henle, ions like sodium, potassium, and chloride are pumped out actively. The filtrate becomes dilute again. However, there is gross reduction in the volume of the filtrate.

Proteins and Peptides

Small-molecular-weight proteins and peptides are filtered in the kidneys to a little extent. The filtered proteins are taken up by endocytosis and degraded. The constituent amino acids are transferred to the plasma. The rate of reabsorption is dependent on the concentration of proteins in the plasma.

Release of myoglobin from damaged muscle and release of hemoglobin during excessive breakdown of red blood cell increases the concentration of small-molecular-weight proteins in the plasma. When the filtered load exceeds the maximum capacity of reabsorption, concentration of protein increases in tubules. This precipitates proteins causing blockage of lumen resulting in renal failure.

Amino Acids

Approximately 98% of filtered load of amino acids is reabsorbed in the PCT. The neutral and acidic amino acids are transported along with sodium ions across the luminal membrane. Normally about 0.5–2.0% of the filtered amino acids are excreted in urine.

Bicarbonate

Carbon dioxide is produced by the brush border of the epithelial cell lining the lumen of the nephron. It combines with water in the presence of the enzyme carbonic anhydrase to form carbonic acid (within the cell). Carbonic acid dissociates into hydrogen ions and bicarbonate ions. Hydrogen ion is extruded into the lumen.

In the lumen of the nephron, filtered sodium bicarbonate splits into sodium ions and bicarbonate ions. The bicarbonate ions combine with the hydrogen ions extruded from the luminal cell to form carbonic acid. This again breaks down into water and carbon dioxide. Carbon dioxide from the lumen diffuses into the cell to form bicarbonate ion.

Applied Physiology

Diabetes Insipidus (Insipid = Tasteless Urine)

Deficiency of ADH results in excretion of large quantities of dilute urine (polyuria). Other features of the disease are polydipsia (excessive intake of water) and dehydration. Dehydration is due to excessive loss of water.

Nephrogenic Diabetes Insipidus

It is the condition in which the kidney fails to respond to ADH. Secretion of ADH is normal.

The loss of water increases sodium retention, resulting in **hypernatremia**.

Aminoaciduria

In this condition a large quantity of aminoacids is excreted in the urine. This condition is due to the deficiency of some specific enzyme or transport process associated with abnormal metabolism of the amino acid. Aminoaciduria is a genetic defect.

Within the cells lining the lumen the following reaction takes place:

$$CO_2 + H_2O \rightarrow H^+ + HCO_3^-$$

$$NaHCO_3 \rightarrow Na^+ + HCO_3^-$$

$$H^+ + HCO_3^- \rightarrow H_2CO_3$$

$$H_2CO_3 \rightarrow H_2O + CO_2.$$

Phosphate

Filtered phosphate is actively reabsorbed in the proximal tubule. Reabsorption involves cotransport with sodium ions. Phosphate acts as an important buffer in the urine. Absorption is inhibited by parathormone.

Sulfate

Most of the filtered sulfate is reabsorbed in PCT by sodium cotransport. A small quantity of sulfate is excreted in urine. Sulfate excretion depends on its concentration in the plasma. There is no hormonal control for sulfate reabsorption.

Chloride

About 99% of filtered chloride is reabsorbed in the nephron. A major part of chloride is passively reabsorbed secondary to absorption of sodium ions. It is also countertransported in exchange for OH^- ions. Chloride is cotransported with sodium ions.

Urea

Urea is reabsorbed passively from the collecting duct. Water is absorbed from the tubule secondary to reabsorption of sodium. Hence, urea concentration in the tubular lumen increases. This creates a concentration gradient for urea. Urea moves along the concentration gradient out of the lumen. However, absorption of urea is less due to lower permeability of the tubular membrane to urea. The remainder of urea in the nephron is excreted through the urine.

Urea absorbed from the nephron contributes for creation of the medullary interstitial concentration gradient.

Uric Acid

Uric acid is the end product of urine metabolism. It is reabsorbed and secreted by the renal tubules. Uricosuric drugs like phenylbutazone used to treat **gout** prevent its reabsorption.

Organic Acids

Metabolic substrates like lactates, acetates, oxalates, and ketoacids are filtered in small quantities and reabsorbed in the PCT. They are cotransported with sodium ions.

In ketoacidosis, plasma concentration of these acids increases beyond the tubular maximum. Hence, the ketoacids escape reabsorption and get excreted in urine. The excreted ketoacids act as additional urinary buffers.

Tubuloglomerular Feedback

The rate of flow of filtrate in the ascending limb of the loop of Henle and the DCT will regulate the rate of filtration in the glomerulus. Macula densa of the DCT will sense the ionic concentration of the filtrate and the rate of flow of the filtrate. Consequently, filtration rate is altered by suitable changes in the size of the afferent arteriole and arteriolar resistance. This feedback will maintain a constant load of filtrate to the DCT. The possible mediators regulating tubuloglomerular feedback are the renin–angiotensin system, adenosine, cAMP, and prostaglandins.

Each nephron regulates its own blood flow by this mechanism. Tubuloglomerular feedback operates through juxtaglomerular apparatus. A change in afferent arteriole alters the resistance and regulates the flow of blood.

Renal vasoconstrictors like prostaglandins (thromboxane) also play an important role in autoregulation in the kidney.

Tubular Secretion

The renal tubules not only absorb physiologically useful substances but also secrete a few substances through the tubular epithelial cells.

The substances secreted in the DCT are

- ammonium ions,
- potassium ions, and
- hydrogen ions.

Ammonium Ions

The tubular cells form ammonium ions by the action of enzyme glutaminase on glutamine. Glutamine enters the cell by sodium-dependent cotransport. It is supplied to the kidney by the liver. The breakdown of glutamine yields ammonium and α-ketoglutarate. Metabolism of α-ketoglutarate consumes hydrogen ions.

Under normal conditions, the proximal tubular cells produce most of the ammonium ions. In the ascending thick loop of Henle, it is reabsorbed in exchange for the potassium ions. The reabsorbed ammonium ions accumulate in the medulla.

As the filtrate passes through the collecting duct, the epithelial cells secrete hydrogen ions. This lowers luminal pH favoring diffusion of ammonia. The ammonium ions formed in the lumen are excreted through the urine.

When the reaction of urine is more acidic, excess of ammonium ions are produced to regulate the acid–base balance.

Potassium Ions

Potassium is secreted in exchange for sodium ions. However, when the hydrogen ion secretion increases, the potassium ion secretion decreases. It is secreted in the thin descending loop of Henle. The principal cells present in the distal tubule and collecting duct also secrete potassium ions. Thus, in a normal individual, potassium excretion depends on the intake and need of the ion.

Hydrogen Ions

Hydrogen ions are also secreted in exchange for sodium ions. They help in retention of sodium ion, which is physiologically important and useful to the body.

Countercurrent Mechanism (Fig. 7.4)

Countercurrent mechanism is a system of U-shaped tubules. In this system, flow of fluid occurs in oppo-

site direction in the two limbs of the tubule. Countercurrent mechanism helps in concentration of urine.

The loop of Henle functions as **countercurrent multiplier system**.

Vasa recta operate as **countercurrent exchanger**.

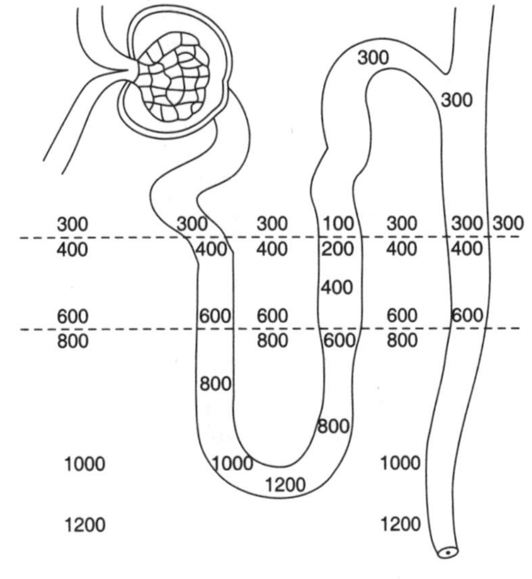

Fig. 7.4 Countercurrent mechanism.

Two important factors that help in the process of concentration of urine are

1. flow of fluid in opposite direction in both nephron and vasa recta;
2. increasing medullary concentration gradient (300 1200 mOsm/L).

The osmolarity of plasma is 300 mOsm/L.

The osmolarity of interstitial fluid in the medulla of the kidney shows a gradual increase from 300 to 1200 mOsm/L.

Factors Influencing the Genesis of Medullary Gradient

Factors influencing the genesis of medullary gradient are as follows:

- Active transport of ions like sodium, potassium, and chloride from the thick limb of the loop of Henle into the interstitium
- Diffusion of urea from the medullary collecting duct into the interstitium

- Reduced water reabsorption in relation to solute reabsorption into the medullary interstitium

Changes to the Filtrate in the Juxtamedullary Nephron

Countercurrent multiplier is formed by the loop of Henle. It is responsible for generation of gradually increasing the medullary concentration gradient.

- As the filtrate passes through the PCT, physiologically useful substances are reabsorbed.

- In the descending limb of the loop of Henle, water moves out of the lumen into the interstitium by the process of osmosis. This change reduces the volume of filtrate and increases its osmolarity.

- The filtrate formed in the PCT has an osmolarity of 300 mOsm/L. The osmotic reabsorption of water increases osmolarity gradually to reach a maximum of 1200 mOsm/L at the tip of the loop of Henle.

- As the filtrate moves up the ascending limb of the loop of Henle, sodium, potassium, and chloride ions are actively pumped out of the lumen. Water is retained in the lumen, as thick limb is impermeable to water. Ions pumped out to interstitium increase the medullary concentration gradient.

- At the beginning of the ascending limb of loop of Henle, osmolarity is around 1200 mOsm/L. As the filtrate passes through the ascending limb the osmolarity gradually decreases to about 150 mOsm/L due to pumping of ions and retention of water.

- As the fluid leaves the ascending limb of the loop of Henle, it is dilute with an osmolarity of about 150 mOsm/L.

- In early part of the distal tubule, fluid gets further diluted due to the active pumping of ions.

- In the remaining part of the distal tubule and collecting duct, the filtrate gets concentrated due to reabsorption of water under the influence of ADH. In the absence of ADH this segment is impermeable to water.

- Urea that is passively absorbed from the tubule contributes significantly in creating the medullary concentration gradient.

Changes in Vasa Recta

The medullary blood flow is low and constitutes about 1–2% of renal blood flow. The countercurrent exchange system of vasa recta regulates the removal of solute from medullary interstitium to maintain the concentration gradient.

- Blood enters the vasa recta and descends down slowly through the long loop.

- Wall of vasa recta is highly permeable. Blood in the descending loop picks up the solute from the medulla and becomes progressively more concentrated.

- There is water loss in this part of the vasa recta by the process of osmosis.

- By the time blood reaches the tip, it has a solute concentration of about 1200 mOsm/L.

- As the blood moves up the ascending part of the vasa recta, it becomes progressively diluted as the solutes diffuse back into the medullary interstitium and water moves into the vasa recta. Flow of blood through the vasa recta does not drain the solutes from the medullary interstitium.

- Thus, the vasa recta helps to maintain gradually increasing medullary concentration gradient.

Unhealthy Kidney and Its Altered Functions

Glomerular Functions

In nephrotic syndrome, the glomerular basement membrane is destroyed. This results in the leakage of protein into the filtrate. The patient has proteinuria. Urinary protein loss is not compensated by its production in liver. This reduces the plasma proteins and, hence, the colloidal osmotic pressure decreases. Reduced colloidal osmotic pressure produces generalized edema and retention of sodium ions.

In chronic renal failure, the glomeruli are destroyed. Urea and creatinine are retained in the body due to decreased GFR.

Tubular Function

In chronic glomerular diseases, the glomerular capillaries are destroyed. The associated peritubular capillaries and nephrons are also destroyed. The remaining nephrons have to handle greater filtered load. The nephrons operate in a state of osmotic diuresis. Hence, ability of the nephron to concentrate or dilute the urine is lost progressively.

An early sign of renal failure is nocturia. This is produced by inability of the kidney to concentrate urine.

Loss of nephrons reduces the excretion of potassium ions resulting in their retention.

Kidney is unable to synthesize bicarbonate ions in sufficient quantities. This results in metabolic (renal) acidosis.

Urinary Bladder

The urinary bladder is a sac of smooth muscle having two parts:

1. body and
2. neck.

The smooth muscle of the bladder is called the **detrusor muscle**. A small triangular area above the bladder neck is called the **trigone**. The ureter enters the bladder at the upper angle of the trigone. The bladder neck has detrusor muscle with elastic tissue forming the **internal sphincter**.

The urethra passes through the urogenital diaphragm. It has a layer of skeletal muscle

---

Applied Physiology

Cystometrogram

It is the graphical representation of relationship between the volume of the urinary bladder and the pressure within it (intravesicle pressure) (Fig. 7.6). It helps to demonstrate the plasticity of the urinary bladder.

A double-barrel catheter is introduced into the urinary bladder. The bladder is emptied and the pressure is measured. Later, the bladder is filled with 50 mL of water or air each time. The corresponding bladder pressure is recorded when the fluid or air is introduced into the bladder. Plot of intravesical pressure against the corresponding volume of the bladder is called **cystometrogram**.

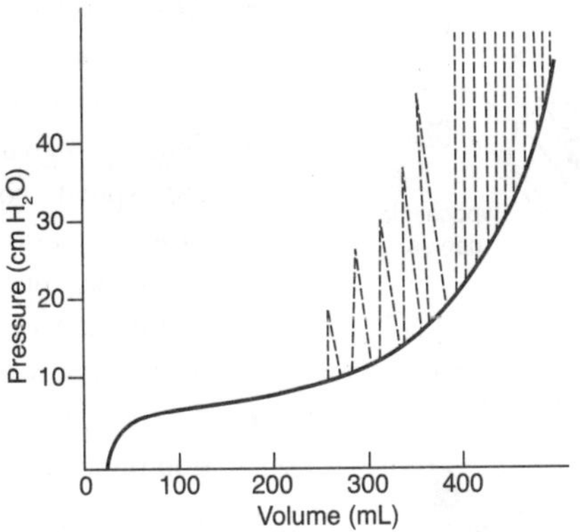

Fig. 7.6 Cystometrogram.

The curve shows three components:

1. a slight increase in the intravesical pressure with an initial increase in the volume;
2. a long, but flat, segment with further increase in the volume;
3. a sudden and sharp increase in pressure as micturition reflex is triggered.

constituting the **external sphincter**. The external sphincter is voluntary and can be used to control micturition.

The contraction of detrusor muscle results in emptying of the bladder and pressure within it increases to 40–60 mm Hg.

The bladder can hold about 300–400 mL of urine with little increase in tension. An increase in the volume of urine beyond this level increases tension. It is appreciated as sensation of fullness of the bladder. If the conditions are suitable, micturition reflex is triggered and urination occurs. First urge to empty the bladder is felt when it contains about 150 mL of urine. An accumulation of urine beyond 600 mL becomes painful.

Urine enters the bladder without a significant increase in pressure (intravesical pressure) within it. The pressure increases only when the bladder is filled up. The bladder muscles exhibit the property of **plasticity**. When the hollow viscus is stretched, initially the tension increases. However, the tension reduces immediately thereafter.

Nerve Supply

Urinary bladder receives both sympathetic and parasympathetic nerve supply (Fig. 7.5).

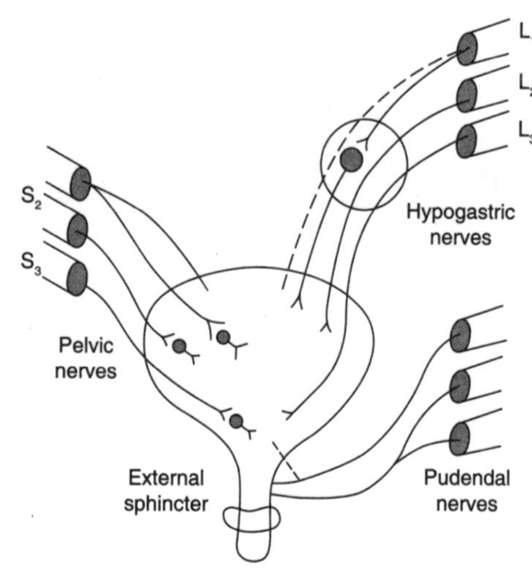

Fig. 7.5   Innervation of the bladder.

Parasympathetic Innervation

Parasympathetic innervation to the bladder arises from the sacral segment of spinal cord (S₂, S₃).

It passes through the pelvic nerves and supplies detrusor muscles of the bladder and the internal sphincter. Stimulation of nerve causes the contraction of bladder muscles and relaxation of the internal sphincter resulting in emptying of the bladder. Hence, it is called the **nerve of emptying**.

Sympathetic Innervation

Sympathetic innervation to the bladder arises from first, second, and third lumbar segments of spinal cord. It relays in the hypogastric ganglion. Postganglionic fibers supply the bladder muscle and internal sphincter. Stimulation of sympathetic fibers influences the blood vessels and alters the blood flow, but has very little role in the bladder muscle contraction.

Pudendal Nerve

It carries motor fibers to external sphincter of the urinary bladder controlling its voluntary activity.

Micturition Reflex

Micturition is the process of voiding of urine. It is a spinal reflex influenced by the higher centers.

- Urine formed in the kidneys dribbles into the bladder continuously.
- If the bladder is partly filled, detrusor muscles relax spontaneously.
- Accumulation of sufficient quantity of urine causes the stimulation of sensory stretch receptors in the bladder.
- Sensory signals reach the sacral segment of the spinal cord through the pelvic nerve. Motor response reaches the bladder through the parasympathetic nerve fibers. This causes contraction of the detrusor muscle resulting in micturition reflex.
- As the bladder gets filled up gradually, micturition reflex becomes frequent.
- When the micturition reflex begins, initial contraction of bladder further stimulates stretch receptors to strengthen the contraction of the detrusor muscles.
- Once the micturition reflex becomes powerful, it reflexly inhibits the external sphincter through the pudendal nerve.
- This causes relaxation of perineal muscles and urine passes through the urethra.

- However, if the condition is not suitable for voiding urine, higher centers exercise an inhibitory control over the lower centers to temporarily postpone micturition.

Influence of Higher Centers

These centers are located mainly in the pons and certain areas of the cerebral cortex.

1. Higher centers exert inhibitory control over the bladder except when micturition is desired.
2. If micturition is desired, the higher centers can facilitate the sacral micturition center to initiate the reflex.

Voluntary Control of Urination

Urination can be commenced, withheld, or postponed by voluntary effort.

During voluntary emptying of the bladder, muscles of the pelvic floor relax. This causes downward tug of detrusor muscle to initiate its contraction.

The contraction of perineal muscles and external sphincter can interrupt the flow and stop urination.

Urination can be postponed by voluntarily contracting the external sphincter.

After urination, female urethra empties due to the influence of gravity whereas the male urethra is emptied by repeated contraction of the bulbocavernous muscles.

Abnormal Functioning

Atonic Bladder

In the atonic bladder, tone of the bladder muscle is lost. It occurs due to a damage to sensory nerve from the bladder to the spinal cord or crush injury to the sacral segment of the spinal cord. Periodic emptying of bladder becomes difficult. There is overflow of urine when the bladder is full, resulting in **overflow incontinence**.

In **tabes dorsalis**, the dorsal roots of sacral nerves are interrupted. Hence, the reflex contraction of bladder is abolished. The bladder becomes thin walled, hypotonic, and distended.

Automatic Bladder

Damage to the spinal cord above the regions of the sacral segment results in automatic bladder. During recovery from spinal shock, micturition reflex is regained but without voluntary control.

There is automatic voiding of urine when small quantities of urine accumulate in the bladder. It is also called spastic neurogenic bladder.

Neurogenic Bladder

Partial damage to the spinal cord or the brainstem produces frequent, uncontrolled urination due to loss of inhibitory control.

Applied Physiology

Renal Failure

It is a condition in which the kidneys stop functioning normally.

Types

It is of two types.

Acute Renal Failure

In this condition, the kidneys stop functioning suddenly. The loss of function could be partial or complete. The renal functions may be restored subsequently.

Chronic Renal Failure

There is progressive loss of renal function with damage to an increasing number of nephrons.

Causes

Renal failure can occur because of reduced blood supply to the kidney (**prerenal cause**), abnormalities of the kidney (**renal cause**), or defective function of the collecting system of the kidney (**postrenal cause**).

Renal failure results in fluid and electrolyte disturbances associated with accumulation of toxic metabolic waste. It causes anemia due to reduced formation of erythropoietin. If it is not treated properly, it can result in death.

Management

Chronic renal failure is managed by

- dialysis and
- renal transplantation.

Dialysis

It is a process by which normal composition of blood is restored. Blood from the patient and dialyzing fluid (fluid having composition similar to that of plasma) are passed on either side of a semipermeable membrane. The metabolic wastes from the blood move into the dialyzing fluid and the physiologically useful substances move from the fluid to the blood. Later, the blood is reintroduced back into the patient. The process of dialysis has to be repeated periodically.

Renal Transplantation

It is a method of long-term management of chronic renal failure. The kidney of the matched donor is transplanted to the recipient. If the organ is well accepted, renal function is restored. However, the common complication is rejection of transplanted kidney. There is need to use immunosuppressants on a regular basis to prevent rejection of transplanted kidney.

Diuresis

Osmotic Diuresis

In this condition the urine output is increased due to the presence of osmotically active particles in the filtrate. *Reducing sugars* in diabetes mellitus produce osmotic diuresis.

Water Diuresis

Increased water intake increases the urine output due to reduced secretion of ADH.

Diuretics

These are substances which increase the output of urine by modifying the functions of nephrons.

Polyuria

It is a condition of increased urine output with reduced solute concentration.

Nocturia

Nocturia is excessive voiding of urine during night. It is a common symptom of diabetes mellitus.

Oliguria

It is reduction in the urine output less than 400 mL/days; it is commonly seen in renal failure.

Anuria

It is the absence of urine output commonly seen in shock and renal shutdown.

Renal Function Tests

Physical Test

Volume	1000–1500 mL/day
Color	Pale yellow
Specific gravity	1.003–1.030
pH	Acidic, 4.5–6
Odor	Aromatic odor in fresh sample

Routine Blood Test

An estimation of serum urea, uric acid, and creatinine gives an indication about the excretory function of the kidney.

Glomerular Function

Glomerular function is assessed by the evaluation of urea, creatinine, and inulin clearance. Creatinine clearance is a more specific test for renal function.

Tubular Function

The concentrating capacity of the kidney gives an idea about the tubular function. Varying quantities of fluid are given to the subject and urine output is estimated. Variation in the urine volume and specific gravity corresponding to changes in the fluid intake indicates normal tubular function.

Measurement of Renal Plasma Flow and Renal Blood Flow

Discussed earlier.

Radiological Investigations

- Ultrasonography
- X-ray
- Intravenous pyelography
- CT and MRI scanning

They help to detect the structural and functional abnormalities in the kidneys.

Urine

Normal Constituents

- **Inorganic:** Sodium, potassium, calcium, and phosphate
- **Organic:** Urea, uric acid, and creatinine
- **Others:** Ammonium chloride, oxalates, and minerals

Abnormal Constituents

- **Proteins:** Presence of protein in urine is proteinuria. Appearance of albumin in urine is albuminuria. Albuminuria is seen in pregnancy and kidney diseases like nephrotic syndrome.

- **Glucose:** Presence of reducing sugars in urine is glycosuria. It is seen in diabetes mellitus and renal glycosuria.

- **Ketone bodies:** Acetone, acetoacetic acid, and beta-hydroxybutyric acid are called ketone bodies. They are present in the urine in uncontrolled diabetes mellitus and during prolonged fasting.

- **Bilirubin:** It appears in the urine in cases of jaundice.

- **Blood:** In diseases of kidney like nephritis, RBC appears in the urine. Hemoglobin appears in the urine in conditions with excessive breakdown of RBC.

- **Creatine:** Creatine appears in the urine whenever there is muscle wasting as in myopathies and starvation.

Acid–Base Balance

The pH of arterial plasma is 7.40. In a normal healthy individual, pH of plasma is slightly alkaline, ranging from 7.35 to 7.45. It is slightly less in venous blood. The pH of water at 25°C is 7.0. The pH of gastric juice is highly acidic (up to 2) and the pancreatic juice is alkaline (up to 8). pH is the negative logarithm of hydrogen ion concentration. Increase in hydrogen ion concentration reduces pH of blood. The condition is called **acidosis**. Decrease in hydrogen ion concentration is termed **alkalosis**. The pH increases in alkalosis.

The maintenance of a stable hydrogen ion concentration is necessary for life. The molecules that donate hydrogen ions are called **acids**, while those that remove the hydrogen ions from solution are called **bases**. HCl is a strong acid and NaOH is a strong base. Strong acids and bases can dissociate completely in water. Most acids and bases in the body are **weak**; hence, they release or take up less hydrogen ions.

The pH of body fluid is stabilized by its **buffering capacity**. A **buffer** is a substance that can bind or release hydrogen ions in a solution. It keeps the pH relatively constant even when a considerable quantity of acids or bases is added.

There are different buffers working in a biological fluid. More than one buffer system act in the body at any give time.

The three main buffers in the body are

- proteins,
- hemoglobin, and
- carbonic acid–bicarbonate systems.

Proteins

Plasma proteins are very effective buffers as their carboxyl and amino groups dissociate.

Hemoglobin

Buffering is provided by hemoglobin by the dissociation of imidazole group of histidine residues. The buffering capacity of hemoglobin is six times greater than that of plasma proteins. Deoxyhemoglobin is a weaker acid and has better buffer than oxyhemoglobin because of its dissociation capacity.

Carbonic Acid–Bicarbonate System

It is one of the effective buffering systems of the body. The dissolved carbon dioxide is handled by respiratory system and bicarbonates are provided by the kidney. Addition of hydrogen ions to blood forms water and carbon dioxide with the help of bicarbonate ions. Carbon dioxide is excreted by lungs. Increase in hydrogen ion concentration increases the rate and depth of respiration eliminating more carbon dioxide.

Carbonic anhydrase present in the RBC facilitates the formation of carbonic acid from carbon dioxide and water.

Hemoglobin present in the blood binds to free hydrogen ions produced during the combination of carbon dioxide and water. The bicarbonate ions formed during this reaction move into the plasma for further buffering action.

Acid–base disorders are of four types:

- respiratory acidosis,
- respiratory alkalosis,
- metabolic acidosis, and
- metabolic alkalosis.

Skin

Skin forms the outer protective covering of the body. It is the largest organ with thickness ranging from 1 to 5 mm.

Layers

It has two layers, outer epidermis and inner dermis (Fig. 7.7).

Epidermis

Epidermis is made of stratified squamous epithelium. It does not contain blood vessels.

It has the following layers:

- **Stratum corneum**: It is the outermost layer. It is made up of dead cells containing keratin.
- **Stratum granulosum**: This is 3–5 layers thick. The cytoplasm has keratohyaline granules.
- **Stratum spinosum**: It contains cells having spine-like processes on their surface.
- **Stratum germinativum**: This layer contains cells which divide by mitosis. The newly formed cells move toward the stratum corneum. These cells contain melanin, a pigment responsible for the color of skin.

Dermis

It has two layers:

1. superficial papillary layer and
2. deep reticular layer.

Papillary Layer

It forms papillae that project into the epidermis. This contains blood vessels, lymphatics, and nerves.

Reticular Layer

It is made up of reticular and elastic fibers along with fat and loose areolar tissue. This layer merges with subcutaneous layer.

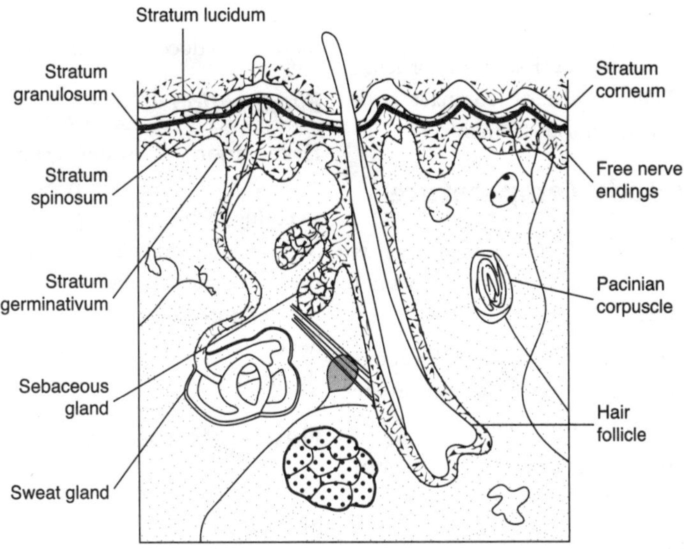

Fig. 7.7   Structure of skin.

Glands

Skin contains two types of glands:

1. sweat glands and
2. sebaceous glands.

Sweat Glands

They are present all over the skin except eardrum and lips.

They are of two types: apocrine and eccrine.

Apocrine glands are present in the axilla, pubic region, and areola of the breast. They become active only after puberty.

Eccrine glands are more numerous and are present all over the body. They secrete a clear watery fluid, sweat.

Sebaceous Glands

They are present in the epidermis of the skin. They develop from hair follicle. Sebum is produced from these glands. At puberty, sex hormones stimulate sebaceous glands leading to development of **acne.**

Functions

- Forms a protective layer around the body.
- Protects the body against infections and UV radiation.
- Regulates body temperature by secreting sweat.
- Is a sensory organ which has specialized receptors.
- Vitamin D_3 is synthesized in the skin.
- Regulates water and electrolyte balance.
- Excretes waste materials like salts and urea.

Appendages

Hairs

Hairs are keratinized thread-like structures that develop from epidermis.

Hair is divided into an outer shaft, root, and hair bulb. The hair bulb is embedded in the hair follicle. Hair follicle is an invagination of the epidermis.

The arrector pili are small smooth muscles attached to hair follicles. Contraction of these muscles brings hairs into vertical position with elevation of epidermis. This is termed **goose flesh** appearance.

Functions

- Help in perception of sensations.
- Thermoregulation.
- Protect against injury to scalp.

Nails

They are homologous to the layer stratum corneum of the epidermis. They consist of compact non-nucleated, keratin-filled squamous filaments.

Regulation of Body Temperature

Normal body temperature (core temperature) is maintained at a constant level irrespective of changes in external temperature.

Normal body temperature is 37°C (98.6°F). It has a diurnal variation of about 0.6°C. It is highest in the evening and lowest in the early morning.

Body temperature is regulated by a balance between heat production and heat loss.

Heat Production

Heat production occurs due to

- metabolic activities of the body,
- food intake (specific dynamic action), and
- muscular activity.

Heat Loss

Heat loss occurs due to

- radiation and conduction (70%),
- vaporization of sweat (27%),
- respiration (2%), and
- urination and defecation (1%).

Heat is lost mainly by radiation, conduction, and evaporation.

Radiation

This loss is in the form of infrared heat rays. The wavelength of these rays is around 5–20 microns. Human body radiates heat in all directions.

Conduction

Heat is transferred from the body to air by conduction. Once the temperature of air adjacent to skin rises to the skin temperature, further loss of heat stops. Conduction is assisted by convection caused by air currents.

When the body is exposed to wind the air present adjacent to the skin is replaced by new air which is cooler. Continuous replacement of air by convection therefore reduces the skin temperature rapidly.

Evaporation

Evaporation of water from the body surface causes heat loss. Even when a person is not sweating, skin and lungs loose water at a rate of 500–600 mL/day. When the temperature of the surroundings becomes greater than the skin temperature, evaporation is the major means of heat loss. Reduction of skin temperature occurs by the mechanism of sweating.

Neural Regulation

Body temperature is regulated by nervous feedback mechanisms. The temperature-regulating centers are present in the hypothalamus.

Heat Loss Center

It is present in the anterior hypothalamus. Stimulation of this center produces cutaneous vasodilation and sweating.

Heat Gain Center

This is present in the posterior hypothalamus. Stimulation of this center causes shivering and rise in the body temperature.

Sweating It is a mechanism that controls the body temperature. Sweat is produced by sweat glands.

Water present in the sweat comes out of the skin through the sweat pore and water vaporizes from the surface of skin. This vaporization of water causes heat loss from the body.

Sweat secretion can increase to very high values of around 1600 mL/h on a hot day and during exercise.

Temperature-Reducing Mechanisms

Heat is lost by

- cutaneous vasodilatation,
- sweating, and
- increased respiration.

Heat production decreases in

- anorexia and
- apathy and reduced activity.

Temperature-Increasing Mechanisms

Heat production increases by

- shivering,
- hunger,
- increased voluntary activity, and

- increased secretion of epinephrine and norepinephrine.

Heat loss is prevented by

- cutaneous vasoconstriction,
- curling up, and
- horripilation (piloerection).

Applied Physiology

Set Point for Temperature Control

The core temperature is maintained exactly at the level of 37.1°C. At temperatures above this level, the rate of heat loss becomes greater than the rate of heat production.

At temperatures below this level, the rate of heat production becomes greater than the rate of heat loss.

Fever

Fever is an increase in the body temperature above normal range. It is commonly caused by bacterial and viral infections.

Cause

The protein breakdown products and toxins released by bacteria cause set point of temperature to rise, resulting in fever. Substances causing this effect are termed **pyrogens**. These pyrogens produce interleukin-1 which on reaching the hypothalamus increases the set point of the temperature.

Hypothermia

Exposure of a person to extreme cold causes drop in the body temperature. The temperature-regulating ability of a person becomes impaired if the body temperature falls below 94°F and the hypothalamus totally fails below 85°F.

Frostbite

This is found in the extremities of persons exposed to extreme cold temperature. The earlobes and digits of hands and feet are affected. Frostbite results in tissue damage and gangrene.

Artificial Hypothermia

The temperature of the person is artificially maintained below 90°F during procedures like heart surgery. Artificial cooling is done to stop the heart beating for 30 min to 1 h without causing damage to the cells.

Central Nervous System

The living beings respond to changes in the external environment. The constantly changing surrounding poses a great threat to homeostasis. Internally, there will be changes to suit the alteration in the exterior. The various systems of the body are controlled by the **nervous** and **endocrine** systems. The regulatory mechanisms are together called **neuroendocrine control**.

The central nervous system (CNS) consists of the brain and spinal cord. It is compared to a supercomputer. However, computer is not a suitable match for the amazing abilities of the human brain. During evolution, there has been an increase in the number of neurons in the brain performing complex integrative functions.

Development of Brain

The earliest phase of brain development starts in a 3-week-old embryo. The ectoderm along the dorsal midline axis of embryo forms the **neural plate**. This plate invaginates to form neural groove with **neural folds** on either side. The superior edge of the neural folds fuses to form the **neural tube**.

The neural tube formed in the fourth week of pregnancy differentiates into the CNS. The anterior part of the neural tube forms the brain and the posterior portion forms the spinal cord.

The nervous system is divided into the following systems:

1. The **central nervous system**, consisting of
    (a)   brain and
    (b)   spinal cord.

2. The **peripheral nervous system**, consisting of
    (a)   12 pairs of cranial nerves and
    (b)   31 pairs of spinal nerves.

3. The **autonomic nervous system** consisting of
    (a)   sympathetic division and
    (b)   parasympathetic division.

The central nervous system is enclosed by

* dura mater,

* arachnoid mater, and

* pia mater.

Parts of Brain

1. Prosencephalon or forebrain
2. Mesencephalon or midbrain
3. Rhombencephalon or hindbrain

The forebrain is divided into **telencephalon** and **diencephalon**. Telencephalon includes cerebral hemispheres, basal ganglia, hippocampus, and amygdala. Diencephalon comprises thalamus, hypothalamus, metathalamus, and subthalamus. The hindbrain is made up of cerebellum, pons, and medulla oblongata.

Cerebral Hemispheres

The cerebral hemispheres occupy a major part of the cranial cavity (Fig. 8.1). They are divided into right and left hemispheres. The two cerebral hemispheres are connected by a bundle of nerve fibers called the **corpus callosum**. The cerebral hemispheres have an outer shell of gray matter, termed the **cerebral cortex**. The cerebral cortex has three kinds of functional areas: motor areas, sensory areas, and association areas. The cells of the cerebral cortex are arranged in six layers. The cortical neurons are made up of pyramidal and nonpyramidal types of cells. The pyramidal cells give major output from the cortex.

The myelinated nerve fibers of tracts form the white matter.

The basal nuclei are the gray matter present deep within the white matter. The subcortical nuclei are called the **basal ganglia**, or basal nuclei.

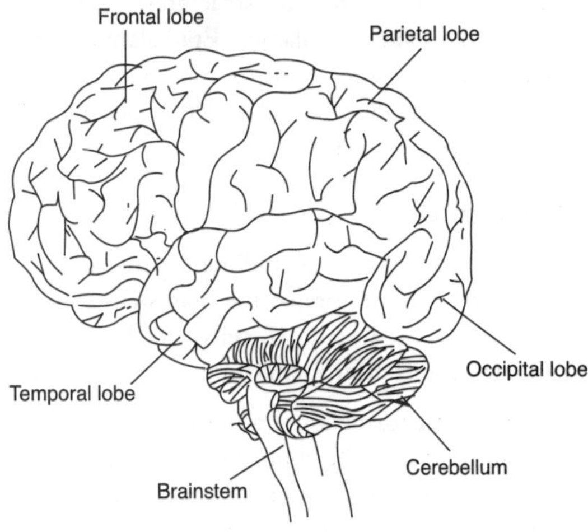

Fig. 8.1   Lateral view of the brain.

Cerebral Ventricles

The ventricles arise from the expansion of lumen of the embryonic neural tube. The brain contains four interconnected cavities lined by ependymal cells (type of neuroglia) called **cerebral ventricles** (Fig. 8.2). They are paired lateral ventricles, third and fourth ventricles. They are filled with circulating cerebrospinal fluid.

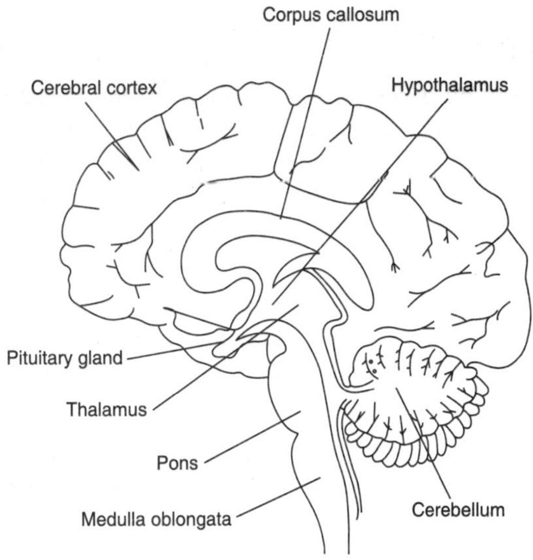

Fig. 8.2   Sagittal section of the brain.

Diencephalon

The diencephalon forms the central core of the forebrain, surrounded by the cerebral hemispheres. It contains three paired structures: thalamus, hypothalamus, and epithalamus. Epithalamus is the most dorsal part of diencephalon and forms the roof of third ventricle. Pineal gland is seen as an extension from its posterior border.

Brainstem

The brainstem consists of midbrain, pons, and medulla oblongata. The core of the brainstem consists of loosely arranged neuronal cells with bundles of axons termed **reticular formation**.

The reticular formation is absolutely essential for life. It is involved in the control of motor functions and cardiovascular and respiratory activities. It regulates the sleep and wakefulness cycle.

Cerebellum

The cerebellum is located posterior and inferior to the cerebrum. It has two cerebellar hemispheres. It is an important center for coordinating movements, controlling posture and equilibrium. It receives information from the muscles, joints, eyes, ears, viscera, and parts of brain involved in the control of movements. The cerebellum not only performs motor functions, but is also involved in the process of learning.

Spinal Cord

The spinal cord is an extension of the medulla oblongata and is located in the bony vertebral column. It has an outer white matter and an inner gray matter. The central canal which is a continuation of the cerebral ventricles passes through the spinal cord.

The cell bodies of the neurons group together in the CNS to form the **gray matter** and the fibers form the **white matter**. In the brain, the gray matter is outside and the white matter is inside.

The cell bodies of the neurons collect together to constitute the **nuclei** and the fibers join to form the **tract**.

The inputs reach the brain through sensory receptors and sensory division of the nervous system. The brain acts as an information-gathering, data-analyzing, and decision-making device. The useful information is stored as memory. The desired response is produced with the help of motor division of the nervous system. It results in the contraction of the muscle or secretion from the gland.

The spinal cord gives out segmental nerves. There are 31 spinal segments with 31 pairs of nerves, which are as follows:

- Cervical   8
- Thoracic   12
- Lumbar   5
- Sacral   5
- Coccygeal   1

A typical spinal nerve is a mixed nerve. It has a sensory division located in the dorsal root. The cell body of the afferent nerve is in the dorsal root ganglion. The ventral division is motor and carries somatic efferent to the muscles. The anterior root of the spinal nerve from T_1 to L_2 segments carries sympathetic efferents. The parasympathetic fibers are carried by the spinal nerves from the S_2 to S_4 segments.

In addition to the neurons, the nervous system has the supporting cells called the **neuroglia**.

The neuron is the structural and functional unit of the nervous system. There are about 100 billion neurons in the CNS.

Synapse

The synapse is a junction between two neurons. The information from the nerve terminal of one neuron is relayed to the other neuron.

The neuron which ends at the synapse is termed the **presynaptic neuron**. The neuron which receives the information is termed the **postsynaptic neuron**.

The electrical activity of the presynaptic neuron influences the activity in the postsynaptic neuron.

There are about 10^{14} synapses in the CNS.

The anatomical types of synapses are

- axoaxonic,
- axodendritic,

- axosomatic, and
- dendrodendritic.

The functional types of synapses are

- electrical and
- chemical.

The electrical synapses have open fluid channels that conduct electricity between the adjacent cells. They have gap junctions and the ions pass through low-resistance bridges. The synaptic cleft is absent.

In the chemical synapse, there is functional continuity but no structural continuity.

Structure (Fig. 8.3)

A typical chemical synapse has the following parts:

1. **presynaptic terminal** with neurotransmitter in the vesicles;
2. **synaptic cleft** or synaptic gutter;
3. **postsynaptic terminal** with receptors for neurotransmitter.

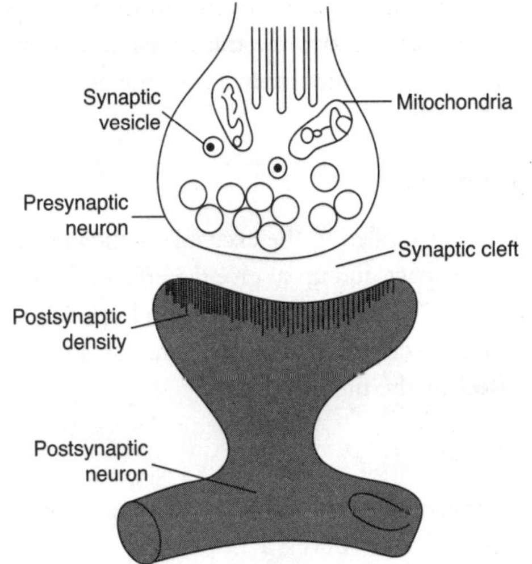

Fig. 8.3   Structure of synapse.

Transmission of Impulse across a Synapse

The impulse (action potential) comes to the nerve terminal. This increases the permeability of the membrane to the calcium ions.

- The calcium ions enter the nerve terminal from the extracellular compartment.

- The calcium ions bind to the protein anchoring the vesicles.
- The release of vesicles from the anchoring protein causes its movement to the presynaptic membrane.
- The vesicles rupture, releasing neurotransmitter into the synaptic cleft.
- The neurotransmitter crosses the synaptic cleft and binds to the receptor on the postsynaptic membrane.
- The neurotransmitter binding to the receptor increases the permeability of the membrane to the sodium ions.
- The entry of sodium ions forms the action potential in the postsynaptic terminal.
- After the impulse transmission is completed, the neurotransmitter is broken down.
- The broken-down products are taken up by the nerve terminal for the resynthesis of the neurotransmitter.

Excitatory Postsynaptic Potential

A single stimulus applied to a sensory nerve results in partial depolarization in the postsynaptic neuron. During this process, the excitability of the neuron is increased to a second stimulus.

Ionic Basis   The excitatory neurotransmitter at the synapse binds to the receptors on the postsynaptic membrane. This triggers opening of the sodium channels. The sodium moves along its concentration gradient. It produces partial depolarization resulting in excitatory postsynaptic potential (EPSP).

The summation of EPSP results in the formation of propagated action potential.

Inhibitory Postsynaptic Potential

A stimulus applied to a sensory nerve can result in hyperpolarization in the postsynaptic neuron. During this potential, the excitability of the neuron to a second stimulus is decreased.

Ionic Basis   The stimulation of the inhibitory synaptic knob at the synapse releases neurotransmitter. This triggers opening of the chloride channels on the postsynaptic membrane. The chloride moves along the concentration gradient. This results in hyperpolarization producing inhibitory postsynaptic potential (IPSP).

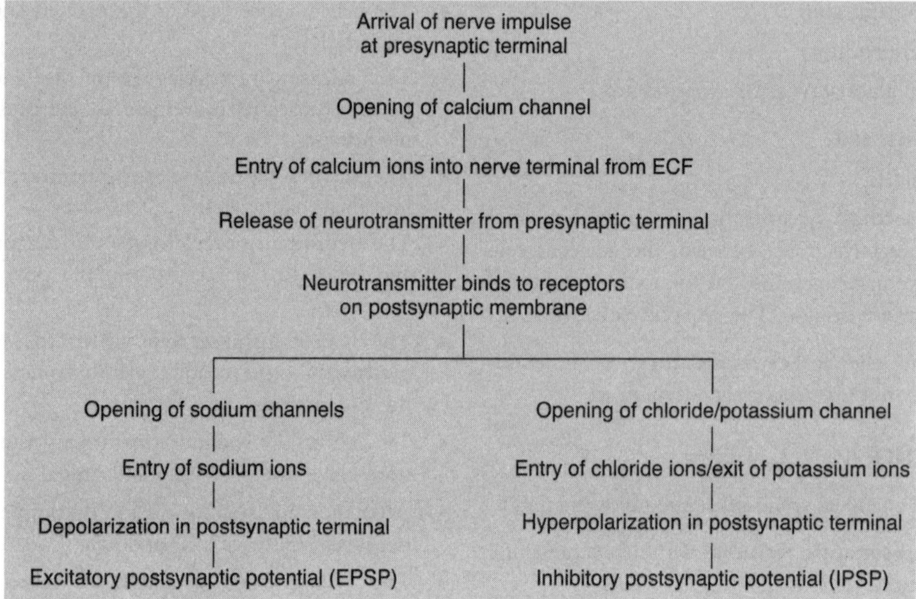

Properties

Synaptic Delay

There is a delay between the application of stimulus in the presynaptic terminal and the onset of response in the postsynaptic terminal. This time interval is called the **synaptic delay**. The normal synaptic delay is about 0.5 ms. This delay is due to the time needed for changes at the synapse during the impulse transmission. It is possible to estimate the number of synapses in a pathway by measuring the synaptic delay.

Convergence and Divergence

If the number of presynaptic terminals ends on a single postsynaptic terminal, it is termed **convergence**. If an axon of the presynaptic neuron makes connection with multiple postsynaptic terminals, it is called **divergence**. Convergence and divergence are structural requirements for the properties like facilitation, occlusion, and reverberation.

One-Way Conduction

The impulse transmission occurs from pre- to postsynaptic terminal. This is due to the specific structure of the pre- and postsynaptic terminals. It must be noted that the transmission of impulse cannot occur in the opposite direction.

Fatigue

The exhaustion or partial depletion of neurotransmitter reduces or stops the transmission of impulse at the synapse temporarily. This phenomenon is called **fatigue**.

Summation

Two stimuli applied to the excitable tissue in relation to time or space add up to give the effect of summation. They are termed **temporal** and **spatial** summation, respectively. The second stimulus potentiates the effect of the first stimulus.

Occlusion

The stimulation of two neurons sharing a common neuronal pool produces a response. The response obtained is less than the sum of responses produced by an individual neuron when they are stimulated separately. This effect is called **occlusion**. It is due to the overlap of neurons.

Habituation and Sensitization

When noninjurious stimuli are repeated, the intensity of response decreases or may even stop. This is **habituation**. When the injurious stimuli are given along with the noninjurious stimulus, it causes increase in the response. This is called **sensitization**. Habituation is due to reduced calcium ions at the presynaptic terminal. Increased entry of the calcium ions at the presynaptic terminal produces sensitization.

Post-Tetanic Potentiation

It is an example of plasticity of the neuron. There is enhanced postsynaptic potential in response to stimulation. It is produced due to the presynaptic accumulation of the calcium ions in response to the tetanizing stimulation. The change lasts for about 60 s.

Synaptic Development

The axons during the formation of synapse exhibit growth cones at their tips, which pass through the tissues. The specialized proteins termed semaphorins influence the migrations of these cones. During the process of development, a large number of synapses are formed. The nonfunctional synapses disappear subsequently.

Synaptic Inhibition

Presynaptic Inhibition (Fig. 8.4)

In this type of inhibition, the inhibitory neuron ends on the presynaptic terminal. The stimulation of presynaptic and inhibitory neurons simultaneously results in a decreased response at the postsynaptic terminal. This is accomplished by reducing the amplitude of the action potential. The mechanisms for presynaptic inhibitions are as follows:

- The hyperpolarization is produced due to the increased efflux of potassium or influx of chloride at the presynaptic terminal. The hyperpolarization at the presynaptic terminal reduces the calcium influx. This in turn reduces the neurotransmitter release.

- The direct reduction in the release of the neurotransmitter is independent of the ionic mechanism.

The first neurotransmitter which has been demonstrated to produce presynaptic inhibition is **gamma-aminobutyric acid** (GABA).

Postsynaptic Inhibition (Fig. 8.4)

The voluntary or reflex contraction of a muscle is accompanied by simultaneous relaxation of the antagonistic group of muscles. This is known as **reciprocal inhibition**. This occurs as a result of the reciprocal innervation. The afferent impulses from the agonist muscle cause **postsynaptic inhibition** of the motor neuron to the antagonistic muscle. The pathway mediating this effect is bisynaptic.

For example, the contraction of biceps muscle causes relaxation of the triceps muscle, resulting in smooth flexion at the elbow joint.

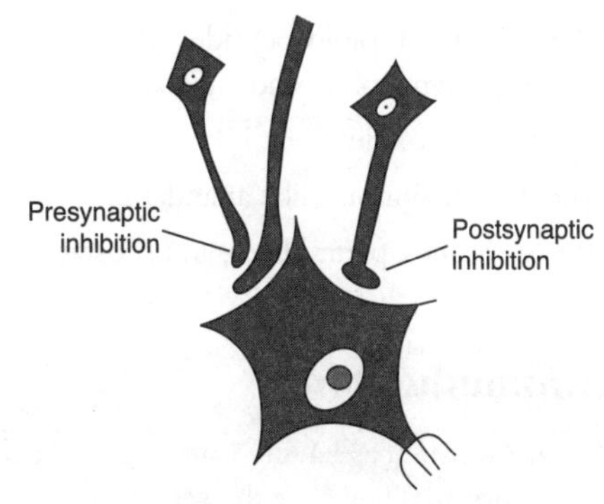

Fig. 8.4   Pre- and postsynaptic inhibitions.

Reciprocal Innervation   The sensory nerve arising from a group of muscles (biceps) makes excitatory connection with the motor neuron for the same muscle. The sensory nerve makes connection with the inhibitory neuron, which ends on the motor nerve to the antagonistic muscle (triceps).

Renshaw Cell Inhibition (Negative Feedback Inhibition)   The axons of the motor neurons give off collaterals as they emerge through the anterior horn of the spinal cord. These collaterals make excitatory synaptic connection with a special group of neurons called the **Renshaw cells**, present in the anterior horn. The Renshaw cells send short axons, making inhibitory synaptic connection with the same motor neuron. These cells are activated when the motor neurons are excited. They have a feedback effect on the same motor neuron, inhibiting their discharge. This is known as **Renshaw cell inhibition**.

Neurotransmitters

Neurotransmitters are the substances that help in the transmission of impulses across the synaptic cleft in a chemical synapse. The proteins needed for the synthesis of neurotransmitter are formed in the cell body and transported to the nerve terminal by the **axoplasmic flow**.

The neurotransmitters are as follows:

- **Acetylcholine**
- **Amines:** Epinephrine, norepinephrine, serotonin, dopamine, and histamine
- **Excitatory amino acids:** Aspartate and glutamate
- **Inhibitory amino acids:** Glycine and GABA
- **Polypeptides:** Opioid peptides like enkephalin, endorphin, dynorphin, and substance P
- **Gases:** Nitric oxide
- **Lipids:** Cannabinoids like anandamide
- **Others:** Purines, pyrimidines, and prostaglandins

Neuromodulators

These are substances having nonsynaptic action on the neurons. They alter the sensitivity of the neuron to synaptic stimulation or inhibition.

Neurotrophins

These are proteins required for the growth, development, and survival of the neurons. They are produced by the muscles, astrocytes, and structures innervated by the neurons.

Receptors

They are modified proteins which act as the binding site for hormones and neurotransmitters. The receptors can be **postsynaptic** or **presynaptic**.

The postsynaptic receptors regulate the response in the postsynaptic neuron in response to the presynaptic stimulation.

The presynaptic receptors or **autoreceptors** inhibit further secretion of the neurotransmitter providing a feedback control.

Reflex Action

The reflex action is an involuntary response to a sensory stimulus, e.g., withdrawal of the hand on touching a hot object.

The reflex action is produced with the help of a reflex arc (Fig. 8.5).

The **reflex arc** consists of

- **receptor**—a modified nerve terminal with a group of special cells capable of receiving different types of stimuli,
- sensory or **afferent nerve**,
- synapse or the **center** present in the spinal cord,
- motor or **efferent nerve**, and
- **effector organ**—muscle or a gland.

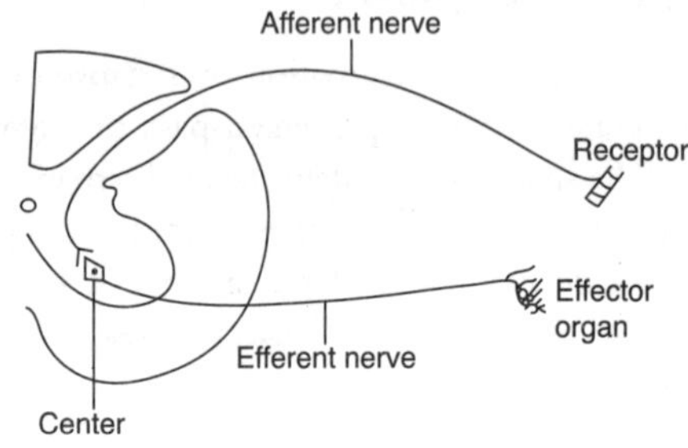

Fig. 8.5 Reflex arc.

Bell–Magendie law

This law states that the dorsal or posterior root entering the spinal cord is sensory, and ventral or anterior root emerging from the spinal cord is motor.

Classification of Reflexes

1. Based on the number of synapses
   - **Monosynaptic reflex:** There is a single synapse in the reflex arc, e.g., stretch reflex.
   - **Polysynaptic reflex:** There is more than one synapse in the reflex arc, e.g., withdrawal reflex.
2. Based on the development
   - **Unconditioned reflex:** It is an inborn reflex or the reflex present since birth; e.g., taste of the food produces salivation.
   - **Conditioned reflex:** It is an acquired reflex or a reflex produced by learning. The conditioned reflex can be produced over an unconditioned response; e.g., thought of favorite food produces salivation.

3. Clinical classification
   - **Superficial reflex:** Example include conjunctival, corneal, and plantar reflexes.
   - **Deep reflex:** Tendon reflexes like biceps jerk and triceps jerk.
   - **Visceral reflex:** Examples include micturition and defecation reflex.

Properties of Reflexes

- **Delay:** The time interval between the application of stimulus and the onset of response is known as delay. This delay is due to the passage of impulse through components of the reflex arc.

- **One-way conduction:** The conduction of impulse occurs in one direction. The conduction is toward the center (centripetal) in the afferent limb and it is away from the center (centrifugal) in the efferent limb.

- **Summation:** A reflex action is capable of being summated. When the summation is related to time it is known as *temporal summation.* In this condition, successive stimuli are given one after the other with a short time interval between them at the same point. The effect of second stimulus potentiates the action of first stimulus to produce a better response.

  If the summation is related to space, it is called *spatial summation.* Two stimuli are given simultaneously close to each other. The local response produced by each of the stimulus adds up to give a summated response. (Summation means to add up.)

- **Occlusion:** The simultaneous stimulation of two nerves sharing a common neuronal pool produces a response. The response obtained would be less than the sum of two individual responses. This occurs as a result of the overlap of two neurons.

- **Facilitation:** The repeated elicitation of the reflex increases the response. This is termed facilitation.

- **Subliminal fringe (subminimal fringe):** The stimulation of a reflex pathway increases the excitability of the associated pathways. As the associated pathway is partially stimulated, it can be activated easily. This increased excitability of the associated pathway is the subliminal fringe.

- **Irradiation:** When the strength of stimulus is gradually increased, the central excitatory state spreads. (Impulses in the spinal cord spread to the segments above and below the level of activation.) Hence, a greater number of nerve fibers and additional groups of muscles take part in reflex response. This is called irradiation.

- **Habituation and sensitization:** When a noninjurious stimulus is applied repeatedly, the intensity of response decreases or may even stop. This is known as *habituation.* On the other hand, injurious stimulus applied repeatedly causes intensification of the response. This is known as *sensitization.*

Types of Reflexes

Conditioned Reflex

The conditioned reflex is a learned or acquired reflex setup by experience. Following are the characteristic features of conditioned reflex:

- Conditioned reflex always develops on the basis of unconditioned reflex.
- Speed of development is fairly quick.
- Unconditioned stimulus must accompany or precede the conditioned stimulus.
- It can be established or abolished.
- It is not transmitted by heredity.

Example   The normal response for presentation of food to an animal is salivation. The conditioned stimulus (ringing the bell) is given along with or immediately before the unconditioned stimulus (presentation of food). When the same procedure is repeated several times, mere ringing the bell (conditioned stimulus) results in salivation. This acquired behavior is a **conditioned reflex.**

Stretch Reflex (Fig. 8.6)

Stretch reflex is an example of a monosynaptic reflex. The stretch of skeletal muscle with intact nerve supply responds by reflex contraction. In this reflex, stimulus is stretch of the muscle. The receptor is muscle spindle. Type Ia and II fibers carry afferent information to the spinal cord. The sensory signals are converted into the motor response at the spinal cord and the neurotransmitter is glutamate. The motor neurons from the center in the spinal cord end on the contractile element (extrafusal fibers) of the same muscle.

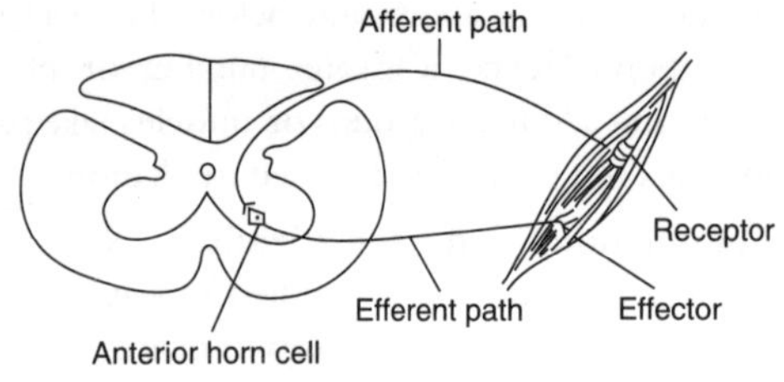

Fig. 8.6   Pathway for stretch reflex.

Inverse Stretch Reflex

The sudden stretch of the muscle results in its reflex contraction. However, when the tension becomes great enough, the contraction suddenly stops and the muscle relaxes. This relaxation in response to a strong stretch is known as **inverse stretch reflex** or **autogenic inhibition**.

Receptor for this reflex is Golgi tendon organ.

Golgi tendon organ regulates the force of muscle contraction.

Withdrawal Reflex

The withdrawal reflex is an example of the polysynaptic reflex. The efferent limb has a varying number of synapses. The polysynaptic path causes prolonged bombardment of the motor neurons supplying the muscle. Hence, a single stimulus produces a prolonged motor response and a sustained contraction of the muscle. There is reflex contraction of the flexor group of muscles and inhibition of the extensor muscles. Thus, the limb is withdrawn from the painful stimulus.

Crossed Extensor Reflex

When a strong painful stimulus is given to the animal, there is flexion and withdrawal of the same limb with extension of the opposite limb. This response is due to **irradiation of the impulses** and **recruitment of the motor units**.

Axon Reflex (Fig. 8.7)

In this reflex, a branch of the sensory nerve returns back to the same area of skin. It innervates the cutaneous arteriole without reaching the spinal cord. Whenever the skin is stroked, it results in arteriolar dilation manifesting as redness at the site of injury (flare). This is known as axon reflex. It is an **asynaptic reflex**.

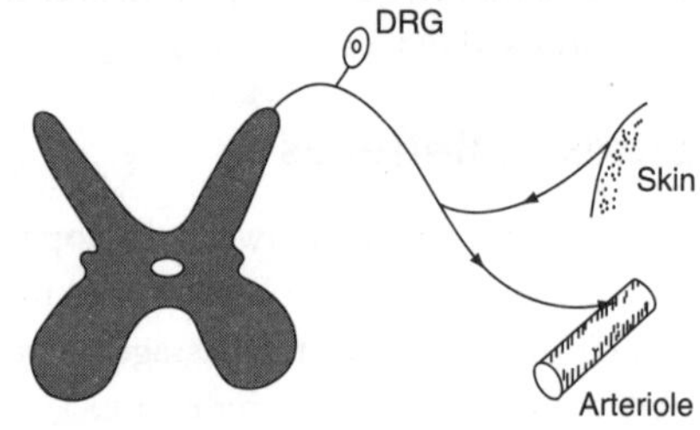

Fig. 8.7   Axon reflex.

Plantar Reflex

When the lateral aspect of the sole of the foot is scratched, it results in plantarflexion and adduction of all the toes. This is the normal flexor response. However, it can be extensor in the upper motor neuron lesion. Then it is termed **positive Babinski's sign**.

In this condition, scratching the lateral aspect of the sole of the foot results in fanning of all the toes, dorsiflexion of great toe, dorsiflexion at the ankle joint, and flexion at knee and hip joints.

An examination of the plantarreflex helps to recognize the upper motor neuron lesion.

In a normal individual, the Babinski's sign can be positive in the following:

- a child below the age of 18 months due to incomplete myelination;
- during deep sleep due to temporary removal of inhibition from higher centers.

Receptors (Fig. 8.8)

The receptors are modified nerve terminals capable of converting different forms of energy into electrical energy.

Classification

1. **Exteroceptors:** These receptors are capable of recognizing changes in the external environment, e.g., receptors for touch, pain, and temperature.

2. **Interoceptors:** These receptors respond to alterations in the internal environment, e.g., baroreceptors and chemoreceptors.

3. **Telereceptors:** These receptors perceive changes in the surroundings from a distance. e.g., receptors for vision and audition.

4. **Proprioceptors:** These receptors provide information about the orientation of different parts of the body in space, e.g., muscle spindle and Golgi tendon organ.

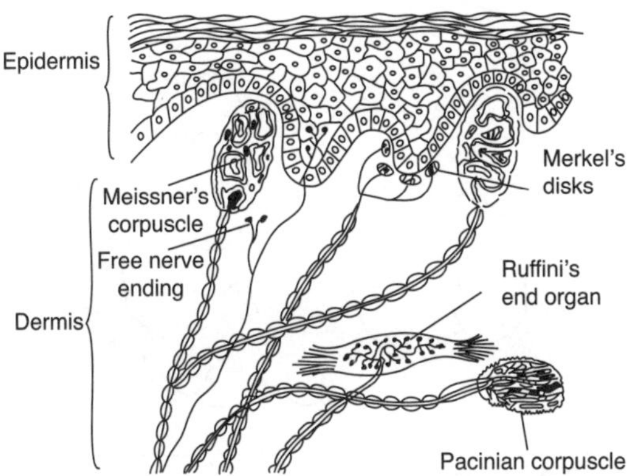

Fig. 8.8   Cutaneous receptors.

Types

General Sensations

1. **Touch and pressure:**
   - *Rapidly adapting:* Meissner's corpuscles and Pacinian corpuscles
   - *Slowly adapting:* Merkel's disk

2. **Pain:** Free nerve endings

3. **Temperature:** Ruffini's end organ

4. **Joint sense:**
   - *Muscle length:* Muscle spindle
   - *Muscle tension:* Golgi tendon organ

Special Sensations

1. **Vision:** Rods and cones
2. **Audition:** Hair cells of the organ of Corti
3. **Taste:** Taste receptor cells of taste buds
4. **Smell:** Olfactory neurons
5. **Linear and rotational acceleration:** Hair cells of vestibular apparatus

Receptor Potential

A low-intensity stimulus to a receptor produces a nonpropagated, depolarizing potential resembling the EPSP. This is called the **generator potential** or the **receptor potential**.

It is produced due to the distortion of receptor and activation of the unmyelinated part of the sensory nerve.

On reaching the firing level, it produces a propagated action potential.

Properties

1. **Specificity:** The sensory receptors respond to a specific type of energy for its stimulation. For example, the chemoreceptors respond to changes in the chemical nature of the blood.

2. **Adaptation:** The stimulation of a receptor with a nonpainful, low-intensity stimuli results in a gradual decline in the response. The receptor may finally stop responding. This is termed **adaptation** or **desensitization**.

   Rapidly adapting receptors are phasic receptors, e.g., touch receptors.

   Slowly adapting receptors are tonic receptors, e.g., muscle spindle and pain receptors.

3. **Law of specific nerve energies:** The stimulation of the receptor or the sensory pathway anywhere along its course produces the same sensation as normally perceived by the stimulation of the receptor.

4. **Law of projection:** The stimulation of the sensory pathway from the receptor to its termination in the cortex gives the sensation as if it is arising from the location of the receptor. If the limb is amputated, stimulation of sensory pathway gives the impression as if the sensation is coming from receptor of the nonexistent limb (**phantom limb**).

5. **Discrimination of intensity:** The intensity of stimulation is appreciated by the brain through
   - changes in the number of action potential produced by the active receptors;
   - number of receptors activated by the stimuli.

The magnitude of the sensation felt depends on the intensity of the stimulus.

Weber–Fechner law

It states that the sensation felt is proportional to the log of the stimulus intensity:

$$R \propto \log S.$$

However, more accurate relationship appears to be the power function:

$$R = KS^A,$$

where R is the sensation felt, S is the intensity of stimulus, and K and A are constants.

6. **Recruitment of sensory units:** A stimulus activates the receptors which are in close contact with it. If the intensity of stimulation is increased, the effect spreads to the surrounding areas activating the receptors in that region. This is termed recruitment of sensory unit. The weaker stimulus activates less number of receptors and those with lower threshold. However, a stronger stimulus activates greater number of receptors including those with higher threshold for stimulation.

Sensory System

The sensory system is responsible for carrying different sensations from all over the body to the CNS. Different types of sensations are perceived by the sensory receptors.

The receptors convert these sensations to electrical signals. The impulses generated at the receptors are transmitted through the sensory tract present in the spinal cord. The sensory tracts finally terminate in somatosensory cortex (Brodmann area 3, 1, 2). The somatosensory area is located in the postcentral gyrus. Understanding the meaning of sensation is termed **perception**. Perception is a result of the neural processing of the sensory information.

Sensory Homunculus (Fig. 8.9)

The body is represented upside down in the sensory cortex. The peripheral parts of the body like hand and finger that perform finer movements have a larger area of representation. However, the trunk

has a smaller area of representation when compared to its size.

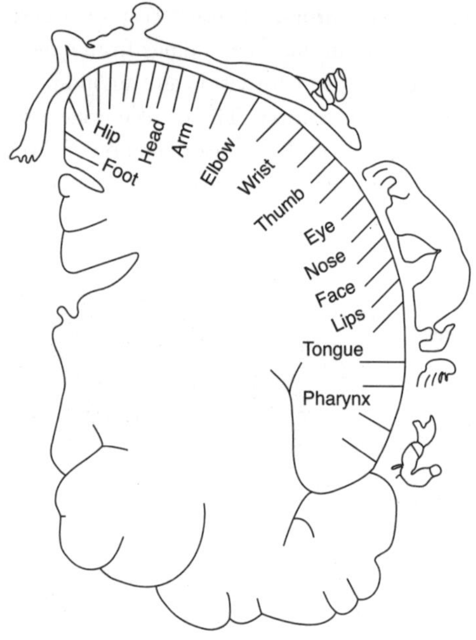

Fig. 8.9   Sensory homunculus.

Sensory Tracts

The neural pathway in the sensory system consists of three or more neurons connected end to end by synapses. The bundle of parallel nerve fibers form the **tract**.

The sensory tracts are present in the spinal cord. These tracts are formed by the sensory fibers from the receptors and reach the higher centers in the CNS. They are also called the **ascending tracts** as they go up to the brain.

The sensory inputs reach the thalamus and cerebral cortex. These are called relay stations. The crude form of sensations and pain are appreciated at the thalamus. This type of sensation is called the **protopathic sensation**.

The finer details of the sensations are perceived by the cerebral cortex. This sensation is termed **epicritic sensation**.

Sensory Unit

A single afferent neuron with all its receptors forms the **sensory unit**. Generally, a single neuron has multiple receptors. Sometimes each neuron can have a single receptor.

Spinal Cord

A section of the spinal cord shows outer white matter and inner gray matter (Fig. 8.10). The central canal passes through the center of the spinal cord.

The white matter has anterior, lateral, and posterior compartments called the **funiculus**.

The **anterior funiculus** contains the anterior spinothalamic tract.

The **lateral funiculus** contains the lateral spinothalamic tract.

The **posterior funiculus** contains the fasciculus gracilis and fasciculus cuneatus.

The gray matter has anterior, lateral, and posterior horns.

The **anterior horn** contains

- alpha motor neurons supplying the skeletal muscles;
- gamma motor neurons supplying proprioceptors in the muscle (muscle spindles);
- interneurons modifying the activity of alpha motor neurons.

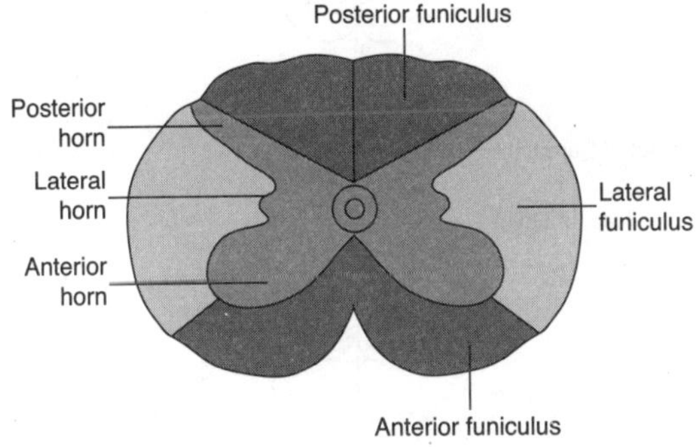

Fig. 8.10   Cross-section of spinal cord.

The **lateral horn** contains preganglionic fibers of the autonomic nervous system. The lateral horns are prominent in the thoracic, lumbar, and sacral segments of the spinal cord.

The **posterior horn** contains the cell bodies of the neurons forming the afferent tract.

The posterior column has several layers of cells. The layers from outer to the innermost are

- substantia gelatinosa of Rolando,
- nucleus of proprius,
- Clarke's column, and
- visceral afferent nucleus.

Rexed Lamina (Fig. 8.11)

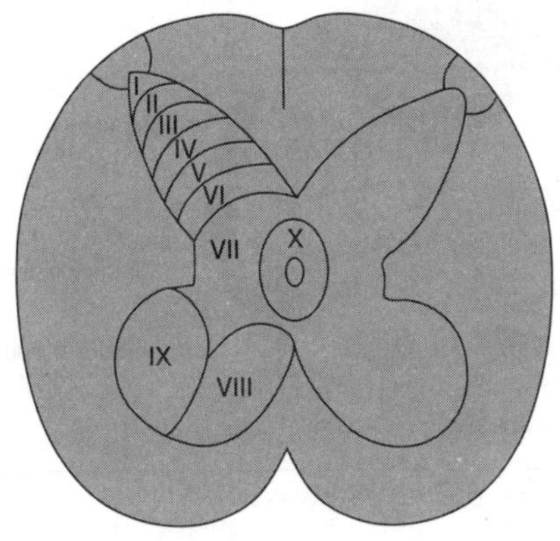

Fig. 8.11   Rexed lamina.

Rexed has identified 10 layers in the spinal cord based on the histological features of the spinal cord. They are numbered from I to X and are called Rexed lamina. The posterior horn of the spinal cord has laminae from I to VI; lamina VII is present in between the anterior and posterior horns. The VIII and IX laminae are present in the anterior horn. Lamina X is present around the central canal.

Spinal Nerve

The spinal cord gives out the spinal nerve in each of its segments. The spinal nerves have anterior and posterior roots. The posterior or dorsal roots contain the sensory fibers entering the CNS. The cell bodies of these sensory neurons are located in the dorsal root ganglion (DRG). The fibers from the ganglion on entering the spinal cord divide into the medial and lateral divisions. The medial division has thicker fibers and carries sensations of fine touch, proprioception, and vibration. The lateral division has thinner fibers carrying pain and temperature sensations.

The anterior root of the spinal nerve has motor fibers. It carries alpha and gamma motor neurons.

Ascending Tracts (Fig. 8.12)

The ascending tracts are sensory tracts. They carry sensation from different receptors all over the body to the CNS.

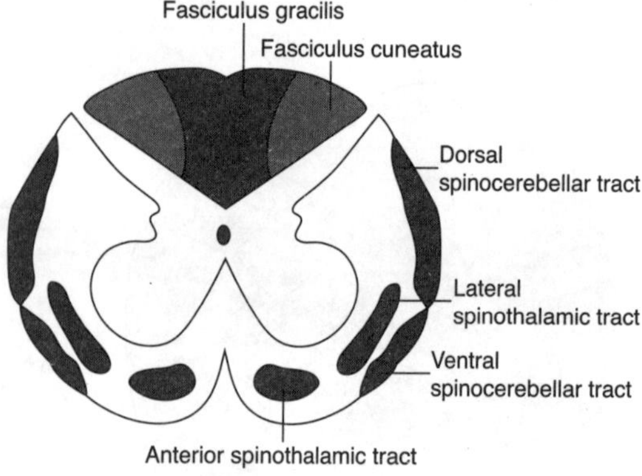

Fig. 8.12   Ascending pathways.

The important sensory tracts are

1. **In the dorsal (posterior) column**
   - Tract of Goll (fasciculus gracilis)
   - Tract of Burdach (fasciculus cuneatus)
2. **In the lateral column**
   - Lateral spinothalamic tracts
   - Dorsal spinocerebellar tract
   - Ventral spinocerebellar tract
   - Spinotectal tract
   - Spino-olivary tract
   - Spinovestibular tract
   - Spinopontine tract
   - Spinoreticular tract
3. **In the ventral (anterior) column**
   - Anterior spinothalamic tract

Tract of Goll and Burdach (Fig. 8.13)

Sensations Carried

- Fine touch
- Proprioception
- Vibration
- Pressure

Pathway

- The first-order neurons arise from the respective receptors and enter the spinal cord through the posterior root.
- It ascends on the same side of the spinal cord to end (relay) in the nucleus gracilis and cuneatus present in the medulla.

   The fasciculus gracilis contains fibers from lower parts of the body (sacral and lower thoracic segments).

   The fasciculus cuneatus contains fibers from the upper part of the body (upper thoracic and cervical segments).

   In the spinal cord, fibers close to midline are from lower parts of the body and lateral fibers are from the upper part.

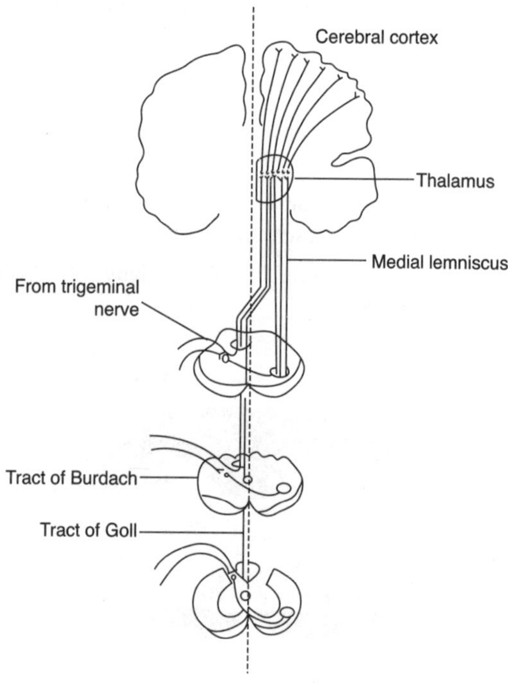

Fig. 8.13   Pathways for touch.

- The second-order neurons arising from these two nuclei cross to the opposite side.

   These crossing fibers are called the internal arcuate fibers.

   The fibers ascend close to the midline forming medial lemniscus (bundle).

- The second-order neurons end in the ventral posterolateral nucleus of the thalamus.
- The third-order neurons arising from the thalamic nucleus end in the sensory cortex (area 3, 1, 2) present in the postcentral gyrus of cerebral cortex.

The tracts of Goll and Burdach do not cross the midline or have a relay at the spinal level.

Anterolateral (Ventrolateral) Spinothalamic Tract (Fig. 8.14)

Sensations Carried

- Pain and temperature (lateral tract)
- Crude touch (ventral tract)

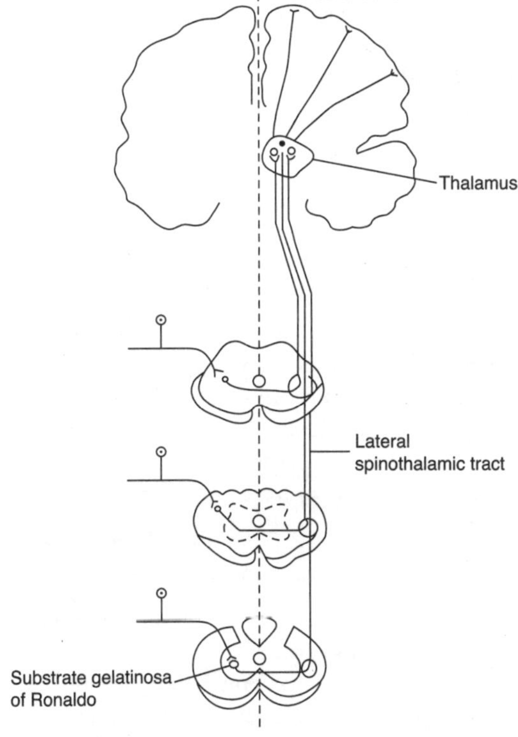

Fig. 8.14 Pathways for pain.

Pathway

- The fibers arising from the receptors enter the spinal cord through posterior or dorsal horn and end in the dorsal horn cells. This forms the first-order neurons.
- The second-order neurons arise from the dorsal horn cells and cross to the opposite side in front of the central canal. They occupy lateral or anterior part of the spinal cord. Axons of second-order neurons from sacral and lumbar segments are pushed laterally after crossing the midline. In the spinal cord, cervical fibers are medial and sacral fibers are lateral.
- The fibers ascend through the segments of the spinal cord, medulla, pons, and midbrain to end in the ventral posterolateral nucleus of the thalamus.
- As the tract ascends through the midbrain, it gives out branches to the reticular formation of the brainstem. Hence, the number of fibers is reduced.
- The third-order neurons from the thalamic nucleus reach the sensory cortex (area 3, 1, 2).

Dorsal Spinocerebellar Tract (Flechsig's Tract; Fig. 8.15)

Sensations Carried

- Unconscious kinesthetic impulses to cerebellum

Pathway

- The first-order neurons arise from the muscle spindle, joints, and skin, and enter the spinal cord through the DRG.
- It terminates in Clarke's column situated at the base of the dorsal horn.
- The second-order neurons arise from Clarke's column and ascend on the same side to the medulla.
- It turns posteriorly to enter the cerebellum through the inferior cerebellar peduncle.

Applied Physiology

The bilateral lesion of this tract results in the loss of crude touch, pain, and temperature sensation below the level of lesion.

The unilateral lesion causes loss of sensation on the opposite side below the level of the lesion.

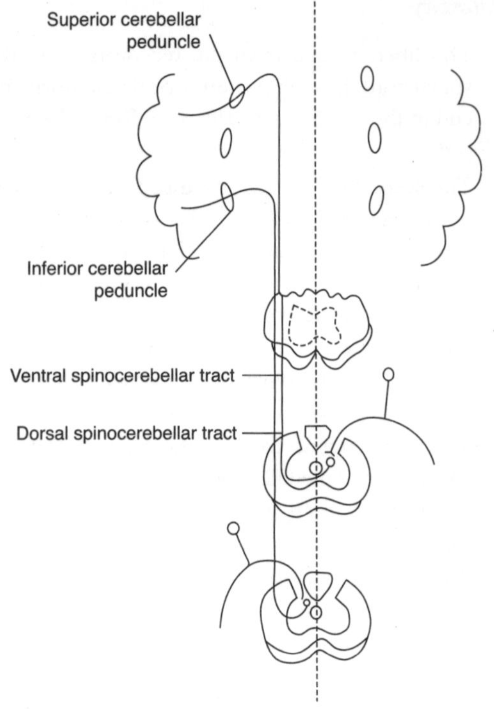

Fig. 8.15   Dorsal and ventral spinocerebellar tracts.

Ventral Spinocerebellar Tract (Gower's Tract; Fig. 8.15)

Sensations Carried

- Unconscious kinesthetic impulses to the cerebellum

Pathway

- The first-order neurons arise from the muscle spindle, joint, and skin.
- They enter the spinal cord through the DRG and relay in the dorsal horn. The second-order neuron arises from rexed lamina V–VII.
- The second-order neurons cross to the opposite side, and proceed through the medulla, pons, and midbrain.
- In the midbrain, the fibers turn posteriorly to enter the cerebellum through the superior cerebellar peduncle.

The spinocerebellar tracts carry impulses from the muscles, joints, and skin like the nonconscious proprioceptive and nonconscious cutaneous sensations.

Synthetic Sense

Synthetic sense is produced due to the combination of two types of basic sensations, which are as follows.

Stereognosis

Stereognosis is the ability to appreciate the size, shape, texture, and weight of the objects by past experience without actually looking at it. It is a complex perception which depends on the synthesis of several somatic sensations.

It is a combination of touch and pressure sensations. It is one of the most sophisticated sensations. An impaired stereognosis is an early sign of damage to the cerebral cortex and a lesion in the parietal lobe posterior to the postcentral gyrus.

Vibration Sense

Vibration sense is also a type of synthetic sensation produced by a combination of touch and pressure sensations.

Two-Point Discrimination

It is the ability to identify two independent points when they are stimulated simultaneously. It depends on touch sensation and the cortical component to identify two different stimuli. The distance of separation for two-point discrimination varies from place to place.

A separation of 2–4 mm can be appreciated at the tip of the tongue and the fingers.

On the back, the distance of separation has to be 5–7 cm to appreciate two distinct points. The distance of separation is least where the touch receptors are present in large numbers.

Pathophysiology of Pain

Pain is an unpleasant, subjective sensation produced due to nerve damage. It warns the organism about the possible damage to the tissue.

The crude sensation of pain can be appreciated at the thalamic level, whereas the finer aspects of it can be perceived at the cortical level.

The sense organs for pain are the free nerve endings present in all the tissues.

Pain is of two major types:

1. A sharp, localized **fast pain** carried by Aδ fibers. These nerve fibers have a diameter of 2–5 μ and conduct impulses at the rate of 15–30 m/s.
2. A poorly localized, dull-aching **slow pain** carried by C fibers. These are unmyelinated fibers having a diameter of 0.4–1.2 μ. They carry impulses at the rate of 0.5–2 m/s.

The sensation of pain is produced by substances like

- prostaglandins,
- bradykinin,
- serotonin,
- potassium ions,
- adenosine, and
- substance P.

Pain is produced due to the following changes in the body:

- inflammation,
- obstruction,
- ischemia,
- distension of hollow viscus,
- muscle spasm, and
- dilation of blood vessels.

Referred Pain (Fig. 8.16)

It is the pain from an internal organ felt in an area of skin away from the site of its production.

Theories of Referred Pain

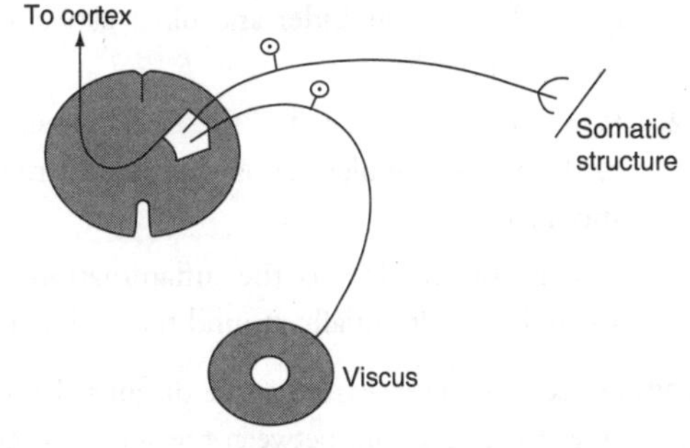

Fig. 8.16   Referred pain.

Dermatomal Rule   Pain is referred to the region of the skin which has developed from the same segment or dermatome from which the internal organ has developed. The organ and region of the skin get nerve supply from the same segment of the spinal cord.

Convergence and Facilitation   The sensory nerve fiber from the skin and the internal organ end on the same dorsal horn cell of the spinal cord. Any irritation in the internal organ causes stimulation of the sensory nerve. The pain gets projected to the region of skin, which has the common nerve supply. Irritation of the

Applied Physiology

Pain Inhibition

The somatic nerve from the skin and the visceral nerve from the hollow viscus end on the same dorsal horn of the spinal cord. Pain signals from the hollow viscus can be blocked by increasing the impulse traffic in the somatic nerve by irritating that region of skin, for example, application of counterirritant balms to get relief from headaches. Thus, the perception of pain is reduced but the basic cause for pain remains untreated.

Anesthetics

These are substances used to block the perception of pain. Anesthetics act on GABA and glycine receptors. The effect is produced by increasing the conductance of **chloride ions**.

Local anesthetics stabilize the activation gates of the sodium channel making it difficult to open the gate. This reduces the excitability of the membrane.

internal organ reduces the threshold for pain sensation. A minor stimulation over skin, which normally goes without notice, is experienced as pain due to lowered threshold. This is called the **subminimal fringe effect**.

Examples

1. Pain produced due to myocardial damage is referred to left shoulder and ulnar aspect of the left upper limb.

2. Pain produced due to the inflammation of liver and gallbladder is felt in the right shoulder.

3. Pain produced due to the inflammation of appendix is felt initially around the umbilicus.

Importance   Some diseases can be diagnosed early by knowing the relationship between the site of origin of pain and the region to which it gets referred.

Endogenous Opioid Analgesic System

It is a pain-inhibiting system present in the body. The pathway contains receptors which can bind to morphine (opioid) and endogenously produced opioids like enkephalins, endorphins, and dynorphins.

The opioids can act at the following sites to inhibit the pain:

- at the site of injury,
- in the dorsal horn where pain fibers synapse with DRG, and
- at rostral sites in the brainstem.

The opioid receptors in the dorsal horn act presynaptically to reduce the release of pain-producing substances.

Pathway for Endogenous Pain Inhibition

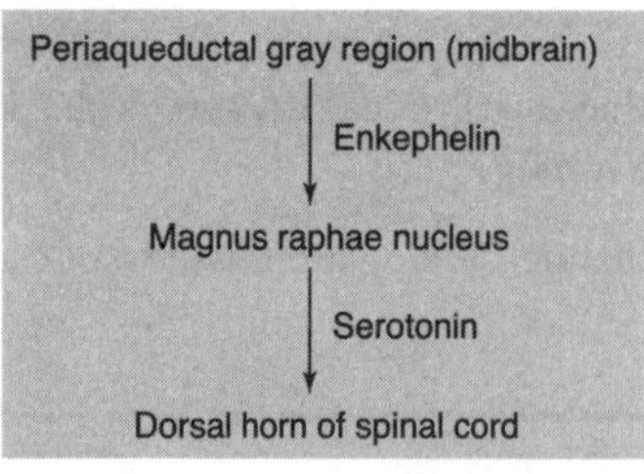

The placebos (tablets having no active medicine, commonly given for psychological satisfaction of the patient) and acupuncture are reported to reduce the intensity of pain by stimulating the release of endogenous opioids.

Gate Control Theory

Transmission of pain impulses can be modified or gated at the posterior horn of the spinal cord. This is achieved by stimulating the inhibitory interneuron in that region.

The counterirritants reduce pain perception by the gate control mechanism.

Motor System

Motor system is responsible for the transfer of information from center to the periphery. The information from center is finally passed on to the glands or muscles called effector organs.

The descending pathways are motor tracts. They are broadly divided into pyramidal and extrapyramidal systems.

Pyramidal System

The corticospinal tract is the main tract of the pyramidal system (Fig. 8.17).

Pyramidal (Corticospinal) Tract

Origin   The pyramidal tract arises from the pyramidal cells in the motor area (4), premotor area (6), and frontal eye field (8). It also gets fibers from the sensory area (3, 1, 2).

Course

- From the cerebral cortex the fibers descend as the corona radiata.

- It passes through genu and anterior two-third of the posterior limb of the internal capsule. (In this region, the fibers are closely packed and hence liable for extensive damage.)

- Then the fibers pass through crus cerebri of the midbrain to enter pons. In pons, the fibers get scattered.

- After leaving the pons, the fibers again become compact in the medulla assuming a pyramidal shape.

- At the lower border of the medulla, the majority of fibers cross to the opposite side forming the crossed pyramidal tract.

- The remaining fibers form the uncrossed pyramidal tract. These uncrossed fibers cross to the opposite side before they end on the anterior horn cell of the spinal cord.

Termination   Fibers of pyramidal tract finally end on anterior horn cell of the spinal cord.

Some fibers of the pyramidal tract while traveling from the cortex to the spinal cord give branches to the cranial nerve nucleus. These are called the **corticonuclear fibers**.

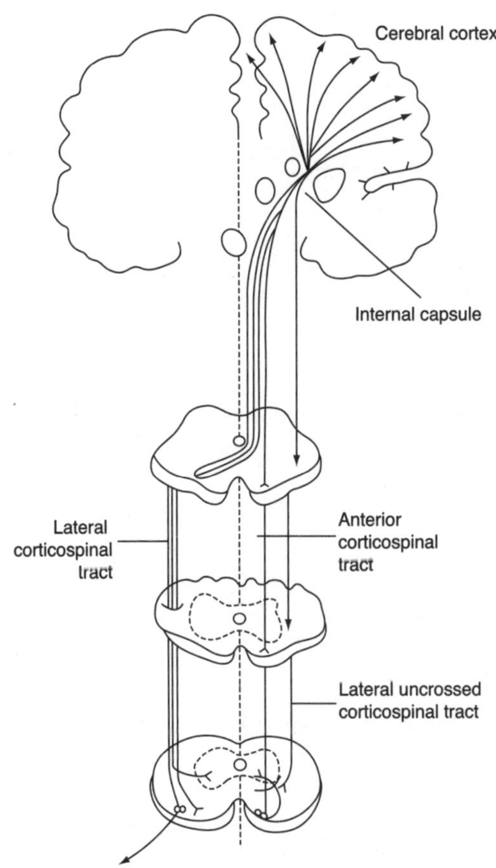

Fig. 8.17   Pyramidal tract.

As the corticospinal fibers descend through the brain from the cerebral cortex, they are accompanied by the **corticobulbar pathway**. The corticobulbar pathway begins in the sensorimotor cortex and ends in brainstem. The corticobulbar fibers control the motor neurons, innervating muscles of the eye, face, tongue, and throat. They are the main source of voluntary control for the muscles of the head and neck.

The pyramidal tract from its origin in cerebral cortex to its termination in the anterior horn cell of the spinal cord forms the **upper motor neuron**.

The fibers from the anterior horn cell of the spinal cord to its termination on the muscle constitute the **lower motor neuron**.

Functions

- Pyramidal tract carries impulses for voluntary movements from the brain to the spinal cord.

- It helps to maintain posture by regulating the action of the trunk muscles.

- It has an influence on the stretch reflex.

Extrapyramidal System (Fig. 8.18)

The extrapyramidal system consists of fibers descending through the brainstem and spinal cord without passing through the pyramids. These fibers are concerned with the control of posture. As there is confusion regarding the precise anatomical division and the functional demarcation of the pyramidal and extrapyramidal systems, it is suggested to drop these terms.

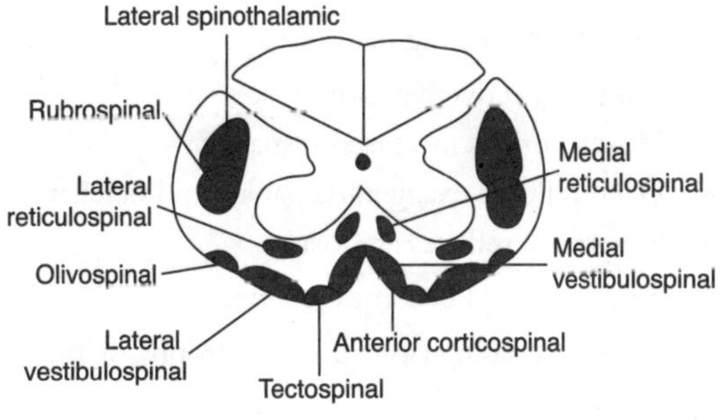

Fig. 8.18   Descending tracts.

Conventionally, fibers in the extrapyramidal system are grouped into following tracts:

- tectospinal tract,

- rubrospinal tract,

- reticulospinal tract,

- vestibulospinal tract, and

- olivospinal tract.

Functions

- Helps in regulation of muscle tone.
- Influences the activity in postural (extensor) muscles.
- Helps in maintenance of posture and equilibrium.
- Facilitates gross postural movements.

Effects of Complete Transection of the Spinal Cord

This can occur in spinal injuries due to accidents. They exhibit the following features:

- immediate and permanent loss of all voluntary movements below the level of lesion;

Applied Physiology

Hemiplegia

Paralysis of one-half of the body.

Paraplegia

Paralysis of both the lower limbs.

Monoplegia

Paralysis of any one limb.

Quadriplegia

Paralysis of all the four limbs.

Upper Motor Neuron Lesion

Damage to the pyramidal tract from its origin in the cerebral cortex to the anterior horn cell is termed **upper motor neuron lesion**.

It has the following features:

- Voluntary movements are lost.
- Muscle tone is increased—spasticity.
- Deep reflexes exaggerated; ankle and patellar clonus present.
- Superficial reflexes are lost.
- Babinski's sign becomes positive.
- In long-standing cases there is atrophy of muscle due to disuse, e.g., hemiplegia.

Hemiplegia

Hemiplegia is the term used to explain the loss of muscle strength on one side of the body, often including the face. This occurs as a result of damage to the pyramidal tract usually at the internal capsule. They have features of the upper motor neuron type of lesion.

Lower Motor Neuron Lesion

Lesion in the anterior horn cell or the nerve from the anterior horn cell to its termination results in the **lower motor neuron lesion**.

It shows the following features:

- Loss of voluntary motor activity.
- Hypotonia—flaccid paralysis.
- Absence of superficial and deep reflexes in the affected segment.
- Muscles supplied by the affected nerves progressively atrophy.
- Fibrillation potential seen in electromyogram.
- Reaction of degeneration present, e.g., poliomyelitis.

- immediate loss of all reflexes below the level of lesion;
- permanent loss of all sensations below the lesion.

Clinically, it has three stages:

1. **Stage of spinal shock**
   - Loss of reflexes due to the removal of supraspinal influences.
   - Loss of voluntary muscle power.
   - All sensations below the level of lesion are lost.
   - There is a sharp fall in the blood pressure due to vasomotor paralysis. Circulation becomes sluggish.
   - Overlying skin and subcutaneous tissue suffer lack of nutrition and are prone to develop bedsores.
   - Urinary bladder muscles become hypotonic or atonic.
   - Bowel becomes hypotonic.

2. **Stage of reflex activity**
   - After a lapse of about 2 weeks, tone of flexor muscle returns giving rise to paraplegia of flexion.
   - Babinski's sign becomes positive.
   - Tendon jerk begins to appear.
   - Mass reflex may appear. (When medial surface of thigh is stroked, there is flexor spasm of lower limb, evacuation of bladder, and bowel associated with sweating. All these changes together constitute **mass reflex**. This reflex is clinically used to periodically evacuate bladder and bowel.

   - Bladder becomes automatic.

3. **Stage of reflex failure**
   Degeneration of the spinal cord and intercurrent infections cause failure of reflex activities. Once again the muscles become hypotonic, mass reflexes disappear, and the patient dies.

Effects of Hemisection of Spinal Cord (Brown Sequard Syndrome)

Above the Level of Lesion

The zone of hyperesthesia limited to one segment.

At the Level of Lesion on the Same Side

1. **Sensory changes**
   - Loss of all sensations (fine touch, pressure, pain, temperature, and vibration).

2. **Motor changes**
   - Lower motor neuron type of paralysis.

Below the Level of Lesion

1. **Sensory changes**
   - Pain and temperature sensations lost on the opposite side.
   - Position sense, fine touch, and vibration sense lost on the same side.

2. **Motor changes**
   - The upper motor neuron type of paralysis on the same side because of damage to the corticospinal tract.
   - On the opposite side, there is minimal motor paralysis following damage to the anterior corticospinal tract.

Applied Physiology

Tabes Dorsalis

It is a condition seen in neurosyphilis. The disease is characterized by progressive degeneration of the posterior nerve root up to the DRG. However, the DRG are not affected.

Manifestations

- Loss of pain, position, and vibration sense.
- Loss of passive movements due to defective kinesthetic sensations.
- Loss of superficial and deep reflexes due to extensive sensory loss.
- Lack of coordination of movements (ataxia).
- Involvement of sacral segments results in loss of micturition reflex and atonic bladder.

Syringomyelia

This condition is characterized by the enlargement of central canal with destruction of the gray matter around the canal. It commonly affects the cervical and thoracic segments.

Manifestations

- Loss of pain, temperature, and crude touch sensation because of damage to the fibers crossing in front of the central canal.
- If anterior gray horn is affected, it results in flaccid paralysis of the muscles.
- Pain sensation is lost in this condition. The withdrawal reflex gets affected. Hence the subject is more prone to injuries.

Poliomyelitis

It is an acute infectious disease characterized by local or widespread muscular paralysis. It is produced by specific neurotrophic virus causing destruction of anterior horn cell of the spinal cord or the corresponding cell in medulla.

Facial Palsy

Facial palsy is produced because of damage to facial nerve.

It can be one of the following three types:

1. supranuclear,
2. nuclear, and
3. infranuclear.

In supranuclear type of facial palsy, one side of the face is affected (unilateral). However, upper part of the face is spared (due to bilateral innervation).

Voluntary movements of facial muscles are affected, but emotional expressions are intact.

In nuclear and infranuclear types, one-half of the face is affected. It may be unilateral or bilateral. There is no impairment of taste sensation.

Features

- Facial muscles are paralyzed on the affected side.

- Eye cannot be closed completely and palpebral fissure is widened. Tears collect in the eye and tend to overflow (epiphora).
- Whenever the individual tries to close the eye, eyeball rolls upward under partly covered eyelid. This is termed **Bell's phenomenon**.
- Angle of mouth is drooping on the affected side and the other angle gets deviated to the normal side.
- Nasolabial fold is lost on the affected side.

Hypothalamus

Hypothalmus is present on the under surface of the brain. It is situated below the thalamus.

It extends from the optic chiasma anteriorly to the mamillary body posteriorly. It weighs about 4 g.

Hypothalamus has the following nuclei.

Anterior Hypothalamus

- Preoptic nucleus
- Paraventricular nucleus
- Supraoptic nucleus
- Suprachiasmatic nucleus
- Anterior hypothalamic nucleus

Medial Hypothalamus

- Dorsomedial nucleus
- Ventromedial nucleus
- Arcuate nucleus

Lateral Hypothalamus

- Lateral hypothalamic nucleus

Posterior Hypothalamus

- Posterior hypothalamic nucleus
- Mamillary nucleus

Connections

Afferent Connections

Hypothalamus receives afferent connections from the following areas:

- cerebral cortex,
- globus pallidus,
- olfactory area,
- amygdala,
- limbic system,
- hippocampus,
- midbrain, and
- reticular formation.

Efferent Connections

Hypothalamus has efferent connections to the following areas:

- anterior thalamic nucleus,
- tegmentum of midbrain,
- brainstem reticular formation,
- frontal lobe of cerebral cortex,
- posterior pituitary,
- limbic system, and
- lateral horn of spinal cord.

Functions

1. **Control of food intake:** Hypothalamus has a feeding center in its lateral part and a satiety center (satisfaction) in the ventromedial part. The coordinated activity of these centers determines the feeding behavior of the animal. The stimulation of the feeding center produces the desire to eat. The stimulation of the satiety center produces a sense of satisfaction. Destruction of the feeding center causes severe anorexia and death. Lesion of the satiety center results in excessive eating producing *hypothalamic obesity.*

   - *Glucostatic hypothesis:* The satiety center has glucostatic cells. The entry of glucose under the influence of insulin stimulates these cells causing a sense of satiety.

   - *Lipostatic hypothesis:* It suggests that the signals are generated in proportion to fat present in the body. These signals influence the hypothalamus to decrease the food intake and increase the energy output.

- *Gut peptide hypothesis:* It proposes that the polypeptides are produced in the GIT by the presence of food. These polypeptides inhibit further intake of food.

- *Thermostatic hypothesis:* According to this theory, a drop in the body temperature below a critical level stimulates the desire to consume food. A rise in temperature above the set point reduces the appetite.

2. **Regulation of water balance:** Hypothalamus has got osmoreceptors. These are capable of detecting osmolarity of the blood. When there is hemoconcentration (decrease in fluid content of the blood), fluid moves out of the osmoreceptor into the blood. This stimulates the cells to increase production of the hormone ADH (antidiuretic hormone).

    ADH enhances water reabsorption and conserves (retain) water by reducing urine output. It also stimulates thirst center, and increases the desire to drink water.

    Hemodilution inhibits ADH secretion and increases urine output.

3. **Control of anterior pituitary:** Hypothalamus produces releasing and inhibiting factors, which regulate the secretion from the anterior pituitary. For example, thyroid-releasing hormone causes secretion of the thyroid-stimulating hormone.

4. **Control of posterior pituitary:** It regulates the formation and release of oxytocin and ADH.

5. **Regulation of body temperature:** Hypothalamus maintains the body temperature within a narrow range of fluctuation. Stimulation of lateral hypothalamus produces vasoconstriction and shivering. These changes increase the body temperature. Stimulation of anterior hypothalamus causes loss of heat by vasodilation and sweating. Hypothalamus acts as a thermostat to maintain the normal body temperature.

6. **Control of autonomic functions:** The stimulation of anterior hypothalamus decreases heart rate, produces vasodilation, and increases movement and secretion of digestive system. These are the effects of parasympathetic stimulation.

    The stimulation of lateral hypothalamus produces vasoconstriction, pupillary dilation, and increase in heart rate.

7. **Control of sleep and wakefulness:** The posterior hypothalamus forms a part of reticular activating system. The stimulation of this system produces wakefulness.

    Activity of anterior hypothalamus produces electrical changes in the brain similar to those seen during sleep.

8. **Control of circadian rhythm:** The body functions exhibit cyclical variation over a period of 24 h. The sleep–wakefulness cycle and the secretion of hormones like cortisol follow the circadian rhythm. This rhythm is maintained by the ventromedial nucleus of hypothalamus.

9. **Control of behavior:** The stimulation of lateral hypothalamus produces fight and flight reactions. The stimulation of ventromedial hypothalamus reduces rage resulting in avoidance reaction. The stimulation of the lateral hypothalamus increases the sex drive. The stimulation of ventromedial nucleus reduces sex drive.

Thalamus (Fig. 8.19)

Thalamus is an oval mass containing groups of nuclei forming the lateral boundary of the third ventricle. It forms partly the floor of the lateral ventricle.

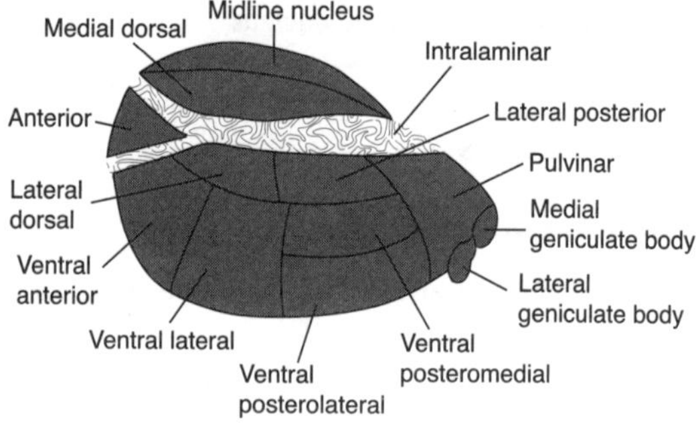

Fig. 8.19   Thalamus.

Nuclei

- Anterior nucleus (A)
- Midline nucleus (ML)
- Intralaminar nucleus (IL)

Dorsal Group

- Medial dorsal nucleus (MD)
- Lateral dorsal nucleus (LD)
- Lateral posterior nucleus (LP)

Ventral Group

- Ventral anterior nucleus (VA)
- Ventral lateral nucleus (VL)
- Ventral posterolateral nucleus (VPL)
- Ventral posteromedial nucleus (VPM)

Posterior Group

- Pulvinar (P)
- Medial geniculate body (MGB)
- Lateral geniculate body (LGB)

Afferent Connections

1. **Medial lemniscus:** It is the continuation of fasciculus gracilis and cuneatus. It conveys fine touch, pressure, vibration, and proprioceptive sensations to ventral posterolateral nucleus.
2. **Spinal lemniscus:** It carries pain, temperature, and crude touch senses to the ventral posterolateral nucleus.
3. **Trigeminal lemniscus:** It carries all sensations from trigeminal area to the ventral posteromedial group.
4. **Sensory visceral fibers from the hypothalamus:** They terminate on the medial part of thalamus.
5. **Cerebellar efferents from the opposite side:** They terminate in the ventrolateral nucleus.
6. **Rubrothalamic tract:** Fibers from red nucleus of the same side terminates on ventrolateral nucleus.
7. **Corticothalamic fibers from different areas of cortex:** They terminate in different nuclei of thalamus.

Efferent Connections

1. Thalamocortical fibers—they are widely distributed to different parts of cerebral cortex.
2. Efferent fibers to caudate nucleus.
3. Efferent fibers to globus pallidus.
4. Efferent intrathalamic connections.
5. Efferents to hypothalamus and midbrain.

Functions

- A sensory relay station; relays general and special sensation except smell sensation.
- Functions as subcortical center for perception of pain sensation.
- Helps in information storage and short-term memory.
- Forms a functional part of reticular activating system responsible for consciousness, sleep, and wakefulness.
- Forms a part of neural circuit (papez) for emotional experience, personality, and social behavior.
- Regulates autonomic functions associated with emotions.
- Forms a part of posture-adjusting system; helps the motor cortex to modify and update signals to perform voluntary motor activity.
- Integrates cortical and subcortical areas for execution of speech.
- Plays an important role in the genesis and synchronization of waves of EEG.
- Forms a link between cerebellum, basal ganglia, and cerebral cortex.

Thalamic Syndrome

Ischemic damage to the posteroventral part of thalamus due to a blockage in the feeding artery produces thalamic syndrome. This condition is characterized by

- loss or alteration in different sensations;
- ataxia—incoordination of voluntary movements due to loss of joint sense;
- astereognosis—it is the inability to identify commonly used objects by the feel of it;
- hypotonia and muscular weakness;
- emotional disturbance;
- increased pain perception.

Medial nucleus of thalamus is not damaged in thalamic syndrome. The pain fibers reach this nucleus. Hence there is dominance of pain sensation over the other sensations.

Basal Ganglia (Fig. 8.20)

The basal ganglia are subcortical structures located lateral to the thalamus, below the lateral ventricle. This is located lateral to third ventricle, consisting of the following nuclear groups:

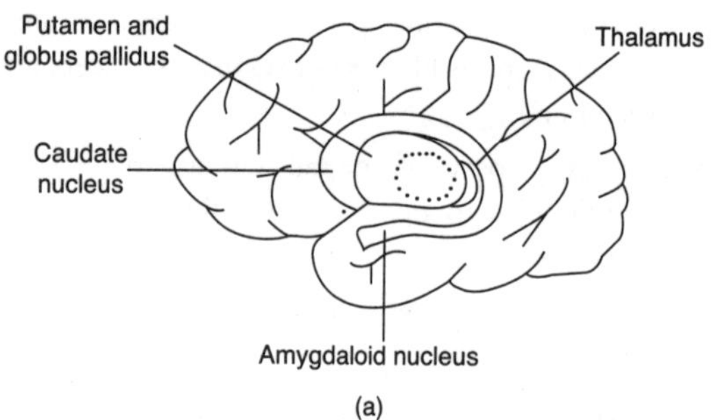

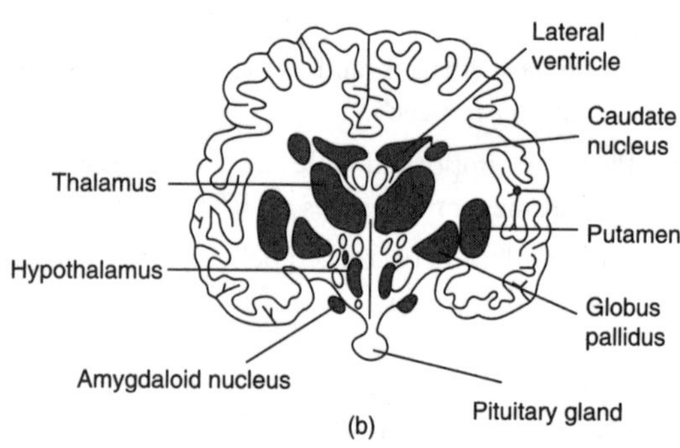

Fig. 8.20   Basal ganglia.

- Caudate nucleus
- Putamen
- Globus pallidus

    External segment

    Internal segment

- Substantia nigra

    Pars compacta

    Pars reticulata

- Subthalamic nucleus (red nucleus)

Caudate nucleus and putamen are together called the **striatum**.

Putamen and globus pallidus are termed the **lenticular nucleus**.

Important neurotransmitters in the basal ganglia are

- dopamine,
- GABA, and
- acetylcholine.

Connections

Afferent Connections

Corticostriate projection—from all parts of the cerebral cortex to the striatum.

Connections within Basal Ganglia

- Nigrostriatal (dopaminergic) projection from pars compacta of substantia nigra to striatum.
- Projection from striatum to pars reticulata (GABAergic) of substantia nigra.
- Projection from caudate nucleus and putamen to both segments of globus pallidus.
- Connection from external segment of globus pallidus to subthalamic nucleus.
- Connection from subthalamic nucleus to substantia nigra and both segments of globus pallidus (opposite direction).

Efferent Connections

- Output from the internal segment of globus pallidus through thalamic fasciculus to thalamus.
- From thalamus, the fibers project to the prefrontal and premotor cortex.

Functions

- Responsible for planning and programming the voluntary motor activity.
- Regulates stretch reflex throughout the body.
- Controls the transfer of information from sensory and association areas to motor cortex.
- Essential for initiation, control, and cessation of muscular activity.
- Provides the necessary muscle tone for skilled movements.
- Coordinates the impulses for skilled motor activity.

- Controls the normal automatic associated movements.
- Regulates the subconscious gross associated movements.
- Intact basal ganglia are necessary for normal degree of tone and posture.

Cerebrum

The cerebrum is the largest part of the human brain. It is divided into right and left cerebral hemispheres separated by the median longitudinal fissure. They are connected in the midline by a thick band of white matter called the **corpus callosum**. The corpus callosum is made up of axons passing between the right and left hemispheres.

Each hemisphere has an outer layer of gray matter that is 5 mm thick. This is termed the **cerebral cortex**. The cerebral cortex has a rich blood supply. It covers thick white matter.

The surface of the cerebral cortex exhibits depressions and elevations, termed **sulci** and **gyri**. Gyri and sulci increase the surface area of the brain. The deeper sulci are called **fissures**.

Applied Physiology

Parkinson's Disease (Paralysis Agitans)

The lesion of the basal ganglia results in Parkinson's disease. In this condition, dopaminergic pathway is damaged. It has both hypokinetic and hyperkinetic features. Akinesia and bradykinesia are the hypokinetic features. Rigidity and tremor are the hyperkinetic features.

Parkinson's disease has the following features:

- rigidity of muscle—lead pipe type/cogwheel type;
- resting tremors (pill-rolling tremors);
- flexed attitude due to increased tone in the flexor muscles;
- difficulty in commencing the movements (akinesia);
- difficulty in execution of movements and slowness of movements (bradykinesia);
- poverty of movements;
- loss of associated movements;
- short shuffling gait (festinent gait);
- autonomic disturbances;
- loss of facial expression—mask-like face.

Disease associated with basal ganglia also produces hyperkinetic movement disorders like chorea, athetosis, and ballism. These are excessive abnormal involuntary movements.

Management

This condition can be managed by administration of L dopa (precursor of dopamine) as dopamine cannot cross the blood–brain barrier.

Resting Tremor (Static Tremor)

Tremor is a rhythmic, alternate contraction of agonistic and antagonistic muscle of a joint.

Tremor in Parkinsonism is seen at rest but disappears during activity. Hence, it is called **resting tremor**. The possible cause for this tremor is damage to feedback circuits through basal ganglia. It might oscillate due to high feedback gain and loss of inhibition.

It can also be seen in thyrotoxicosis, anxiety states, mercury poisoning, and chronic alcoholics.

Intention Tremor

These tremors appear when the subject intends to do some work. It is seen in cerebellar lesion. This is due to failure of the system to dampen motor activity.

The white matter has axons connecting different parts of the brain with the cerebral cortex. It has lesser blood supply. The white matter of each hemisphere has a large collection of cell bodies forming the basal ganglia.

The cerebral cortex is made up of the following six layers:

1. molecular or plexiform layer,
2. external granular layer,
3. outer pyramidal cell layer,
4. inner granular layer,
5. inner pyramidal cell layer, and
6. fusiform cell layer.

Cerebral cortex is anatomically divided into the following lobes:

1. frontal lobe,
2. parietal lobe,
3. temporal lobe, and
4. occipital lobe.

Brodmann has divided cerebral hemisphere into functional areas (Fig. 8.21).

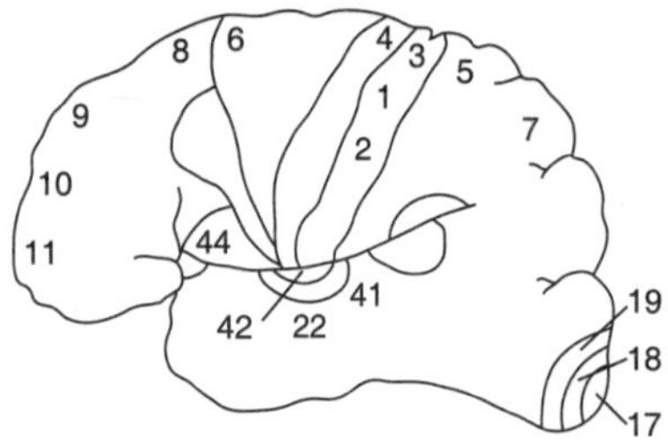

Fig. 8.21   Brodmann areas of cerebral cortex.

The major areas are as under:

1. Frontal lobe

- *Area 4:* It is the primary motor area. It lies in front of the central sulcus. This area helps to initiate voluntary movements. The axons from the primary motor cortex pass through the brainstem and spinal cord. They synapse with motor neurons at different segments of the spinal cord.

  Motor homunculus—the body is represented upside down. Stimulation of the medial part causes movement of toes and lower limbs. Stimulation of the lateral part causes movement of tongue. Arrangement of different parts of the body in motor cortex is termed motor homunculus.

- *Area 6:* It is the premotor area. Fibers to the pyramidal tract also arise from this region.

  It is connected with skilled movement. It coordinates the actions initiated by area 4.

- *Area 8:* It is frontal eye field area.

  It helps in voluntary and conjugate movements of the eye. It also controls the movement of eyelids, size of pupils, and lacrimation.

- *Area 44:* This is Broca's speech area. It is present in dominant hemisphere.

  It helps in vocalization by controlling the movement of lips, tongue, and larynx.

- *Prefrontal cortex: Areas 9, 10, 11, 12, 13, 14, 29, 32:* Prefrontal cortex present in the anterior part of the frontal lobe is the most complicated cortical region. It is connected with complex learning abilities, intelligence, personality, recall of information, production of abstract ideas, reasoning, judgment, long-term planning, and conscience.

  Prefrontal cortex matures slowly, and depends on positive and negative feedback during its development.

  It is connected to limbic system which caters to emotional functions of the brain. It plays an important role in mood and intuitive judgment.

  Lesion of the prefrontal cortex results in mental and personality disorders.

  The other manifestations are mood swings, loss of judgment, and attentiveness. The affected individual is unmindful of social restraints.

2. Parietal lobe

- *Areas 3, 1, 2:* The primary sensory cortex (somatosensory area) present in the postcentral gyrus.

  They receive information from receptors in the skin, joints, and muscles.

  They are also connected with integration of sensory information.

- *Areas 5, 7:* These are sensory association areas. They are concerned with the synthesis and interpretation of the information received by somatosensory cortex.

3. Occipital lobe

- *Area 17:* It is primary visual area. It is concerned with processing visual information.

- *Areas 18, 19:* These are visual association areas. They are concerned with the interpretation of visual information received by primary visual cortex. They are also responsible for the movement of eyes.

4. Temporal lobe

- *Areas 41, 42:* These are the primary auditory areas. They are responsible for the perception of auditory information.

- *Area 22:* This is Wernicke's area. It is concerned with the interpretation of auditory information.

Cerebellum (Fig. 8.22)

It is the part of the CNS located posterior and inferior to the cerebral hemispheres. It is divided into right and left cerebellar hemispheres. It is connected to the brainstem through superior, middle, and inferior cerebellar peduncles.

Classification

Anatomical Division

- Flocculonodular lobe
- Anterior lobe
- Posterior lobe

Phylogenetic Division

- Archicerebellum
- Paleocerebellum
- Neocerebellum

Functional Division

- Vestibulocerebellum
- Spinocerebellum
- Cerebrocerebellum (neocerebellum)

Nuclei

- Nucleus globosus
- Nucleus emboliformis
- Nucleus fastigius
- Nucleus dentatus

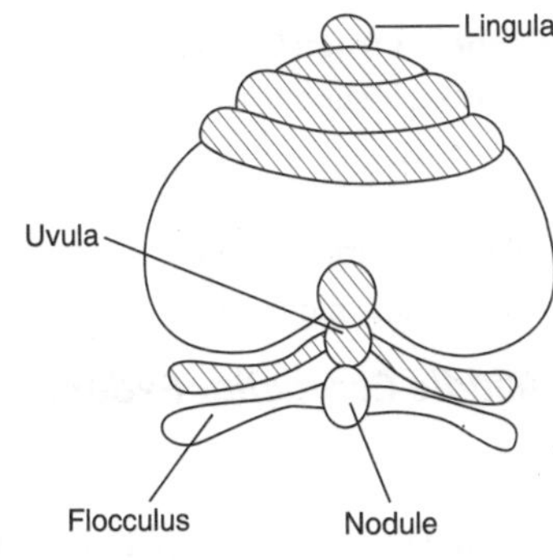

Fig. 8.22   Cerebellum.

Input to the Cerebellar Cortex

The cerebellum receives inputs through

- climbing fibers and
- mossy fibers.

Climbing fibers arise from the region of inferior olive in the medulla. They make synaptic connections with Purkinje cells. The climbing fibers produce high-frequency bursts or **complex spikes**. They play a major role in motor learning.

Mossy fibers arise from different centers in the brainstem and spinal cord. They make synaptic connection with Purkinje cells. They produce **simple spikes**.

They also synapse with granular cells. Axons of granular cells bifurcate. They excite the Purkinje cells (through parallel fibers) and also inhibitory interneurons.

Output from Cerebellar Cortex

Output of the cerebellar cortex is from Purkinje cells. These outputs are always inhibitory.

GABA is the neurotransmitter. The output projects to deeper cerebellar nuclei and vestibular nucleus. The inhibitory inputs influence the output from the cerebellum to regulate range, direction, and rate of movement.

Connections

Through Superior Cerebellar Peduncle

Afferent

- **Ventral spinocerebellar tract:** Carries proprioceptive impulses from the trunk and limbs
- **Tectocerebellar tract:** Carries visual and auditory impulses through superior and inferior colliculi

Efferent

- Dentatothalamocortical tract
- Dentatorubrothalamic tract

Through Middle Cerebellar Peduncle

Afferent

- **Pontocerebellar tract:** Impulses from the opposite motor cortex via pontine nucleus
- **Cerebellocerebellar tract:** Fibers from dentate nucleus of one cerebellar hemisphere to that of the opposite side

Efferent

- Cerebellocerebellar tract

Through Inferior Cerebellar Peduncle

Afferent

- **Dorsal spinocerebellar tract:** Carries proprioceptive sensations from trunk and limbs of the same side
- **Olivocerebellar tract:** Proprioceptive impulses from all over the body relayed through inferior olive
- **Vestibulocerebellar tract:** Carries impulses from vestibular apparatus from the same side of the body
- **Cuneocerebellar tract:** Carries proprioceptive impulses from the arm and neck from the same side of the body
- **Reticulocerebellar tract:** Impulses from brainstem reticular formation

- **External arcuate fibers:** Originating from nucleus gracilis and cuneatus
- **Fibers arising from fifth, ninth, and tenth cranial nerves**

Efferent

- Fastigiobulbar and fastigiovestibular tracts
- Cerebello-olivary tract

Functions

Vestibulocerebellum (Archicerebellum)

- Concerned with maintenance of balance and equilibrium
- Responsible for regulating the stability of head and body in space
- Adjusts the tone of the trunk muscle and controls the ocular movements and other postural reflexes.

Spinocerebellum (Paleocerebellum)

- Maintains the posture and helps in execution of gross movements
- Controls the interplay between the agonist and antagonist group of muscles
- Essential for the control of rapid muscular activities like running and talking

Cerebrocerebellum (Neocerebellum)

- Controls fine, highly precise, and coordinated movements
- Involved in programming of voluntary and skilled movements
- Plays a major role in the timing of the motor activities and rapid progression from one movement to the next

Servo Control Mechanism

The cerebellum acts as a comparator-and-error detector. It compares the information coming from the cortical regions involved in programming and execution of movements with that coming from periphery (joints, muscles, and skin). If there is any difference between the two informations, cerebellum adjusts the activity in descending pathway to correct the ongoing movement. It sends an error signal to the motor cortex and subcortical structures for modification of program.

Effects of Cerebellar Lesions

- Ataxia—incoordinated, intermittent jerky movements with drunken gait
- Hypotonia or atonia—reduced or absence of muscle tone
- Dysmetria—inability to judge the force and range of movement resulting in past pointing
- Dysdiadokokinesia—failure to perform rapid alternating movements
- Decomposition of movement—lack of smooth flow of movement
- Speech defect—staccato speech or slurring speech
- Pendular knee jerk (a feature of hypotonia)
- Intention tremors
- Nystagmus (jerky movements of the eye)

Electroencephalogram

Electroencephalogram (ECG) is the electrical potential of brain. It is recorded from the surface of the scalp by using electrodes. An electroencephalogram recorded with electrodes in direct contact with the brain is called **electrocorticogram** (Fig. 8.23).

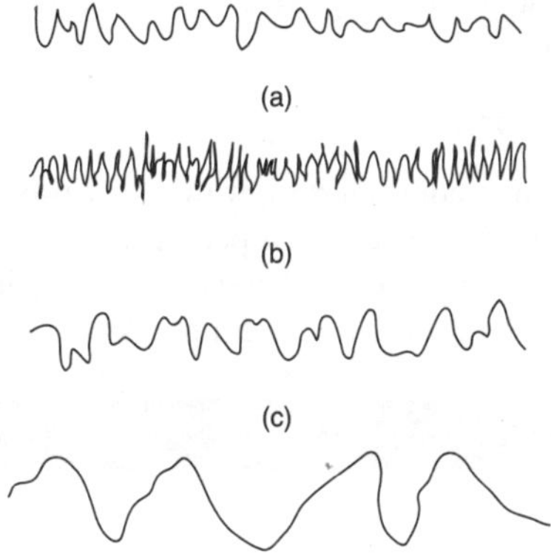

Fig. 8.23   Waves of EEG: (a) alpha, (b) beta, (c) theta, and (d) delta.

EEG waves have two variables; amplitude and frequency. The **amplitude** indicates the quantum of electrical activity beneath the recording electrode. It is measured in microvolts (μV).

The **frequency of wave** indicates the number of waves per unit time. It is measured as Hertz (Hz or cycles/s).

EEG was first analyzed systematically by a German psychiatrist Hans Berger. Hence, it is also called Berger's rhythm.

It has four different waves:

1. **Alpha-wave:** It has a frequency of 8–12 Hz with an amplitude of 50–100 μV. It can be recorded mainly from occipital region, also from frontal and parietal regions.
2. **Beta-wave:** It has a frequency of 18–30 Hz with lower amplitude. It is recorded from parietal and frontal regions.
3. **Theta-wave:** This is large-amplitude, regular wave with a frequency of 4–7 Hz. Theta-wave appears in children. It is recorded from parietal and temporal regions.
4. **Delta-wave:** This is a large slow wave with a frequency of less than 4 Hz. It appears in deep sleep, infancy, and serious organic brain disease.

Uses

- EEG is a widely accepted and reliable method of studying electrical changes occurring in brain during normal and abnormal conditions.
- It is helpful in localizing cerebral tumors and abscesses.
- It is of special importance in the diagnosis of epilepsy and other types of fits. In epilepsy there is excessive discharge of signals from the cerebral cortex.
- It is helpful in the diagnosis of various diseases of cerebral cortex and impaired cerebral function.

Sleep

Sleep is a reversible state of altered consciousness characterized by diminished excitability of the brain and reduction in physiological functions.

Mechanism

- Activity of ascending reticular activating system (ARAS) leads to awakening. Conversely, inhibition of ARAS promotes sleep. Lesion of RAS produces coma.

- Serotonergic fibers arise from raphe nucleus of pons. Stimulation of these fibers induces sleep.
- Sleep-promoting peptide and sleep peptides (muramyl peptides) accumulate during wakefulness. When its concentration in the brain increases, it promotes sleep.

Physiological Changes during Sleep

The heart rate, blood pressure, and respiratory rate decrease. The blood vessels to the skin dilate. There is a decrease in the excitability of the nervous system. The sympathetic activity decreases and the parasympathetic activity increases. There is muscle relaxation. The net effect aims at restoration of the natural balance among the neuronal centers.

Types

- Nonrapid eye movement (NREM) sleep
- Rapid eye movement (REM) sleep

Nonrapid Eye Movement Sleep

- It is a slow-wave sleep.
- There is no rapid movement of the eyeball.
- It occupies a major part of sleeping time.
- Each cycle lasts for about 70 min.

Rapid Eye Movement Sleep (Paradoxical Sleep)

During REM sleep there is increased eye movements. Each cycle of REM sleep lasts for about 5–30 min. It alternates with NREM sleep.

- It is associated with dreaming.

- During this phase, it is difficult to arouse the person.
- Muscle tone is exceedingly depressed.
- Heart rate and respiration are irregular, but the brain is highly active.
- Overall metabolism is increased by 20%.
- This is not restful form of sleep.
- EEG shows wave pattern similar to that seen during wakefulness. Hence, it is called **paradoxical sleep**.

Importance

- REM sleep produces muscle relaxation due to activity in pontine reticular formation.
- It helps in consolidation of memory.
- It helps in restoration of neuronal balance.

EEG Changes from Alert State to Deep Sleep

Alert and awake person has **beta-wave**.

If person is awake, relaxing with eyes closed, **alpha-waves** are seen.

When the individual becomes drowsy and falls asleep, alpha-waves are replaced by slower and larger **theta-waves**.

During deep sleep very large irregular **delta-waves** are seen.

Alpha-Block

In a normal adult relaxing with eyes closed, alpha-waves are recorded. On opening the eyes, alpha-waves are replaced by low-voltage, fast, irregular waves. This is known as **alpha-block**.

Applied Physiology

Disorders of Sleep

Insomnia

It is a condition of insufficient and nonrefreshing sleep in spite of an opportunity to sleep.

Insomnia is temporarily managed by using benzodiazepines (sleeping pills). Prolonged use of these drugs can result in addiction and can adversely affect the performance of the individual.

Somnambulism

It is also called sleepwalking. It is common in children than in adults. They walk with eyes open but cannot recollect the incident when awakened. Somnambulism occurs during slow-wave sleep.

Narcolepsy

It is a disease characterized by irresistible urge to sleep during daytime associated with sudden loss of muscle tone. The condition is characterized by sudden onset of REM sleep. Human subjects with narcolepsy have a low level of **orexins** (hypocretin) in CSF. Orexins (hypocretin) is a polypeptide secreted from neurons of lateral hypothalamus which regulates food intake and sleep.

REM Behavior Disorder

In this condition, hypotonia is not seen during REM sleep. The subject reacts physically during dream. Jumping out of the bed or fighting with an imagined aggressor is a common feature. The condition is managed by benzodiazepines.

Reticular Formation

Reticular formation is a diffuse network of neurons and discrete collection of nuclei. It occupies the midventral portion of the medulla, pons, and midbrain.

The nerve fibers of RAS are multisynaptic. They begin at the medulla and receive numerous collaterals from specific sensory tracts like the spinothalamic and trigeminal tracts. They relay at the thalamic nuclei. Further-order neurons terminate on parts of the cerebral cortex. Some fibers may bypass the thalamic region and terminate in the cerebral cortex.

These fibers carry nonspecific impulses concerned with alertness, wakefulness, and consciousness to the cerebrum and activate whole of the cerebral cortex.

Reticular formation has

- ascending reticular activating system (ARAS) and
- descending reticular activating system.

Ascending Reticular Activating System

It is a polysynaptic pathway extending from lower pons to the thalamus. It mainly has cholinergic fibers.

Connections

The cholinergic fibers from the midbrain and pons project to the cerebral cortex passing through the thalamus. The adrenergic fibers from all over the reticular formation project to the cerebral cortex. The serotonergic neurons from the raphe nucleus project to the thalamus, hypothalamus, cerebral cortex, and limbic system. It regulates sleep, wakefulness, and consciousness.

Descending Reticular System

The reticular fibers descending to spinal cord form the descending reticular system. This system has both facilitatory and inhibitory projections.

Connections

The pontine and medullary reticulospinal tract project to spinal cord. The noradrenergic fibers from different parts of the reticular formation project to the cerebellum. The dopaminergic fibers from midbrain reticular formation project to the basal ganglia. The serotonergic neurons in the raphae nucleus of the medulla project to the spinal cord.

The descending reticular formation controls the tone of the extensor muscles.

The projections from reticular formation help to regulate respiratory, cardiovascular, and vasomotor functions.

The sensory inputs to the reticular formation come from the areas connected to the reticular formation by the projection. There is extensive sensory input from the fibres carrying slow pain.

The reticular formation has four distinct systems with specific neurotransmitter. The neurotransmitters are

1. acetylcholine,
2. norepinephrine,
3. serotonin, and
4. dopamine.

Functions of Reticular Formation

- ARAS is responsible for arousal and wakefulness.

- Reticular facilitatory and inhibitory areas influence the spinal motor neurons to excite or inhibit them.
- Several important autonomic centers like cardiovascular and respiratory centers are located in reticular formation.
- It helps in the modulation of sensory impulses.
- Many behavioral functions are mediated through reticular formation.
- Descending reticular activating system controls muscle tone.

Sedatives and hypnotics prevent synaptic transmission in RAS to produce their effect.

Limbic System

Limbus means rim. The limbic system or limbic lobe consists of cortical tissue around the hilum of cerebral hemisphere. It consists of parts of frontal and temporal lobes on either side, namely, hippocampus, septal nucleus, cingulate gyrus, anterior thalamic nucleus, and amygdala.

The **cingulate gyrus** lies around the corpus callosum.

The **hippocampus** lies on the medial wall of the temporal lobe.

The amygdala lies in front of the hippocampus.

The septum lies in midline anterior to the hypothalamus.

The limbic cortex is the oldest part of the cerebral cortex. It is made up of primitive cortical tissue called the **allocortex**. The transitional cortex which forms the second ring is termed the **juxtallocortex**. It is observed that the size of allocortex and juxtallocortex has not changed significantly with evolution.

Connections of Limbic System (Papez Circuit)

The neocortical activity influences the emotional behavior. However, the connection between limbic cortex and neocortex is limited.

Duration of emotions cannot be regulated by conscious effort. Emotional responses are prolonged due to prolonged after-discharges in the limbic cortex. The response exceeds the duration of the stimulus producing it.

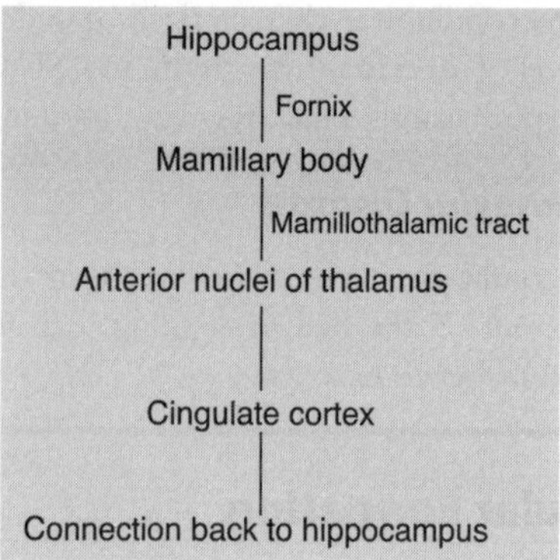

Functions

- Controls emotions of rage, fear, and motivation.
- Regulates the sexual behavior in association with hypothalamus.
- Plays a role in the process of olfaction.
- Connected with autonomic responses
- Plays an important role in memory.

Amygdala controls the choice of food and time of consuming it.

Septal nucleus regulates taste preference, and controls food intake and metabolism.

Limbic system generates emotional tone. Manifestation of emotional expression is by hypothalamus with the help of autonomic and somatic nervous system.

Emotions

Emotion is strong feeling as anger or joy. It is also described as instinctive feeling as distinguished from reasoning. Emotions have two components, namely,

1. mental and
2. physical.

The *mental component* involves

- **Cognition:** It is awareness of the sensation and cause for that sensation.
- **Affect:** It is the feeling produced by the sensation.
- **Conation:** It is the desire to take action.

The *physical component* involves an increase in blood pressure and heart rate associated with sweating.

Types

Motivation, Reward, and Punishment

It is reason behind one's action or behavior. It is the enthusiasm to perform a task. Behavior is motivated by stimulation of the **reward system** with a reduction in unpleasant effect by inhibition of the **punishment system**.

The stimulation of dopaminergic pathway of the ventral tegmentum to nucleus accumbens produces pleasurable sensation. Hence, it is called a **reward** or **approach system**.

The stimulation of lateral part of posterior hypothalamus, dorsal midbrain, and entorhinal cortex produces sensation of fear or terror. This area is termed **punishment** or **avoidance system**.

Fear

Fear is an unpleasant emotion caused by threat of danger, pain, or harm. It is the likelihood of something unwelcome happening. Stimulation of hypothalamus and amygdaloid nuclei produces the reaction of fear. Fear reactions to auditory and visual inputs disappear with destruction of amygdala.

Anxiety

It is a normal emotional response. However, excessive anxiety is considered abnormal. During anxiety reaction, there is increased blood flow to the anterior end of the temporal lobe. Anxiety is mediated by α_2-GABA receptors. It is relieved by benzodiazepines. They bind to GABA receptor and increase conductance to chloride ions.

Rage and Placidity

Rage is an emotional condition where a minor stimulus evokes a violent response.

Placidity is a condition in which anger-provoking and traumatic stimuli fail to disturb the animal.

Removal of neocortex and destruction of ventromedial nucleus of hypothalamus produce rage in animals.

Lesion to amygdaloid nucleus produces placidity.

Addiction

It is the repeated compulsive use of a substance in spite of its negative effect on the health. Addiction is associated with reward system in the brain especially with nucleus accumbens. Exogenous opiates

Applied Physiology

Hydrocephalus

It is a condition of increased intracranial pressure due to defective absorption or circulation of CSF. Baby shows enlargement of the cranial cavity and associated damage to the brain because of pressure effect.

It is of two types:

1. external or communicating hydrocephalus;
2. internal or noncommunicating hydrocephalus.

In communicating hydrocephalus, a large quantity of CSF accumulates due to defective reabsorption by arachnoid villi.

Blockage of foramens of Magendie and Luschka results in accumulation of CSF proximal to the block, distending the ventricles. This results in noncommunicating hydrocephalus.

Lumbar Puncture

It is a procedure by which CSF is taken out from the subarachnoid space. Normally, CSF is drawn by introducing a needle between third and fourth lumbar vertebrae. Histological and biochemical study of CSF gives an indication about various disease processes affecting the CNS.

CSF changes in common disorders are as follows:

- **Pressure:** Pressure is increased in subarachnoid hemorrhage, acute bacterial meningitis, and tuberculous meningitis.
- **Color:** It is blood stained in subarachnoid hemorrhage and cloudy in acute bacterial meningitis and tuberculous meningitis.
- **RBC:** RBC count is increased in subarachnoid hemorrhage.
- **Glucose:** It is decreased in acute bacterial meningitis and tuberculous meningitis.
- **Proteins:** Proteins are increased in subarachnoid hemorrhage, acute bacterial meningitis, viral meningitis, multiple sclerosis, and tuberculous meningitis.
- **Microorganisms:** Microorganisms are demonstrated in infective meningitis.

are addictive drugs. They increase the amount of dopamine to act on D_3 receptors in nucleus accumbens. Prolonged use of addicting drugs produces tolerance and withdrawal resulting in withdrawal symptoms.

Cerebrospinal Fluid

Cerebrospinal fluid (CSF) is a specialized extracellular fluid. It is present in the ventricles of brain, central canal of the spinal cord, and subarachnoid space.

Formation and Circulation

The choroid plexus of lateral and third ventricle of brain forms CSF by the processes of filtration and secretion. It passes through fourth ventricle, and central canal in spinal cord. CSF in the ventricles flows through the foramens of Magendie and Luschka to the subarachnoid space. It gets absorbed through the arachnoid villi present in sagittal sinus.

Composition and Properties

It is a colorless transparent fluid with a specific gravity of 1005.

It is alkaline in reaction.

The volume of CSF is about 150 mL. (About 500 mL of CSF is produced per day.) Normal CSF pressure is 5–15 mm Hg.

CSF contains 99% water and 1% solids.

The organic constituents are amino acids, sugar, proteins, cholesterol, urea, uric acid, and creatinine.

The inorganic constituents are sodium, calcium, potassium, magnesium, chlorides, bicarbonates, and phosphates.

Functions

- Acts as a cushion between the brain and the rigid cranium.
- Supports the weight of brain. Net weight of brain in CSF is about 50 g as compared to its weight of 1400 g in air.
- Distributes force of blows on the head.
- Maintains intracranial pressure by balancing the volume of blood and CSF.
- Drains metabolites from the brain.
- Supplies nutrients and oxygen to the brain.

Blood–Brain Barrier

It is a hypothetical barrier present between the brain and the blood. It selectively permits the passage of substances from blood to brain and vice versa.

Oxygen, carbon dioxide, glucose, water, amino acids, electrolytes, and drugs like sulfonamides and tetracycline cross this barrier.

Structure

- Capillaries of the brain consist of endothelial lining which have tight junctions. These junctions close the pores in blood vessels.
- Astrocytes completely cover the capillaries and make it less porous.
- Blood vessels in the brain have a thick basement membrane. They prevent the passage of substances across them.

Functions

- Maintains constancy of environment for the neurons in CNS.

- Protects brain from the effect of endogenous toxins.
- Prevents the escape of neurotransmitters from the CNS.

Inflammation, irradiation, and tumors destroy the blood–brain barrier. This permits free entry to the substances, toxins, and drugs that do not cross the barrier under normal conditions.

Lipid-soluble drugs cross the blood–brain barrier more freely when compared to water-soluble drugs.

Circumventricular Organ

The areas of brain located outside the blood–brain barrier are called circumventricular organs, which are as follows:

- posterior pituitary,
- median eminence of hypothalamus,
- subfornical organ,
- area postrema, and
- organum vasculosum of lamina terminalis.

Regulation of Tone, Posture, and Equilibrium

Tone is resistance offered by the muscle against passive stretch. Alternatively, tone is the partial contraction of the muscle at rest.

Muscle tone is influenced by intact nerve supply (alpha motor neuron activity), viscosity, and elasticity. The resting length of muscle is regulated by muscle tone.

Muscle tone is necessary for smooth and effective contraction.

Muscle tone is tested by performing passive movement of the limb.

It is maintained by structure in the muscle called **muscle spindle**.

Structure of Muscle Spindle (Fig. 8.24)

The skeletal muscle contains two types of fibers:

1. **Extrafusal fibers:** These are regular contractile units of the muscle.
2. **Intrafusal fibers:** About 10 intrafusal fibers enclosed in connective tissue capsule form the muscle spindle. Intrafusal fibers are parallel to the extrafusal fibers. The two ends of intrafusal fibers are striated and have limited ability to contract.

   Intrafusal fibers are of two types:

   (a) *Nuclear bag fibers:* It has a bulged central portion containing nuclei in it.
   (b) *Nuclear chain fibers:* It contains the nuclei arranged in a single row.

They are connected to the spinal cord by sensory nerves.

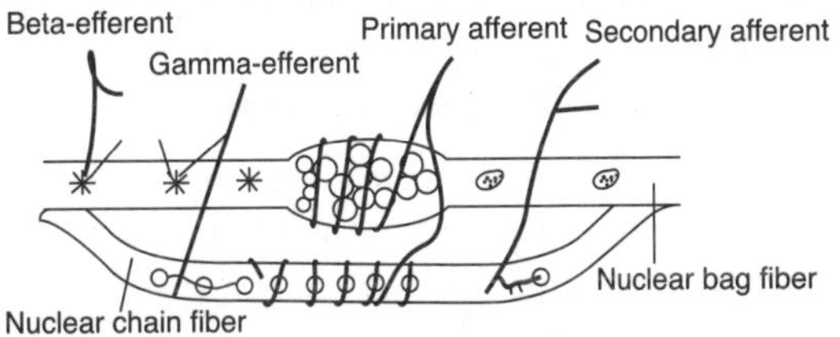

Fig. 8.24 Muscle spindle.

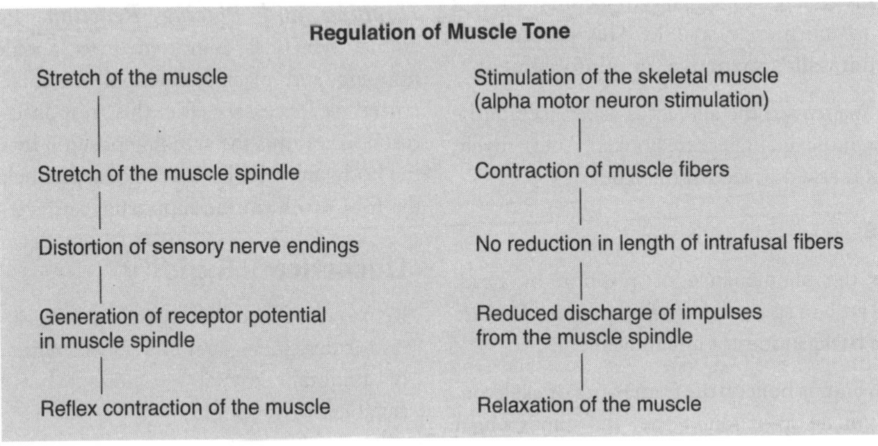

Regulation of Muscle Tone	
Stretch of the muscle	Stimulation of the skeletal muscle (alpha motor neuron stimulation)
↓	↓
Stretch of the muscle spindle	Contraction of muscle fibers
↓	↓
Distortion of sensory nerve endings	No reduction in length of intrafusal fibers
↓	↓
Generation of receptor potential in muscle spindle	Reduced discharge of impulses from the muscle spindle
↓	↓
Reflex contraction of the muscle	Relaxation of the muscle

Group IA fibers arise from **primary** or **annulospiral ending** in the central portion of both types of fibers.

Group II fibers arise from **secondary** or **flower spray endings** of nuclear chain fibers (located near the end of fibers).

Motor Connection

Gamma efferent (motor) fibers end on the striated portion of the intrafusal fibers. They control the sensitivity of the spindle.

Functions of Muscle Spindle

Muscle spindle is stimulated by stretch giving rise to stretch reflex. This forms the basis for control of muscle tone.

Nuclear bag fibers respond to rapid stretch of the muscle (dynamic response).

Nuclear chain fibers respond to sustained stretch (static response).

Gamma efferent system is regulated by descending tracts. Stimulation of gamma efferent nerve causes contraction of the contractile end of intrafusal fibers. This stretches the nuclear bag fibers. The annulospiral ending is distorted. There is increased number of impulses generated in the muscle spindle. Consequently, there is contraction of extrafusal fibers.

Anxiety increases gamma efferent discharges. Hence, tendon reflex becomes hyperactive in anxious patients.

Voluntary muscle contraction anywhere in the body increases the sensitivity of tendon reflex (stretch reflex). This is due to enhanced gamma efferent discharge to the muscle spindle. This procedure is termed **Jendrassik's maneuver** or **reinforcement**.

In this maneuver, the subject is asked to pull the hand when the flexed fingers are hooked. Alternatively, the subject is asked to clench the teeth.

Posture

Posture is the maintenance of position of head, trunk, and limb in space for a period of time. Posture serves as a background for any movement.

Human body is built on the framework of skeleton. Skeleton is made up of long bones and spines which have multiple joints. The major problems faced in the maintenance of posture are to

- maintain balance in upright position;
- balance the tall structure on a relatively small base;
- keep the body erect against forces of gravity;
- counter the effect of center of gravity which is located very high.

The problems faced in the maintenance of posture are overcome by postural reflexes.

The afferent input to these postural reflexes comes from eyes, vestibular apparatus, and somatic receptors.

Alpha motor neurons to the skeletal muscles form the efferent pathway. These reflexes are generally integrated at brainstem and spinal cord.

Simple reflexes are integrated at the spinal level. However, more complex reflexes such as **anticipatory postural adjustments** involve the cerebral cortex.

Some parts of brain appreciate the position and orientation of body in space. This mechanism helps in planning and executing motor action.

Postural Reflexes

Postural reflexes are integrated at different levels.

Cortical Integration

Optical Righting Reflex   This reflex is observed in animals with intact cerebral cortex. Visual signals to the animals activate the optical righting reflex to bring about the righting response. This reflex operates even in the absence of labyrinthine or body stimulation.

Hopping and Placing Reaction   Pushing an animal which is blindfolded to a side exhibits hopping and placing reaction. An intact cerebral cortex is necessary for this response. Hopping reaction restores the standing position by supporting the body on its limbs. Placing reaction helps to place the foot firmly on the supporting surface.

Decorticate Rigidity

Removal of cerebral cortex produces minimal motor deficit. In such individuals, reflex patterns of midbrain animal are present but they are capable of movement.

Integration at Midbrain Level

Righting Reflexes   These reflexes help to maintain the normal position of the animal and keep the head upright.

There are four types of righting reflexes:

1. **Labyrinthine righting reflex:** This type of reflex can be demonstrated in the midbrain of the animal. The midbrain of the animal is held by its body and moved from side to side. In spite of the movement, position of head is maintained by this righting reflex. Tilting of the head stimulates otolithic organs. It results in contraction of the neck muscles to maintain the level of head.
2. **Body on head righting reflex:** When the animal is placed on its side, pressure on side of the body initiates righting reflex. The animal tries to restore its normal position. Reflex righting of the head is functional even when the labyrinths have been destroyed.
3. **Neck righting reflex:** Righting of the head by above two mechanisms leaves the body in a tilted position. This stretches the neck muscles. Contraction of neck muscle rights the thorax and initiates stretch reflex passing down the body to right the abdomen and hind parts.
4. **Body on body righting reflex:** Pressure on the side of the body can initiate body righting reflex even when the head is prevented forcibly from righting.

Midbrain Animal

In this animal, a section is made in the neural axis at the superior border of midbrain. Extensor rigidity is seen when the animal lies on its back. The midbrains animal can stand, walk, and right themselves.

Integration at Medullary Level

Tonic Neck Reflex   Tonic neck reflex is initiated by stretch of proprioceptors in the upper part of neck.

Turning the head to one side results in extension of the limb on the same side with increased rigidity.

Flexion of head results in flexion of forelimbs and extension of hindlimbs.

Extension of head causes extension of forelimbs and flexion of hindlimbs.

Tonic Labyrinthine Reflex   This reflex is produced due to action of gravity on vestibular apparatus. It is seen in decerebrate animal. The pattern of rigidity varies with position.

Placing the animal on its back results in extension of all the four limbs.

Rigidity decreases when the animal is turned toward any side.

Rigidity is minimal in prone position.

Decerebrate Rigidity (Effects of Section of Brain at Midcollicular Level)   This is a type of rigidity produced in experimental animals by making a section between superior and inferior colliculus. The animal shows increased tone in antigravity muscles. All the four limbs become rigid like pillar; tail and neck are hyperextended. Decerebrate rigidity is due to the removal of inhibitory influences from higher centers. Brainstem and vestibular nucleus normally send facilitatory impulse to spinal center.

In decerebrate preparation, such facilitatory impulses are exaggerated or remain unopposed due to removal of cortical inhibition.

Integration at Spinal Level

Stretch Reflex   Stretch of the muscle results in its reflex contraction. This forms the basic mechanism in maintenance of posture. Receptor for this reflex is the muscle spindle.

Positive Supporting (Magnet) Reaction   Stimulation of sole or palm by contact causes the extension of same limb to support the body. Since the extending limb appears to follow the object touching it, this response is also termed **magnet reaction**.

Negative Supporting Reaction   Positive supporting reaction is lost by excessively stretching the limb.

These reflexes are demonstrated in spinal animal.

Vestibular Apparatus and Equilibrium (Fig. 8.25)

Vestibular apparatus are concerned with the maintenance of balance. They are made up of bony and membranous labyrinth. In between the bony and membranous labyrinth a fluid called **perilymph** is present.

The membranous labyrinth has three semicircular canals and two large chambers termed **utricle** and **saccule**. Utricle and saccule are together called **otolith organs**. Membranous labyrinth contains the fluid endolymph. The three semicircular canals are lying in three planes at right angles to each other. Crista ampullaris are the end organs in semicircular canals. Macula is the end organ of utricle and saccule.

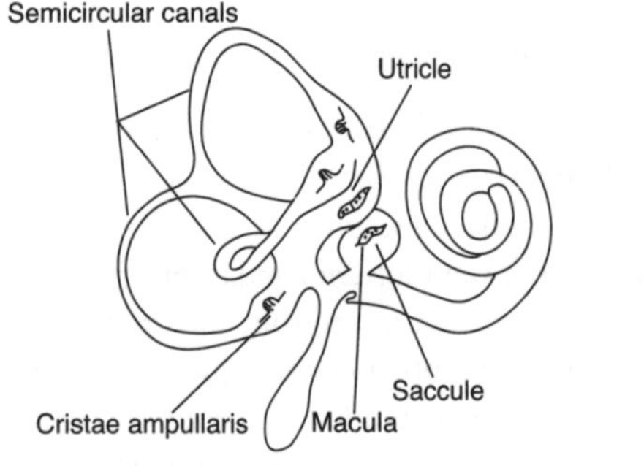

Fig. 8.25   Vestibular apparatus.

Neural Pathway

The cell bodies of neurons supplying crista and macula are present in the vestibular ganglion.

The vestibular nerve ends in vestibular nucleus and flocculonodular lobe of the cerebellum. The vestibular nuclei also project to thalamus and somatosensory cortex.

Crista Ampullaris

Hair cells are the receptors. They are present on a ridge called **crista**. The hair cells of the vestibular apparatus have two types of hair or cilia. Kinocilium is long and located at one end on the hair cell.

Stereocilia shows a gradually increasing length toward the kinocilium. Bending of stereocilia toward the kinocilium results in depolarization and the movement in opposite direction causes hyperpolarization in the hair cells.

Applied Physiology

Abnormal Muscle Tone

Hypertonia

There is increased resistance to passive stretch of the muscle. Hypertonia is due to increased alpha motor neuron activity. This keeps the muscle in a contracted state in spite of effort of the subject to relax.

Hypertonia is commonly seen in disorders of descending tract. The inhibitory influence of descending tract on the motor neuron is decreased.

Spasticity

It is a form of hypertonia in which the muscle develops an increased tone on stretching. There is an initial increase in the tone followed by reduced tone for a brief period. This is observed in **clasp-knife phenomenon**.

Rigidity

It is a type of hypertonia in which resistance to passive stretch is constant and the muscle contraction is prolonged.

Brief contraction of multiple muscle groups is called **spasm**.

Prolonged and painful contraction of muscle is termed **cramps**.

Hypotonia

It is a condition of abnormally low muscle tone associated with weakness and atrophy of the muscle. Hypotonia is common in disorders of alpha motor neurons and cerebellar disease.

Hypotonic muscles which are soft and weak are often described as **flaccid**.

Semicircular Canals

They give information about degree, direction, and plane of the movement of head. In humans they are stimulated by angular acceleration.

When the individual rotates, bony labyrinth and the attached structures move. But the endolymph lags behind. Therefore, hairs in crista move toward the midline in one semicircular canal and away from the midline in the other. This bending of hair causes activation of hair cells and stimulation of the vestibular nerve. If the individual continues to rotate, the endolymph also starts moving and the hair cells regain their initial position as seen at rest. Now the action potential in the vestibular nerve stops. But on stopping the rotatory movement, hair bends in the opposite direction to stimulate the cell again. Thus the direction of rotatory movement can be appreciated.

Utricle and Saccule

These are sac-like structures forming a part of membranous labyrinth. They communicate with each other through ductus endolymphaticus and contain the fluid endolymph.

Otolith Organ

Hair cells, the receptors of otolith organ, are present over the ridge. Cilia are embedded in a jelly-like substance called **otolith membrane**. The membrane has deposition of calcium carbonate crystals termed **otolith**. This membrane is rigid.

Applied Physiology

Motion Sickness

It is produced by stimulation of vestibular apparatus due to jerky movement of the vehicle. The conflicting stimuli about movement within and outside the vehicle cause motion sickness in susceptible individuals. The subject has headache, giddiness, nausea, and vomiting. The manifestations are due to the stimulation of vagus nerve, which lies close to the vestibular apparatus.

Meniere's Disease

It is a disease affecting the vestibular apparatus. The condition is characterized by sudden giddiness, ringing sound in the ear, vomiting, and temporary loss of hearing. The condition is produced due to differences in vestibular input from both the ears.

Nystagmus

It is the jerky back-and-forth or oscillatory movement of eyeballs in response to unusual vestibular inputs. It is a reflex which helps to fix the gaze on an object when the body moves. During movement, eye moves slowly in the direction opposite to that of the body. After reaching the maximum limit, it quickly moves back to the point of new fixation. Slow movement of the eye is influenced by impulses from the labyrinths. The quick component is triggered by brainstem. Nystagmus is of different types. The types are

(a)   horizontal,
(b)   vertical, and
(c)   rotatory.

The direction of eye movement in nystagmus is determined by the direction of quick component.

Nystagmus is seen at rest in patients with lesions of brainstem.

Vertigo

It is the sensation of rotation experienced by an individual in the absence of actual rotation. Inflammation of one of the labyrinth causes vertigo.

Saccules respond to vertical acceleration. It is stimulated by side-to-side movement of the head. When the individual is in erect position, saccules are stimulated due to the effect of gravity. It gives information regarding the position of head in lateral plane.

Utricle responds to horizontal acceleration. Anteroposterior movement of the neck stimulates the hair cells. Utricle gives information about the position of head in anteroposterior plane.

Higher Functions

Memory

It is the ability to store learnt or acquired information and to recollect the same when it is needed.

Memory is of two types:

1. **Explicit memory or declarative or recognition memory:** It is a memory associated with awareness or consciousness. For retention of this memory, hippocampus and medial temporal lobe of the brain are necessary.
2. **Implicit memory or nondeclarative or reflexive memory:** It is associated with the acquired skills and habits which become unconscious and automatic.

Memory involves the following.

Short-Term Memory

This type of memory lasts for few seconds to few hours.

Hippocampus processes the information and converts it into long-term memory. Short-term memory is likely to be lost during damage to the brain.

Long-Term Memory

This type of memory stores the information for years. Long-term memory is stable and is not susceptible for loss in brain damage.

Working Memory

Information is retained only for a short duration when a decision has to be made based on the information.

Mechanism

Memory is dependent on alteration in the synaptic connection involving protein synthesis or activation of related gene. Hippocampus, parahippocampal area of medial temporal cortex, and prefrontal cortex are connected with different aspects of memory.

Learning

It is alteration in the behavior of an individual based on experience and information acquired.

It can be

1. **Associative learning:** In this form of learning, person appreciates the relationship between two stimuli given.
2. **Nonassociative learning:** It is the process of learning about a single stimulus.

Habituation and sensitization are simple forms

Applied Physiology

Amnesia

Amnesia is loss of memory.

Retrograde Amnesia

It is the inability to recall recent memories. It occurs in damage to the brain.

Anterograde Amnesia

It is a condition in which the subject is unable to establish new long-term memory.

Alzheimer's Disease and Senile Dementia

It is a condition with progressive loss of short-term memory followed by loss of other functions of the brain. This disease is common in middle age. It is associated with damage to hippocampus and entorhinal cortex. Histopathologically, neurofibrillary tangles and senile plaques are seen.

of learning. Habituation is a form of nonassociative learning and sensitization is associative learning.

Example

An unconditioned (inborn) response like salivation on giving the food is paired with a conditioned stimulus (acquired) of ringing the bell to produce a conditioned reflex. By this process of learning, animal salivates on ringing the bell even without giving the food.

Operant Conditioning

Animal is taught to perform a task to get a reward or to avoid punishment.

Conditioned Avoidance Reflex

It is the motor response of an animal to avoid an unpleasant sensation.

Speech

Speech is the ability to express oneself with the help of words.

Mechanism

- Wernicke's area located at the posterior end of superior temporal gyrus comprehends the auditory and visual information. (The angular gyrus behind Wernicke's area processes the information about the words which are read.)
- The information is fed to Broca's area of speech through arcuate fasciculus.
- Broca's area analyzes the information received and prepares a pattern for vocalization.
- The pattern is conveyed to motor cortex through speech articulation area in the insula.
- Motor cortex brings about the necessary movements of larynx and lips to produce speech.

Applied Physiology

Aphasia

It is a condition of defective speech without a defect in vision, audition, or motor system.

Nonfluent Aphasia

Defect is in Broca's area. Speech is slow and difficulty is experienced in producing the words.

Fluent Aphasia

Lesion is in the Wernicke's area. Patient has difficulty to understand the spoken and written words. Speech is fluent but with little sense.

Anomic Aphasia

It is the difficulty to understand the written language and pictures due to lesion in angular gyrus of the categorical hemisphere. The visual information is not analyzed and transmitted to Wernicke's area.

Global Aphasia

It is a condition in which Wernicke's area and Broca's area are damaged. Individual lacks the ability to speak, write, or understand the language.

Dyslexia

It is an inherited abnormality characterized by impaired ability to read. The subject has a reduced ability to recall speech sounds or has trouble in translating mentally into sound units.

Slurring or Scanning Speech

It is seen in conditions of cerebellar dysfunction. There is a defect in skilled movements involved in production of speech.

Autonomic Nervous System

The autonomic nervous system (ANS) controls visceral functions of the body.

It has two anatomic divisions:

1. sympathetic nervous system and
2. parasympathetic nervous system.

Organization of Autonomic Outflow

The ANS consists of the preganglionic and post-ganglionic neurons. The cell bodies of preganglionic neurons are located in the intermediolateral gray column of the spinal cord and motor nuclei of the cranial nerves. Axons are myelinated and they synapse with cell bodies of postganglionic neurons located outside the CNS.

Sympathetic Division (Fig. 8.26)

The sympathetic fibers arise from thoracolumbar regions. Axons of the preganglionic sympathetic fibers leave the spinal cord through ventral root. They pass through white rami communicantes to reach paravertebral ganglion chains. In the ganglion, they make synaptic connections with cell bodies of post-ganglionic neurons. The postganglionic neurons pass through sympathetic nerves to reach the viscera.

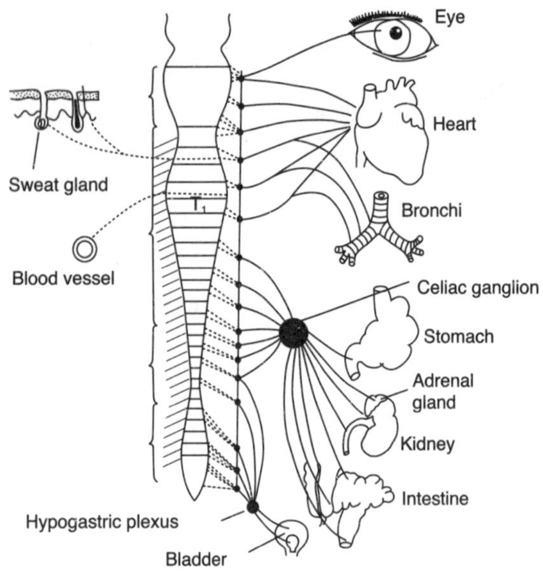

Fig. 8.26 Sympathetic nervous system.

Parasympathetic Division (Fig. 8.27)

The parasympathetic fibers come from craniosacral regions. The preganglionic fibers end on short postganglionic neurons present on or near the viscera.

The cranial division supplies the visceral structures in head, thorax, and upper abdomen through the facial, glossopharyngeal, and vagus nerves.

The sacral division supplies pelvic viscera through the pelvic branches of sacral nerves.

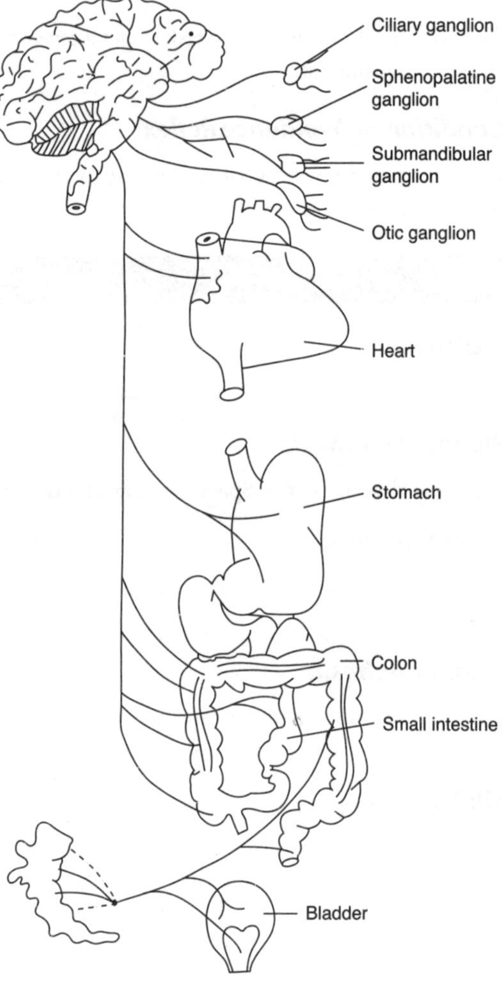

Fig. 8.27 Parasympathetic nervous system.

Neurotransmitters in ANS

Transmission of impulse across pre- and postganglionic neurons, between postganglionic neuron and the effector organ, occurs with the help of a chemical mediator.

Based on the chemical mediator released, ANS is divided into

(a) cholinergic division and
(b) adrenergic division.

The principle neurotransmitters of the ANS are acetylcholine, norepinephrine, and dopamine.

The cholinergic neurons are

- all preganglionic neurons;
- parasympathetic postganglionic neurons;
- sympathetic postganglionic neurons innervating the sweat gland;
- sympathetic neurons innervating the blood vessels to skeletal muscle. Stimulation of these fibers produces vasodilation.

Acetylcholine has two types of receptors, namely,

1. nicotinic receptors and
2. muscarinic receptors.

The neurotransmitters bring about the desired response by acting on the respective receptors.

The adrenergic neurons are postganglionic sympathetic neurons except for the locations mentioned above.

Adrenergic Receptors

α_1 **Receptors**   Located on vascular smooth muscle of skin, GIT, bladder sphincter, and radial muscle of iris.

α_2 **Receptors**   Located at presynaptic nerve terminal, platelet, and walls of GIT.

β_1 **Receptors**   Located in SA node, AV node, and ventricular muscles of the heart.

β_2 **Receptors**   Located at vascular smooth muscle supplying skeletal muscle, bronchial smooth muscle, wall of GIT, and bladder.

α and β_1 receptors are sensitive to epinephrine and norepinephrine.

β_2 receptor is more sensitive to epinephrine.

Stimulation of α_1 and β_1 receptors produces excitation. Stimulation of α_2 and β_2 receptors produces inhibition and relaxation.

Effect of Stimulation of ANS

The smooth muscles of the viscera and internal organs are supplied by cholinergic and noradrenergic divisions. The stimulation of one of the divisions increases the activity in the same division and reduces the activity in the other division. Thus, there is delicate balance between the activities in both the divisions of the ANS.

Cholinergic Division

The stimulation of cholinergic fibers increases the activity of GIT in terms of secretion and motility. This favors digestion and absorption. Hence, cholinergic division is also called **anabolic nervous system**.

Action of acetylcholine, the mediator of cholinergic division, is localized and lasts for a short duration.

Adrenergic Division

This division is activated during fight or flight reactions. It prepares the individual to face the emergencies. The stimulation of noradrenergic division brings about the following changes in the body:

- dilation of pupil for better vision;
- increased heart beat and blood pressure for better tissue perfusion;
- sustained discharges to arterioles to maintain blood pressure;
- reduced threshold in reticular formation for enhancing arousal and alertness;
- increased plasma glucose and fatty acids for improved supply of energy.

Norepinephrine has a widespread action as compared to acetylcholine. Its actions are prolonged. The neurotransmitter and its metabolites are present in the plasma. A part of norepinephrine and dopamine comes from adrenal medulla. Adrenal medulla acts as sympathetic ganglia without the postganglionic fibers.

Autonomic Pharmacology

An alteration in the autonomic function is possible by manipulation of the junctions or pathways by suitable drugs. Drugs are used to influence the neurotransmitter synthesis, storage, release, and binding with the receptors.

The drugs which produce effects similar to sympathetic and parasympathetic stimulation are called **sympathomimetic** and **parasympath-omimetic drugs**.

The sympathetic and parasympathetic blockers prevent the action of respective neurotransmitter at the target site by blocking the receptors.

Some important actions of autonomic nervous system are given in the following table:

Organ	Parasympathetic Stimulation	Sympathetic Stimulation
Eye		
Iris	Pupillary constriction	Pupillary dilation
Heart		
SA node	Decreased heart rate	Increased heart rate
Atria	Decreased contrac-tility	Increased contrac-tility
AV node	Decreased conduc-tion	Increased conduc-tion velocity
Ventricles	Decreased contrac-tility	Increased contrac-tility
Arterioles		
Coronary	Dilation	Constriction/dilation
Skeletal muscle	Dilation	Constriction/dilation
Cerebral	Dilation	Constriction
Lungs		
Bronchial muscle	Contraction (bron-choconstriction)	Relaxation (broncho-dilation)
GIT		
Motility	Increased	Decreased
Sphincter	Relaxation	Contraction
Secretion	Increased	Decreased
Detrusor muscle	Contraction	Relaxation
Sphincter	Relaxation	Contraction

9

Special Senses

The normal functioning of the body is influenced by changes in the external environment. These changes are perceived by the sensory system.

The sensations are of two types:

1. general sensations involving the appreciation of touch, pain, and temperature;
2. special sensations.

The receptors for general sensations are present all over the body and respond to different types of stimuli.

The receptors for special sensations are located in regions close to the central nervous system. They respond to one type of stimulus.

The special sensations are functionally important as they can appreciate the stimulus from a distance.

The special senses are

- vision,
- hearing or auditory sense,
- taste,
- smell or olfaction, and
- skin.

Vision

The eye is the receptor organ for vision. The visual stimuli provide information about the world around us. Vision is a process by which the brain creates representation of the external world. A relatively large area of the brain is involved in perception and interpretation of the visual information. This clearly emphasizes the importance of vision.

Anatomy of Eye (Fig. 9.1)

The human eye is present in the orbit. The orbit is a bony structure which protects the eyeball.

Eyes have evolved from the light-sensitive spot present in invertebrates.

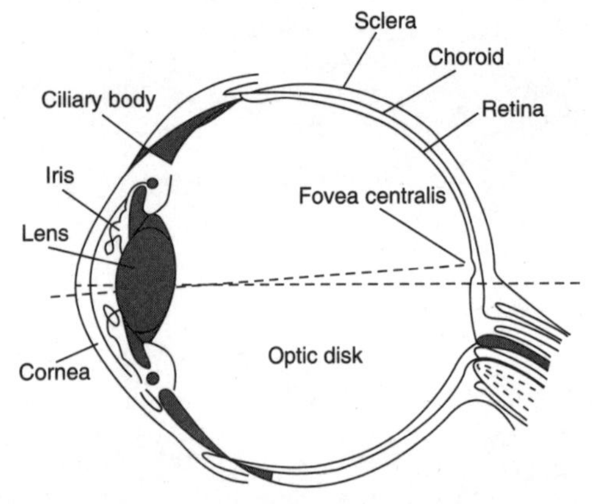

Fig. 9.1   Structure of the eye.

Each eye has

- layer of light-sensitive receptors,
- lens system to focus light on these receptors, and
- system of nerves to carry impulses from receptors to the brain.

Wall of the eyeball is made up of three layers, namely,

1. sclera (outer layer),
2. choroid (middle layer), and
3. retina (inner layer).

Sclera

It is a tough white fibrous layer which continues as the transparent cornea anteriorly. The cornea is an avascular structure (i.e., it has no blood supply). Light passes through the cornea to enter the eye.

Cornea

This is a transparent structure present in the anterior part of the eyeball. It is around 11 mm in diameter and 0.5–1 mm in thickness.

It has a rich nerve supply. The free nerve endings in the cornea carry sensory information of pain, touch, and temperature.

It is avascular. Nutrition is provided by the lymph and aqueous humor.

It has a refractive index of 1.38.

The cornea plays an important role in focusing light on the pigment layer, the **retina**. The major part of bending of the light ray occurs as it passes from air into the cornea.

The cornea is a curved structure. The light originating from a source reaches the cornea at different angles. It gets bent to varying extent to be focused on the most sensitive part of the retina, the **fovea centralis**. The image formed on the retina is upside down with respect to the object.

The cornea contains the following layers:

- corneal epithelium,
- Bowman's membrane,
- substantia propria,
- Descemet's membrane, and
- corneal endothelium.

Applied Physiology

Corneal Grafting

Blindness due to opacities in cornea is treated by replacing the defective cornea with a healthy cornea taken from a donor (eye donation). The procedure is termed **corneal grafting**. Cornea is an avascular structure; hence, the chances of graft rejection are very low. Rejection of a graft or transplanted organ is common in other location due to vascularity and immune reactions.

The corneal endothelium maintains the transparency of cornea.

The cornea is transparent because of

- unique architecture of the collagen fibers,
- lack of blood vessels, and
- presence of active mechanism that prevents the accumulation of water.

The epithelial layer can repair minor injuries to the surface of cornea. However, deeper corneal injuries result in the development of opacities.

Lens

The lens is the main refracting medium of the eye situated between the iris in front and the vitreous humor behind.

It is a transparent, elastic, biconvex structure. It is encased by a capsule held in place by the lens ligament (zonule). It is attached to the thickened anterior part of the choroid termed the ciliary body. The contraction of the ciliary body decreases tension in the ligament and the anterior surface of the lens bulges.

The lens has a refractive index of 1.4 at the center and less at the periphery.

It is made up of ribbon-like transparent fibers arranged in concentric lamella. The peripheral part is nucleated, while the central part is non-nucleated.

Functions

The lens helps in the refraction of light to focus it on the retina.

Choroid

It is the vascular layer which forms the iris and the ciliary body anteriorly. The blood vessels in the choroid nourish structures in the eye.

Choroid is a thin, deeply pigmented layer consisting of blood vessels and connective tissue network.

Anteriorly, the choroid continues as uvea which thickens to form the **ciliary body**.

The ciliary body is made up of ciliary muscle which helps in adjusting the curvature of the lens.

The anterior one-third of ciliary body forms the ciliary process. It is involved in the production of aqueous humor.

From the ciliary body projects a thin contractile tissue called the **iris**. The iris is highly pigmented and is responsible for the color of the eye.

The central aperture of the iris is called the **pupil**. The iris contains the sphincter pupillae and dilator pupillae muscles which help to change the size of the pupil.

Applied Physiology

Cataract

The opacity of the lens is termed **cataract**. The cataract that develops during the old age is **senile cataract**. An injury to the lens can also cause opacity. This is called **traumatic cataract**.

The persons exposed to the ultraviolet rays and heat are at a greater risk of developing cataract. An alteration in the ionic environment surrounding the lens is the cause for cataract. There is an increase in the water content, sodium, and calcium ion, which is associated with a decrease in the potassium ion concentration. An increase in the calcium ion concentration enhances the accumulation of high-molecular-weight lens proteins. An aggregation of insoluble lens protein disturbs the arrangement of the protein molecules rendering the lens opaque.

Treatment

The treatment of cataract is removal of the opaque lens. Nowadays, **synthetic intraocular lens** is inserted to improve the vision.

Functions of Iris

- Adjusts the amount of light falling on the retina.
- Improves the clarity of image by cutting the peripheral rays of light.
- Increases the depth of the focus.

Retina

It is a layer containing the visual receptors, rods and cones. It stops short anteriorly near the ciliary body.

Retina is the light-sensitive portion of the eye (Fig 9.2). It converts the visual stimuli into nerve impulses and transmits it to the central nervous system.

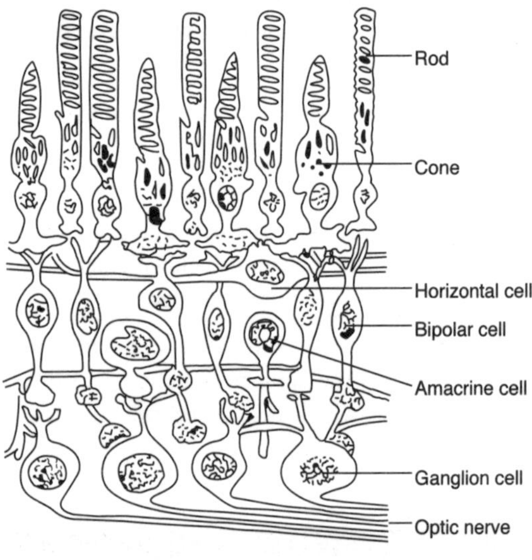

Fig. 9.2   Retina.

Layers

The retina is organized into ten layers. The layers from outside to inside are as under:

1. pigment epithelium,
2. rods and cones,
3. outer limiting membrane,
4. outer nuclear layer,
5. outer plexiform layer,
6. inner nuclear layer,
7. inner plexiform layer,
8. ganglion cell layer,
9. layer of optic nerve fibers, and
10. inner limiting membrane.

The rods and cones are the visual receptors. In addition to rods and cones, the retina contains bipolar cells, amacrine cells, horizontal cells, and ganglion cells.

The rods and cones synapse with bipolar cells and bipolar cells synapse with ganglion cells. The ganglion cells send axons which form the optic nerve. The horizontal cells connect the receptor cells to one another in the outer plexiform layer. The amacrine cells connect the ganglion cells to one another in the inner plexiform layer.

The light entering the eye first passes through the inner limiting membrane and then through all other layers finally to reach the layer of rods and cones.

The receptor layer of the retina rests on the pigment epithelium. The pigment layer absorbs the light and prevents its reflection. The reflection of light results in blurring of the visual images.

The optic nerve is formed by the axons of the ganglion cells. It leaves the eye and the retinal blood vessels enter at a point 3 mm medial and slightly above the posterior pole of the eyeball. This region is the **optic disk**. There are no visual receptors in the optic disk and hence this forms the **blind spot**.

At the posterior pole of the eye there is a yellowish pigmented spot called the **macula lutea**.

The central part of the macula is the **fovea centralis**. It is a minute area occupying about 1 mm^2. This area has only cones. Each cone synapses with a bipolar cell which in turn synapses with a ganglion cell. It provides direct pathway to the brain. The blood vessels, ganglion cells, and other layers are all displaced to one side, allowing the light to pass undisturbed to the cones in this region. The color vision and bright-light vision are best in this area. When attention is fixed on the object, the light rays coming from the object get focused at the fovea centralis.

Extrinsic Eye Muscles

The movements of the eyeball are controlled by six extrinsic muscles. They originate from the bony orbit and get inserted into the outer surface of the eyeball. The four rectus muscles originate from the tendinous ring called the annular ring at the back of the orbit, run straight, and get inserted on the eyeball. The superior oblique muscle originates with the rectus muscle and gets inserted to the superolateral surface of the eyeball. The inferior oblique muscle originates from the medial surface of the orbit and gets inserted to the inferolateral surface of the eyeball.

The extrinsic muscles of the eye are the most precisely and rapidly controlled skeletal muscles. Each motor unit has 8–12 muscle cells.

These muscles

- help the eye to follow moving objects,
- maintain the shape of the eyeball, and
- hold the eyeball in the orbit.

Name of the Muscle	Action	Nerve Supply
Lateral rectus	Lateral movement of eye (abduction)	VI (abducens)
Medial rectus	Medial movement of eye (adduction)	III (oculomotor)
Superior rectus	Elevates the eyeball	III (oculomotor)
Inferior rectus	Depresses the eyeball	III (oculomotor)
Inferior oblique	Elevates and turns the eye laterally	III (oculomotor)
Superior oblique	Depresses and turns the eye laterally	IV (trochlear)

Blood Supply

The internal layers of the retina are supplied by branches of the central retinal artery. The rods and cones layer of the retina is dependent on diffusion from the choroid for their nutrition. Therefore, the retinal detachment causes degeneration of the retina and blindness.

Electroretinogram

Electroretinogram (ERG) is the recording of electrical activities from the eye. One electrode is placed over the cornea and the other over the skin of the head. A flash of light produces electrical activity in the eye. A typical recording shows rapid a- and b-waves due to the electrical activity in the retina and a slower c-wave produced by the pigment epithelium.

Uses

- To diagnose diseases in conditions where the retina cannot be visualized
- To detect congenital retinal dystrophy (in these conditions the retina appears normal by ophthalmoscopic examination)

Critical Fusion Frequency

Critical fusion frequency (CFF) is the rate at which the visual stimuli presented to the eye are appreciated as separate stimuli. The stimuli presented at a higher rate than CFF are appreciated as continuous stimuli. In motion pictures, frames are projected at a rate greater than CFF.

Intraocular Fluid

The eye contains two types of fluids:

1. **Aqueous humor:** Lies in front of the lens and behind the cornea
2. **Vitreous humor:** Lies between the lens and the retina

Aqueous Humor

It is a clear watery fluid occupying both anterior and posterior chambers of the eye.

It is produced by the ciliary body by diffusion and active transport. It flows through the pupil to fill the anterior chamber of the eye. It is absorbed through a network of trabeculae into the canal of Schlemm, a venous channel at the junction of the iris, and the cornea.

Properties

Reaction	Alkaline
Specific gravity	1.002–1.004
Refractive index	1.34

Aqueous humor closely resembles CSF in its chemical composition.

Functions

- Maintains intraocular pressure and shape of the eyeball
- Acts as a refractive medium
- Supplies nutrition and drains metabolites from surrounding structures

Regulation

- Parasympathetic stimulation: ↑ secretion
- Sympathetic stimulation: ↓ secretion
  Normal intraocular pressure is 12–20 mm Hg.

Vitreous Humor (Vitreous Body)

It is a jelly-like substance present in vitreous chamber. Vitreous humor is present between the lens anteriorly and the retina posteriorly. It holds the retina over the choroid, providing an even surface for the reception of light. Vitreous humor is formed during embryonic life and does not get replaced later. It contains phagocytic cells which remove the debris.

Lacrimal Apparatus

Lacrimal apparatus consists of lacrimal glands present in the upper and outer part of the orbit. It secretes a watery fluid called tears.

The tears spread over the eyes by blinking. They collect at inner angle of the eye. The tears then pass through the following structures:

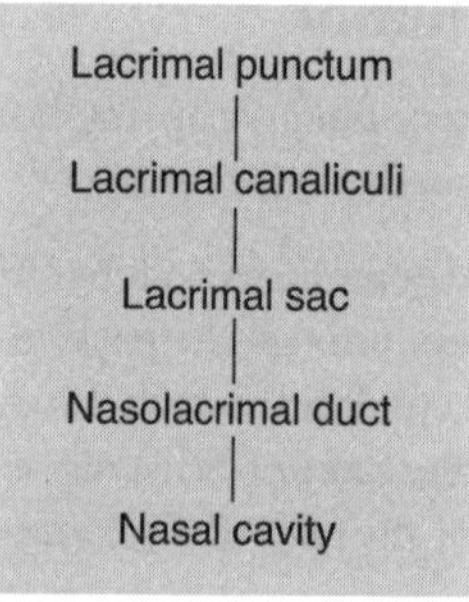

Functions of Tears

- Keep the exposed surface of eye moist
- Protect the eye from microbes and irritant substances

Principal of Optics

The passage of light rays from one medium to other medium with different optical densities results in its bending. This is termed **refraction**. When the gaze is fixed at a distant object, the light entering the eye gets bent and comes to focus on the retina. A major part of refraction occurs at the air corneal interface.

The refracting media of the eye are

- cornea,
- aqueous humor,
- lens, and
- vitreous humor.

Principal Focus (Focal Point)

It is the point at which the parallel rays of light striking a convex lens are brought to focus.

The light rays coming from an object placed at a distance of more than 6 m (20 ft) are considered parallel. Hence, the charts to assess distant vision are placed at a distance of 6 m from the patient.

The rays coming from an object closer than 6 m are divergent.

Focal Length

It is the distance between the principal focus and the center of curvature of the lens.

Applied Physiology

Glaucoma

Glaucoma is a pathological condition in which normally the intraocular pressure is increased.

It is caused by a defective absorption of the aqueous humor due to obstruction at the trabeculae or the canal of Schlemm.

The causes for obstruction are

- decreased permeability through the trabeculae (open-angle glaucoma);
- forward movement of iris closing the angle (angle-closure glaucoma).

This leads to compression of the optic disk and blindness.

Principal Axis

It is the line passing through the centers of curvature of lens. Principal focus is located on principal axis.

Diopter

The refractive power of the lens is expressed as diopter (D). The greater the curvature of lens, greater is the refractive power. It is reciprocal of the focal length in meters:

$$\text{Diopter} = \frac{1}{\text{Focal length (in meters)}}.$$

Convex lens is positive. It converges the light rays.

Concave lens is negative. Biconcave lens diverges the light rays.

The normal human eye has a refractive power of about 60 D. The cornea contributes a refracting power of about 45 D, whereas lens provides about 15 D.

Reduced Eye

The refraction of light at different refracting media of the eye before it comes to focus on retina is complex. Hence, a simplified model to explain optics of the eye was developed by Listing. This is called the **reduced eye**.

The reduced eye has a single refracting surface. This is resultant of all refracting surfaces of the eye. The center of the optical system, termed the **nodal point**, is located 1.5 mm behind the anterior surface of the cornea.

The focal length of reduced eye is 17 mm and the refractive power is about 59 D.

Emmetropic Eye

Parallel rays of light are focused on the retina. This is a normal eye.

Errors of Refraction (Fig. 9.3)

Ametropic Eye

Parallel rays of light are not focused on the retina. The errors of refraction are

- myopia,
- hypermetropia,
- presbyopia, and
- astigmatism

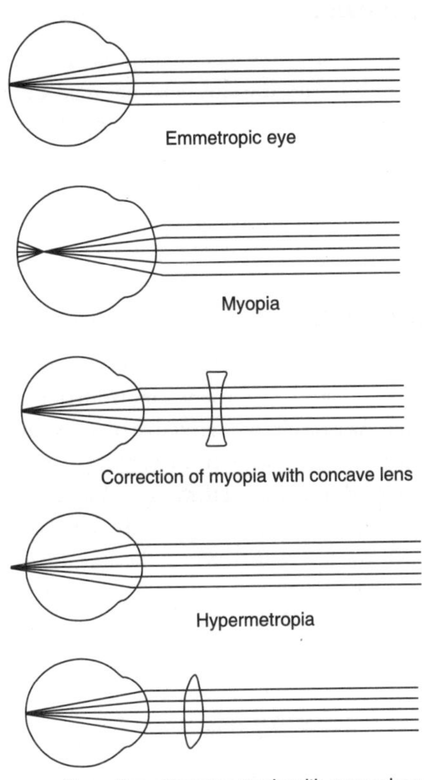

Fig. 9.3   Errors of refraction.

Myopia (Short-Sightedness)

In myopia, the person is unable to see the distant objects clearly. The defect is due to elongation of the eyeball (increase in anteroposterior diameter) or increased curvature of the cornea. Image of the distant object is focused in front of the retina. It is corrected by concave lens (diverging lens).

Myopia is seen in younger individuals. The defect increases as the age advances due to increase in the size of the eyeball.

Hypermetropia (Long-Sightedness)

In hypermetropia, the person is not able to see the nearby objects clearly. It is due to a decrease in the anteroposterior diameter of the eyeball. The light rays from the nearby objects are focused behind the retina. The correction is made by a convex lens (converging lens).

Presbyopia

Presbyopia is an adult type of hypermetropia. After the age of 40 years, the lens becomes rigid and hence there is a decrease in the power of accommodation. Such persons are not able to see the nearby objects and letters clearly at the usual distance for reading. This is corrected by using a convex lens (bifocal lens).

Astigmatism

In this condition, the curvature of the cornea and rarely the curvature of the lens vary from one plane to the other. As a result, the refractive power is different in different planes. Image from all parts of the object is not properly formed on the retina. A clear image of the object from the vertical and horizontal axes does not form on the retina. When the image from the horizontal axis is clear, image from the vertical axis is not clear. The defect is corrected by a cylindrical lens.

Visual Pathway (Fig. 9.4)

The visual pathway conveys the visual signal from the eye to the CNS.

The receptors for vision are the rods and cones. They synapse with the bipolar cells. The bipolar cells synapse with the ganglion cells. Axons of the ganglion cells form the optic nerve.

The fibers of each optic nerve decussate (crossover) partially at the optic chiasma. The fibers from the nasal half of each retina cross to the opposite side, but those from the temporal halves do not cross.

After the decussation, optic tract is formed. The fibers of the optic tract end in the lateral geniculate body.

From the lateral geniculate body, the neurons proceed as the optic radiation (geniculocalcarine tract) to terminate in the primary visual cortex (Brodmann's area 17).

Lesions (Fig. 9.5)

(a) **Lesion of the optic nerve:** *Blindness* of the corresponding eye

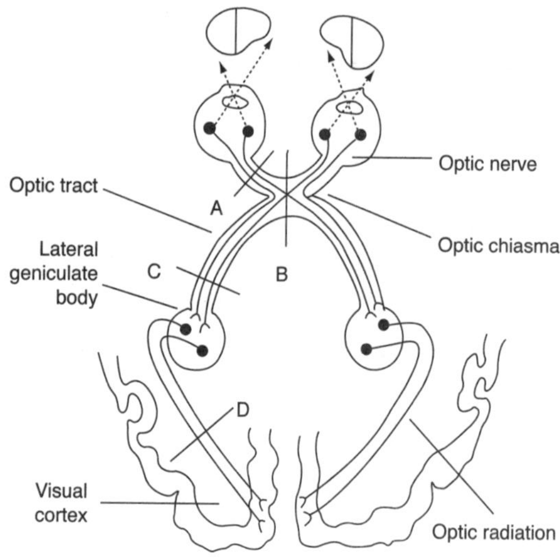

Fig. 9.4 Visual pathway.

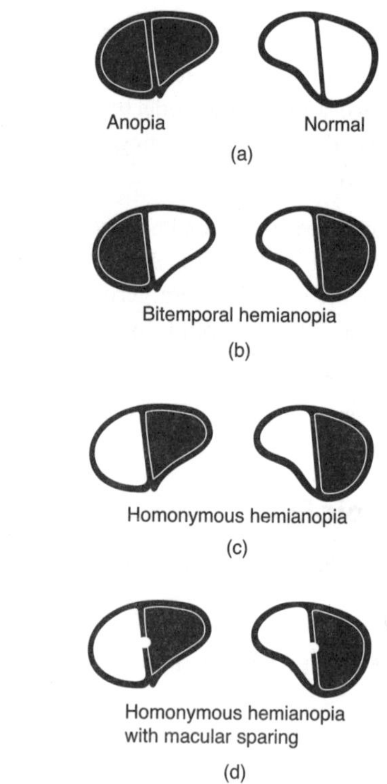

Fig. 9.5 Lesions at different levels of visual pathway.

(b) **Lesion in the midline at the optic chiasma:** *Bitemporal hemianopia* (hemi, one-half, anopia, blindness; hemianopia is blindness in one-half of the eye. In this condition, temporal halves of both the eyes are blind.)

   Lesion of the lateral portions of the optic chiasma: *Binasal hemianopia*

(c) **Lesion in the optic tract:** *Homonymous hemianopia* (lesion of the right optic tract results in left-sided homonymous hemianopia). The blindness is present in corresponding half of each eye. Nasal side of right eye & temporal side of left eye are blind.

(d) **Lesion in the optic radiation:** *Homonymous hemianopia with macular sparing* (vision in the region of macula lutea is retained)

   Lesion in the occipital cortex: *Scotoma* in the opposite eye

Macular Sparing

It is a condition characterized by loss of peripheral vision with an intact macular vision. The macular sparing is common in the occipital lesions. The macular representation in the visual cortex is very large and separate from that of the peripheral fields.

An extensive damage to the occipital cortex results in the loss of both peripheral and macular vision.

Bilateral destruction of occipital cortex results in subjective blindness. There is still a residual response to a visual stimuli. It is termed **blindsight**.

Anopia

The loss of vision in one eye is termed anopia.

Hemianopia

The loss of vision in one-half of the eye is termed hemianopia.

Homonymous Hemianopia

The loss of vision in the nasal half of one eye and the temporal half of the other (loss of vision in the corresponding half of the eye) is termed homonymous hemianopia.

Lateral Geniculate Body

It relays the visual information from the optic tract to the visual cortex by way of the optic radiation.

It has six layers:

- Layers I and II contain large neurons and are called **magnocellular layers**.
- Layers III–VI have small- to medium-sized neurons and are called **parvocellular layers**.

The magnocellular pathway carries signals for the detection of movement, depth, and flicker.

The parvocellular pathway carries signals for color vision, texture, shape, and finer details of the object.

Visual Cortex

It is located in the occipital lobe. It is divided into primary visual cortex and secondary visual cortex.

Primary Visual Cortex

It lies in the calcarine fissure. The signals from the macular area of the retina terminate near the occipital pole, whereas signals from the peripheral areas terminate in the concentric circles around it.

It corresponds to area 17 of the Brodmann's cortical area.

Secondary Visual Cortex

The visual association areas surround the primary visual cortex. The signals transmitted to these areas are for visual interpretation. It corresponds to areas 18 and 19 of the Brodmann's cortical area.

Light Reflex

It is a change in the size of the pupil as a reflex in response to a change in illumination.

When a beam of light is shone into the eye, it results in constriction of the pupil.

The change noted in the same eye is called the **direct light reflex**.

The corresponding change seen in the other eye is called the **indirect light reflex**.

Pathway

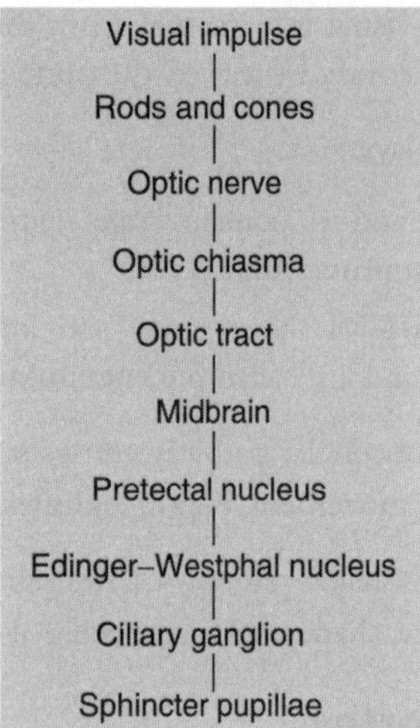

Functions

- Adjusts the amount of light entering the eye
- Prevents spherical aberration by cutting off the peripheral rays
- Increases the depth of focus

Accommodation

It is the adjustment of the visual apparatus to focus image of the near objects on the retina.

Changes during accommodation are

- convergence of eyeball,
- constriction of pupil, and
- change in anterior curvature of the lens.

Mechanism

Convergence of the Two Optical/Visual Axes

This is brought about by internal rotation of the eyeball due to contraction of the medial rectus. This effect is also mediated by III cranial nerve (oculomotor).

Constriction of Pupil

This effect is caused by contraction of sphincter pupillae. The action is mediated by III cranial nerve.

Change in Curvature of Lens

At rest, suspensory ligament of the lens is tense. Traction on the capsule of lens causes flattening of the anterior surface of the lens. When the eye gets accommodated to near vision, ciliary muscle contracts causing relaxation of the suspensory ligament. Natural elasticity of the lens makes it more convex. More spherical shape of the lens provides additional bending of the light ray which is necessary to focus nearby objects on the retina.

Pathway for Accommodation Reflex

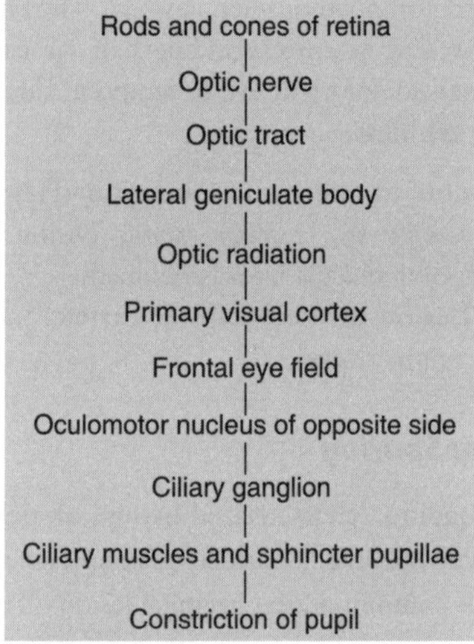

Change in Curvature of Lens

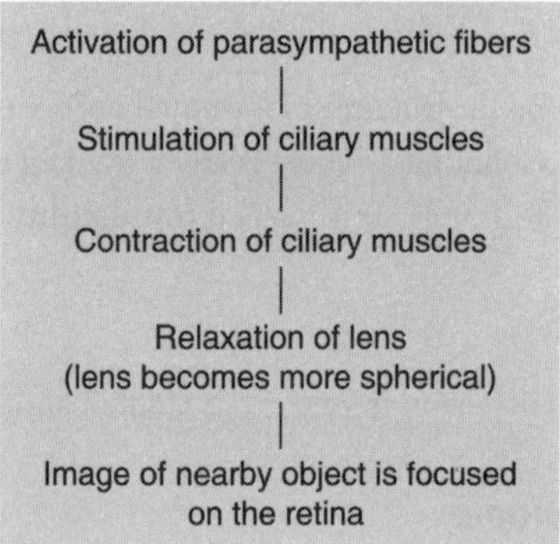

Near Point

It is the nearest point to the eye at which an object placed can be brought into clear focus by accommodation.

Near point is about 9 cm at the age of 10 years. It recedes as the age advances, reaching about 83 cm at the age of 60 years.

Recession in near point of vision is due to increase in hardness of lens and loss of accommodation.

Purkinje–Sanson Images

The Purkinje–Sanson images help to demonstrate that the anterior curvature of the lens increases during accommodation.

When a lighted candle is held in front of the eyes with subject looking at a distant object, three images of the candle are seen:

1. bright, upright image formed by anterior surface of the cornea;
2. large, upright image produced by anterior surface of the lens;
3. bright, smaller inverted image formed by posterior surface of the lens.

When the subject looks at a nearby object, there is no change in the position of images 1 and 3. However, image 2 becomes smaller and moves toward image 1, indicating that the anterior curvature of the lens has increased.

Argyll Robertson Pupil

In this condition, the light reflex is lost but the accommodation reflex is retained.

Site of Lesion

Damage to the fibers from pretectal nucleus to Edinger–Westphal nucleus

This occurs in syphilitic lesion of the CNS.

Visual Acuity

Visual acuity is the ability of the eye to identify two points separated in space as two distinct points.

It indicates the clarity of vision.

The two points of an object can be seen separately as two distinct points when they form an angle of 1 min or more (visual angle) at the nodal point of the eye.

Snellen's chart or **Landolt C chart** is used to test the visual acuity for distant vision. The chart contains letters/numbers/objects of different sizes.

Applied Physiology

Squint or Strabismus

It is a condition where the visual axes of the two eyes are not parallel.

Types of squint are

1. convergent squint and
2. divergent squint.

Based on the development it is classified as

1. **Congenital squint**: It is present since birth. There is no paralysis of the extraocular muscles. It is commonly seen in subjects with uncorrected refractive errors.
2. **Paralytic squint:** It is due to paralysis of the extraocular muscle. Damage to III cranial nerve results in a lateral squint. Double vision (diplopia) is a prominent feature of this condition.

Development of Squint

The formation of visual images in noncorresponding points on the retina results in double vision or diplopia. In children below the age of 6 years, diplopia is compensated by suppression of one of the defective images. The visual axis of the defective eye is moved away from the line of focus. The deviation of defective eye results in the development of squint.

The suppression of one of the images results in the suppression scotoma. Uncorrected suppression of the image can result in permanent blindness. The loss of vision in these cases is called **amblyopia** (anopia).

Treatment for squint must be started before the age of 6 years for best results.

The topmost row has the biggest size and a normal man can see it from a distance of 60 m. The second line on the chart should be seen from a distance of 36 m. The subsequent lines should be seen from the distances of 24, 18, 12, 9, and 6 m, respectively.

The subject is seated at a distance of 6 m (20 ft) from the chart. At this distance the eye receives the parallel rays of light. The normal visual acuity is expressed as 6/6. The numerator indicates the distance between the subject and the chart. The denominator indicates the distance from which the letter should be read by a normal person.

The numerator is constant and the denominator varies.

The near vision is tested by using **Jaeger's test chart** held at a distance of 30 cm. The normal individual is able to read the smallest type with each eye separately.

Other Tests

The perception of light, hand movements, and finger-counting tests are used to assess the retinal function.

Photochemistry of Vision

Rods and cones (Fig. 9.6) are the receptors for vision. The rods are narrower and longer than the cones. The outer segment of the cone is conical in shape.

Structure of Rods and Cones

The rods and cones contain the following:

(a) **Outer segment:** Rods are modified cilia and are made up of regular stacks of flattened saccules or disks. There are around 1000 disks in each rod or cone. They contain visual pigments.

(b) **Inner segment:** It consists of usual cytoplasm of the cell with its organelles. Mitochondria play a major role in providing energy for the function of photoreceptors.

(c) **Nucleus:** It is similar to the nucleus of other cells in structure and function.

(d) **Synaptic body:** It connects visual receptors with other retinal cells.

There are approximately 3 million cones and 120 million rods in each eye and 1.2 million nerve fibers in each optic nerve.

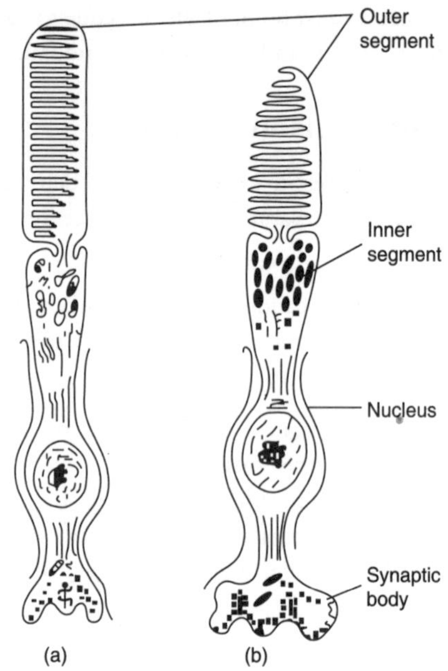

Fig. 9.6   Structure of (a) rods and (b) cones.

Both rods and cones contain chemicals that decompose on exposure to light. Rods contain rhodopsin (scotopsin and retinal). Cones contain cone pigments (photopsin and retinal).

Rhodopsin

It is the light-sensitive visual pigment present in the rods. It is a combination of the protein scotopsin and 11-*cis*-retinal.

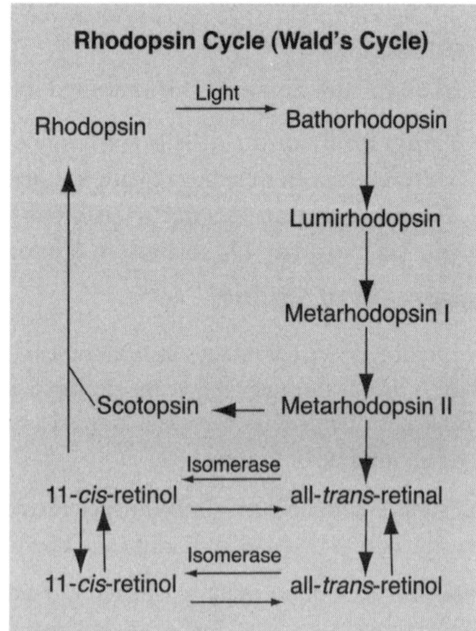

Metarhodopsin II activates the rods and transmits visual impulses to the CNS. The synthesis of visual pigment requires vitamin A. Vitamin A is present in the cytoplasm of the rods and in the pigment layer of retina as all-*trans*-retinol. This is used to produce new retinal whenever needed. When there is excess retinal it is converted back to vitamin A.

Night-Blindness (Nyctalopia) This occurs in persons with severe vitamin A deficiency. The nonavailability of vitamin A leads to decreased formation of rhodopsin. The amount of light available in the night becomes too little to permit satisfactory vision.

Electrical Activity in Rods The membrane potential inside the rods is about −40 mV. The inner segment of rod continuously pumps out sodium creating a negative potential in the inner segment. The outer segment is leaky to sodium and, therefore, sodium ions continuously leak into the rods.

When rhodopsin in the outer segment is exposed to light, it begins to decompose. 11-*cis*-retinene gets converted to all-*trans*-retinene. There is a change in the configuration of opsin. This activates a G-protein, transducin. These changes in turn activate cGMP phosphodiesterase. Phosphodiesterase reduces the concentration of cGMP, which acts directly on the sodium channel and keeps it closed.

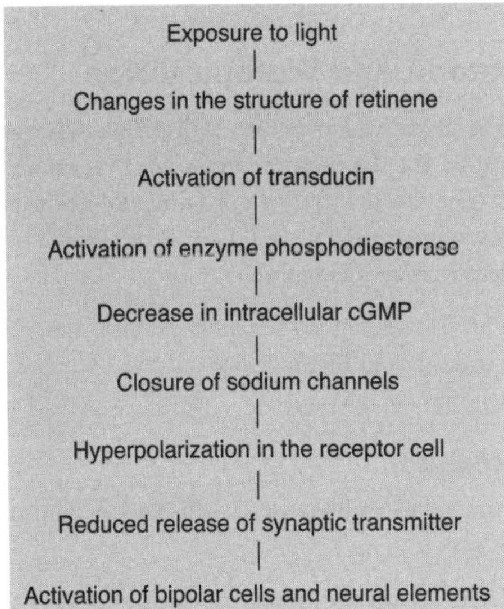

Subsequently, the conductance of sodium ions in the outer segment is reduced even though sodium ions are pumped out of the inner segment. This creates increased negativity inside the rods leading to hyperpolarization. Hyperpolarization reduces synaptic transmitter release. The response is produced in the bipolar cells and other neural elements.

Duplicity Theory

The CNS receives two kinds of inputs from the eye. The inputs are from rods and cones. Two kinds of inputs working maximally at different intensities of illumination is called the **duplicity theory**.

Dark Adaptation

When a person moves from a brightly lit area to a dark area, the retina becomes more sensitive to light and visual threshold decreases. This is known as **dark adaptation**. These changes help in better visibility in the dark.

The perception of bright light and color vision is due to cones. When the subject enters a dark room the rod vision takes over.

During the dark adaptation there is regeneration of the rhodopsin pigment and the scotopic vision becomes possible.

The gain of optical system increases due to summation. The efficiency of the visual apparatus increases. It gives an increased response to low-intensity stimulation.

The dark adaptation occurs in 20 min and is completed by about 40 min.

The dark adaptation time can be reduced by wearing red goggles when the subject is in bright light.

The subjects with vitamin A deficiency are susceptible to night-blindness and have a poor dark adaptation.

Light Adaptation

When a person coming from a dark area is suddenly exposed to bright light, he/she requires some time to adjust to this bright light. The change in the visual apparatus to suit the altered condition is called the **light adaptation**. Exposure to bright light results in instantaneous breakdown to photopigments in both the rods and the cones. This increases signals generated at the retina producing glare.

During light adaptation,

- the sensitivity of retina is decreased drastically and
- the retinal neurons adapt rapidly, switching from rods to cones system. The cones are stimulated in about 60 s to take over the bright-light vision.

The visual acuity and color vision improve over the next 5–10 min. During light adaptation, retinal sensitivity (function of rod) is reduced but the visual acuity is increased.

Field of Vision

The part of space seen by each eye at a given instant is called the field of vision.

The field of vision is not conical in cross-section.

It measures as follows:

- medially—60°,
- superiorly—50°,
- laterally—100°, and
- inferiorly—75°.

The medial parts of the visual field of each eye overlap. Both the eyes see objects in this part of the visual field. This is called binocular field of vision. The binocular field of vision is helpful for depth perception.

The field of vision is restricted on the superior side by the orbital ridge, medially by the bridge of the nose, and inferiorly by the maxillary prominence. The lateral field of vision is the greatest because there is no obstruction.

Damage to the optic nerve fibers from the peripheral retina due to pressure near the optic disk results in reduced field of vision termed the **tubular vision**.

Types of Vision

Binocular Vision

The central part of visual fields of both the eyes overlap. The objects located in this region are appreciated by both the eyes. This is termed the **binocular vision**. Impression of a single object is formed by fusion of retinal images from both the eyes at the cortical level. If the images are not formed at the corresponding points on the retina of both the eyes, fusion becomes defective. This results in **diplopia** or **double vision**.

Binocular vision is helpful in perception of depth.

Color Vision

The ability of a person to identify different colors by a light-adopted eye is called **color vision**. The colors that we appreciate are related to the wavelength of light reflected, absorbed, or transmitted by the objects around us.

The color of the object is appreciated as red when the light of longer wavelength (red) is reflected by the object. The white light is a mixture of lights of all wavelengths.

The absence of all types of light gives the perception of black.

Primary colors of vision are

- red,
- green, and
- blue.

A normal eye can see all wavelengths of light between violet and red.

Photopic and Scotopic Vision

The scotopic vision is dim light vision. The visual receptors for the night and dim light vision are the rods. The scotopic visual apparatus are not capable of resolving the details and boundaries of the object or determining their color.

The visual receptors for photopic vision are cones. The cones have a higher threshold and a better acuity of vision.

Mechanism

Young and Helmholtz described the mechanism of color vision.

There are three different types of cones for three primary colors. The colors other than primary colors are appreciated by the differential stimulation of these cones.

Three types of cones are as follows:

1. **Red-sensitive:** Maximum sensitivity at 580 nm
2. **Green-sensitive:** Maximum sensitivity at 535 nm
3. **Blue-sensitive:** Maximum sensitivity at 440 nm

The pigments in the retinal cones that are sensitive to red, green, and blue range of colors in the spectrum are **erythrolabe**, **chlorolabe**, and **cyanolabe**, respectively.

When a strong red light falls on the eye, only red cones are stimulated and the individual appreciates red color.

When any color other than the primary colors is seen, three types of cones get activated to a varying extent. The summated response results in perception of a nonprimary color.

The visual impulses from different cones are carried to the occipital cortex. It is this area where differentiation of the visual impulses takes place and there is perception of various colors along with the complimentary colors. The color vision is grossly affected when this part of the cerebral cortex is damaged.

Color-blindness

The subnormal or total absence of color vision is called color-blindness.

Color-blindness is inherited as a X linked recessive character. Males have color-blindness if their X chromosome has the abnormal gene. However, females exhibit the defect if both their X chromosomes have defective genes. X-linked color-blindness skips generations and appears more commonly in males of every second generation.

Types

Monochromats

They have one type of cone. They are color-blind. But the condition is rare.

Dichromats

They have two types of cones. One type of cone is absent.

- **Protanopia:** Red color-blindness
- **Deuteranopia:** Green color-blindness
- **Tritanopia:** Blue color-blindness

Trichromats

They have all three types of cones but one of them is weak. They have subnormal color vision.

Tests for Color Vision

- **Color-matching test (Holmgren's wool test):** The subject is given a set of colored wool. He has to match the given sample color by selecting colored wool from the given set.

- **Ishihara's chart (pseudoisochromatic test):** Test consists of specially designed cards containing a number or letter on a colored background. The normal person identifies the designated number or letter and the color-blind individual will identify it wrongly. The key given with the chart can be used to confirm the correctness of identification.

- **Edridge–Green lantern:** In this test, the different colors are focused through a small illuminated area and the subject identifies the same. This test is commonly used for testing the color vision of drivers.

- **Spectroscopic test:** In this test, the subject identifies the colors in the spectrum, their limit, and position.

Perception of an Image

When we look at an object, the light rays from it pass through the refracting medium of the eye, namely, cornea, aqueous humor, lens, and vitreous humor. During the passage of light through these refracting media, the light rays bend to varying degree forming an inverted image on the retina. Image of the object is formed in the corresponding parts of both the eyes. Images formed in both the eyes are superimposed in the visual cortex to produce a single final image.

If images in both the eyes are not formed in the corresponding parts, then superimposition of images becomes defective, resulting in double vision (diplopia).

In order to avoid defective superimposition as in uncorrected refractive errors, visual axis of one eye could be deviated from the line of focus, resulting in a squint.

In the perception of an image, the visual information reaching the eye is processed and it forms images at three different stages. The first image is formed by the action of light on the rods and cones. The second image is formed in the bipolar cells modified by the horizontal cells. Third image is formed in the ganglion cells modified by the amacrine cells. Impulses generated in the ganglion cell reach the lateral geniculate body and then the visual cortex (occipital lobe) with little modifications. ·

The visual cortex is divided into primary and secondary visual areas. The primary visual area corresponds to area 17 and secondary area corresponds to area 18. The visual cortex is organized into vertical columns which represent the functional unit. In between these vertical columns are specialized columns called **color blobs**.

The images in the cortex are perceived by contrast in the object. The intensity of neuronal stimulation depends on difference in the intensity of contrast. Borders, lines, and their direction are detected by simple cells (layer 4). Further processing of these signals is performed by complex cells. The progressive processing of visual signals helps in appreciating the finer details of the object.

Hearing

The sense of hearing is based on sound. Sound is produced by vibration of objects. It causes alternate compression (molecules come close to each other, pressure increases) and rarefaction (molecules get widely separated, pressure decreases) of air present in front of the vibrating object. Sound is transmitted through gas, liquid, and solid medium with different velocities of conduction. Sound is not transmitted through vacuum. The character of sound is determined by the amplitude and frequency of the sound wave.

Amplitude

It is the extent of displacement of molecules during vibration. It is determined by difference between the pressures of molecule in the zone of compression (increase in the density of medium) and rarefaction (decompression–reduction in the density of the medium). The amplitude influences the loudness of the sound. Greater the amplitude, greater is the loudness.

Frequency

Frequency is the number of sound waves occurring in unit time. It is the number of compression and rarefaction in a given time. Frequency determines the pitch of the sound. Greater the frequency, higher is the pitch of sound.

Audible Frequency

The human ear can appreciate the sound with a frequency between 1000 and 4000 Hz (cycles per second). The audible frequency ranges from 20 to 20,000 Hz. About 4,00,000 different sounds can be distinguished by the human ear.

Ear

The ear is divided into (Fig. 9.7)

- external ear,
- middle ear, and
- internal ear.

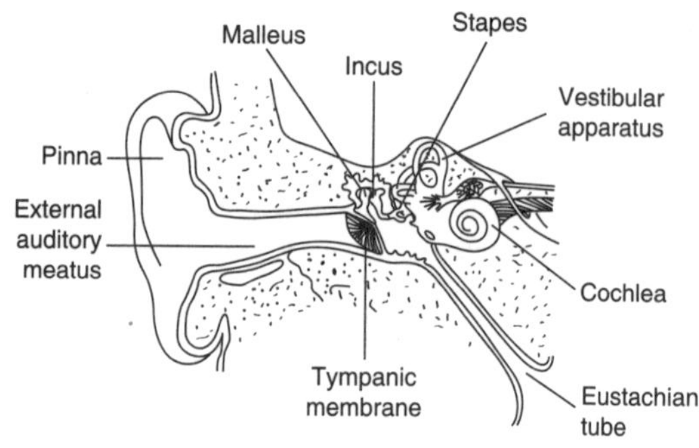

Fig. 9.7   Structure of the ear.

External Ear

The external ear has two parts:

1. pinna and
2. external auditory meatus.

Function

The external ear collects the sound and conducts it to the tympanic membrane.

Middle Ear

The middle ear or tympanic cavity is an air-filled cavity in the petrous part of the temporal bone lined by the mucosa. Laterally, it has the ear drum or tympanic membrane.

The medial side of the middle ear contains a bony wall with two openings. The superior opening is oval and inferior opening is round window.

- **Oval window:** The foot plate of the stapes is attached to it.
- **Round window:** Closed by the secondary tympanic membrane.

  The anterior wall has two canals:

  1. Upper one contains the tensor tympani muscle.
  2. Lower one is called Eustachian tube.

Middle ear contains three small bones called ossicles. They are

1. malleus,
2. incus, and
3. stapes.

It also contains two small muscles:

1. tensor tympani and
2. stapedius.

Functions

- The ossicles of the middle ear conduct the sound from the external ear to the internal ear. They also amplify the sound.
- They provide impedance matching for the sound waves in air and vibrations in cochlear fluid.
- The small muscles, tensor tympani, and stapedius help in protecting the auditory receptors against loud sound (**tympanic reflex** or **attenuation reflex**).
- Eustachian tube helps to equalize the pressure on either side of the tympanic membrane.

Tympanic Reflex

It is a protective reflex which prevents strong sound waves from causing excessive stimulation of auditory receptors resulting in its damage. The loud sound initiates reflex contraction of the tensor tympani and the stapedius muscle present in the middle ear. This is known as **tympanic reflex**. The contraction of tensor tympani and stapedius pulls the handle of the malleus inward and foot plate of the stapes outward. This decreases the sound transmission. The reaction time for this reflex is 40–60 ms. The tympanic reflex fails to protect the auditory receptors against gunshot sound which has a shorter reaction time.

Impedance Matching

The ossicles amplify the sound during conduction of sound. The arrangement of ossicles increases the sound pressure by about 1.3 times. The difference in size of the tympanic membrane and the base of stapes increases the sound pressure by about 20 times.

The effective increase in sound pressure is 30–40 times. This amplification is required to overcome the resistance offered by the fluid in the internal ear for the movement of the base of stapes. This is called **impedance matching**.

Inner Ear

Inner ear is made of two parts:

1. bony labyrinth and
2. membranous labyrinth.

The **bony labyrinth** is a series of channels in the petrous part of the temporal bone. Inside these channels is the membranous labyrinth. The fluid surrounding it is called the **perilymph**.

The **membranous labyrinth** is filled with the **endolymph**.

The perilymph resembles the CSF and the endolymph resembles the ICF.

Inner ear has

- vestibular apparatus (for equilibrium) and
- cochlea (for audition).

Cochlea (Fig. 9.8)

This is a system of coiled tubes 35 mm long. It makes 2 ¾ of a turn.

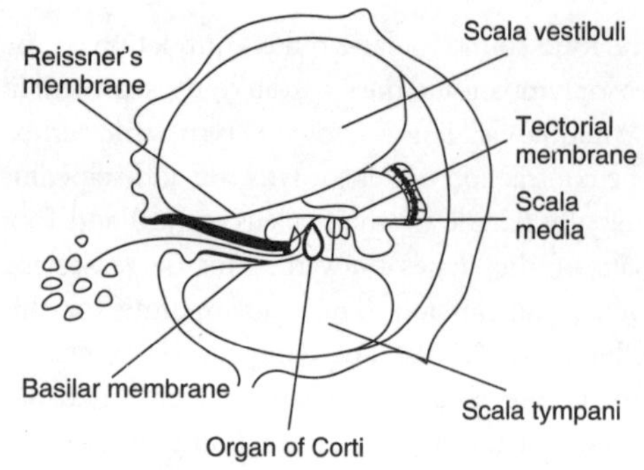

Fig. 9.8   Structure of Cochlea.

It consists of three tubes lying side by side:

1. scala vestibuli,
2. scala media, and
3. scala tympani.

Scala vestibuli and scala tympani contain perilymph. They communicate with each other at the apex of cochlea through a small opening called **helicotrema**.

Scala media contains endolymph.

Scala vestibuli has an oval window which is closed by foot plate of the base of stapes.

Scala tympani ends at the round window. It is covered by secondary tympanic membrane.

Scala vestibuli and scala media are separated by **Reissner's membrane**. Scala media and scala tympani are separated from each other by **basilar membrane**.

On the surface of the basilar membrane lies the organ of Corti containing hair cells.

Organ of Corti (Fig. 9.9)   It is the receptor organ that generates the nerve impulses in response to vibration of the basilar membrane.

The receptors of the organ of Corti are hair cells. They are of two types: external hair cells and internal hair cells.

The external hair cells are arranged in three rows. The internal hair cells form a single row.

The hair cells are covered by a thin viscous elastic membrane called the **tectorial membrane**.

The base and sides of the hair cells synapse with a network of nerve endings of the cochlea. The nerve

fibers from these endings lead to spiral ganglion of Corti which lies in the modiolus of the cochlea. The spiral ganglion in turn sends axon to the cochlear nerve.

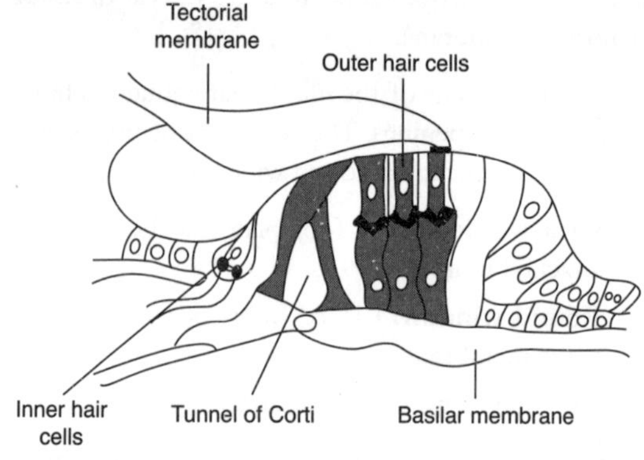

Fig. 9.9   Organ of Corti.

Hair Cells (Fig. 9.10)   They are embedded in the epithelium made up of supporting cells. The basal part is in contact with the afferent neurons.

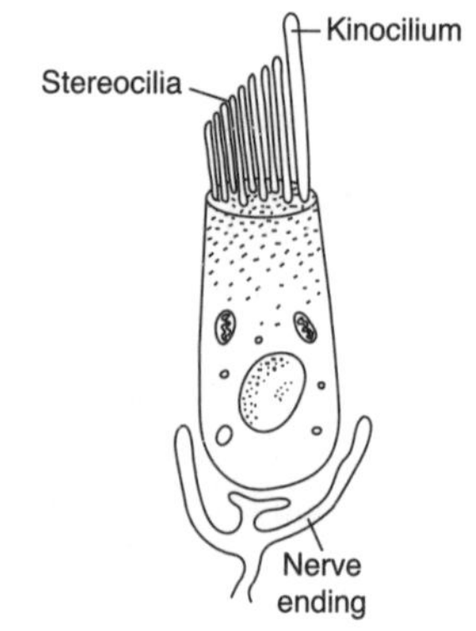

Fig. 9.10   Hair cell.

The apical part contains rod-shaped processes called hairs. They are called the **stereocilia**. These stereocilia are covered by thin, viscous but elastic tectorial membrane.

The RMP of hair cells is –60 mV.

Appreciation of Sound

The human ear can best appreciate the sound waves in the frequency of 1000–4000 Hz. However, the audible frequency range is 20–20,000 Hz.

- Sound waves cause the vibration of the tympanic membrane.

- These vibrations are amplified and transmitted by a chain of ossicles of the middle ear.

- Base of stapes moves forward and backward in the fluid of scala vestibuli setting up a wave. These waves cause the displacement of the basilar membrane.

- Auditory receptors, hair cells, are located on the basilar membrane. Hair cells on the basilar membrane move up and down along with the membrane. In the upward movement, cilia of the hair cell touch the rigid tectorial membrane and get bent.

- Bending of cilia activates the cell by producing a receptor potential.

- This in turn activates cochlear nerve endings that synapse with the base of the hair cells.

- Action potential produced in the nerve travels along the auditory nerve.

- High-frequency sound produces maximum vibration of the basal part of the basilar membrane which is thin and narrow. Low-frequency sound produces maximum vibration of apical part of the basilar membrane.

- Different regions of basilar membrane vibrate maximally to different frequency sounds. This property helps in discrimination of pitch of the sound.

Mechanism of hearing and pitch discrimination is explained on the basis of **traveling wave theory**.

Traveling Wave Theory

The movement of the footplate of stapes causes displacement of the perilymph in the scala vestibuli. The movement of perilymph in the scala vestibuli displaces the fluid in scala media. This movement of fluid produces a wave in the basal portion of the basilar membrane. The wave setup at the base of the basilar membrane travels toward the apex. As the wave travels along the basilar membrane, it becomes strong at one part of the membrane causing significant vibrations at that region, called the **resonance point**. The wave does not travel beyond the resonance point on the basilar membrane. Traveling wave helps in appreciating sound of a particular frequency by vibrating specific part of the basilar membrane.

Endolymphatic Potential

It is the potential difference between the perilymph and the endolymph. The potential difference is 80 mV, the endolymph being positive with respect to perilymph. The endolymphatic potential is due to an increased level of potassium ions produced by the activity of the striae vascularis.

Cochlear Microphonic Potential

It is a potential developed in the cochlea due to auditory stimulation.

It is a nonpropagated (not transmitted) graded potential which depends on the intensity of stimulation.

It has no latent period. The cochlear microphonic potential progresses to form an action potential.

Action Potential in Cochlear Nerve

The stimulation of hair cells releases the chemical mediator glutamate. It activates the auditory nerve to set up the action potential after a brief latent period. Type of action potential depends on the character of the sound.

Auditory Pathway (Fig. 9.11)

The nerve fibers from hair cells of the organ of Corti end in the spiral ganglion of Corti.

The fibers from the spiral ganglion of Corti pass to the dorsal and ventral cochlear nuclei located in the upper part of the medulla.

Second-order neurons pass to the opposite side of the brainstem to terminate in the superior olivary nucleus. Some fibers also pass to the superior olivary nucleus of the same side.

From the superior olivary nucleus the fibers pass through the lateral lemniscus and few fibers terminate in the nucleus of the lateral lemniscus. The remaining fibers bypass this nucleus and reach the inferior colliculus (through cochlear nerve).

From the inferior colliculus fibers pass to the medial geniculate body where all the fibers synapse.

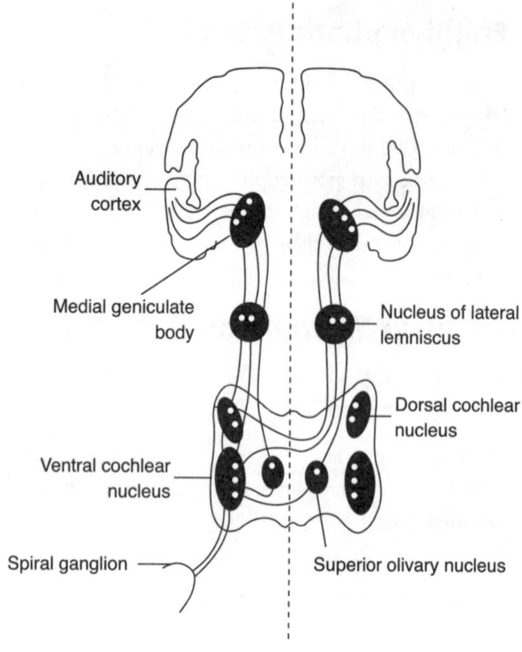

Fig. 9.11   Auditory pathway.

The pathway then proceeds through the auditory radiation to the auditory cortex area 41 and 42 (superior gyrus of temporal lobe).

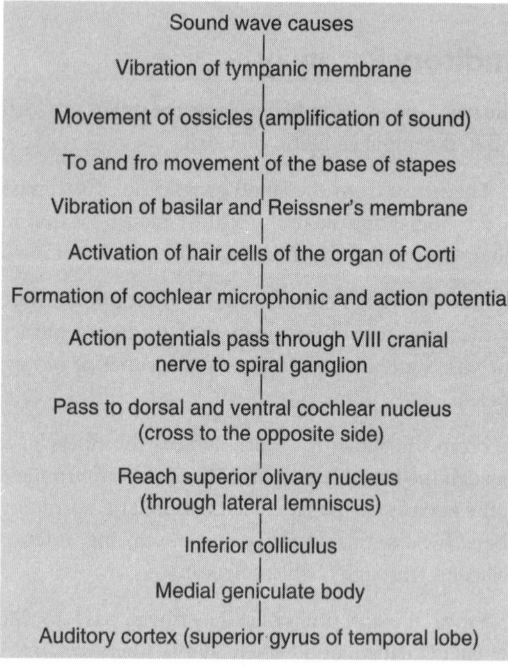

Intensity of Sound

The intensity of sound is measured in decibel scale. Bel is the logarithm of the ratio of intensity of given sound to that of the standard sound. A decibel (dB) is 1/10 bel. Intensity of 0 dB sound corresponds to the intensity of standard sound. It does not mean the absence of sound. Discomfort is experienced at an intensity level of 120 dB or above. The higher intensity sounds can damage the organ of Corti.

Masking

Masking is the decreased ability of a person to appreciate one sound fully in the presence of another sound (with different intensities). It is due to refractoriness (unresponsiveness to further immediate stimulation) of the receptors and the nerve by the earlier stimulation. The extent of masking of one tone over the other depends on the pitch of the sound.

Localization of Sound

The sound waves traveling in the horizontal plane reach right and left ears at different times. This difference in the arrival of sound at each ear helps to determine the direction of sound. Secondly, ear closer to the source of sound perceives it louder than the other ear. The cortical interpretation of loudness and time difference in perception of sound by both the ears help to determine the direction of sound.

Tests for Hearing

Watch Test

The subject is asked to appreciate the tick sound by keeping the watch at a reasonable distance. This is compared with the sound perception of the examiner.

Rinne's Test

The base of vibrating tuning fork (256 or 512 Hz) is kept on the mastoid process to study the bone conduction. When the subject ceases to appreciate the sound, vibrating prong of the tuning fork is held in front of the external auditory meatus (air conduction).

In a normal person, air conduction is better and longer than bone conduction. If the bone conduction is better, it indicates conductive deafness or middle ear deafness.

Weber's Test

In this test, the base of vibrating tuning fork is placed on the vertex of the skull or on the forehead. In a normal person sound is heard equally in both ears.

In middle ear deafness and blockage in the external auditory meatus, sound is better heard on the defective side.

In unilateral nerve deafness, sound is better heard on the normal side. Weber's test is of no value in bilateral nerve deafness.

Absolute Bone Conduction (ABC) Test

The external auditory meatus of the subject and examiner are occluded. Vibrating tuning fork is placed on the subject's mastoid bone. When the subject stops hearing the sound, tuning fork is placed on the examiner's mastoid bone. If the examiner continues to hear the sound for a longer duration than the subject, the subject has reduced absolute bone conduction. This indicates nerve (sensorineural) deafness.

Applied Physiology

Deafness

Inability to appreciate sounds is called deafness.

If deafness is present since birth, individual is unable to speak (deaf mute). Hence to have the ability to produce sound, person has to hear the sound.

Types of deafness are as under.

Conductive Deafness

It is caused due to impaired sound transmission in the external or middle ear.

Causes

- Wax or foreign body in the external ear
- Otosclerosis in the middle ear
- Rupture of tympanic membrane

Nerve (Sensorineural) Deafness

It is caused by damage to auditory receptors in the inner ear or auditory pathway.

Hearing Aids

These are electronic devices that compensate for the loss of hearing due to the damage in middle ear, cochlea, and neural structures. Hearing aids amplify the incoming sound and transmit the sound in the normal route of its perception. The cochlear mechanism to appreciate the sound remains the same as in a normal person.

Cochlear Implants

Cochlear implants are used when the damage to the auditory apparatus is extensive and the loss of hearing is significant. The implants directly stimulate cochlear nerve with small currents in response to sound. The sound signals are transmitted directly to the auditory nerve without the involvement of cochlea.

Audiometry

In this test, sounds of different frequencies and loudness produced by an instrument are presented to the subject through earphones. The threshold of hearing at each frequency for air conduction and bone conduction is plotted. The graph obtained is an audiogram. The extent of hearing loss is evaluated by comparing recorded values with the standard values obtained for normal subjects.

Types of audiometry are

- pure tone audiometry,
- speech audiometry,
- impedance audiometry, and
- evoked response audiometry.

Taste (Gustation)

The primary taste sensations are sweet, salt, sour, bitter, and umami.

Taste Sensations

Sweet

- It is best appreciated at the tip of the tongue.
- It is produced by organic substances.
- Polysaccharides, glycerols, alcohols, ketones, chloroform, and amides of aspartic acid also produce sweet sensation.

Salt

- It is produced by ionizing substances releasing Na^+ ions.
- It is best appreciated on lateral margin of the tongue.

Sour

- It is produced by acids which release H^+ ions.
- It is best appreciated on lateral margin of the tongue.
- Sourness depends on the hydrogen ion concentration in the given acid. Organic acids are more sour when compared to mineral acid with similar hydrogen ion concentration because they penetrate the cells more rapidly than mineral acids.

Bitter

- It is best appreciated at the back of the tongue.
- It is produced by alkaloids like quinine.
- Organic compounds like morphine, caffeine, urea, inorganic salts of magnesium, ammonia, and calcium also taste bitter.
- The bitter taste is due to cations.

Umami

- It is a pleasant and sweet taste sensation different from standard sweet taste.
- It is produced by monosodium glutamate (MSG).

Taste Buds (Fig. 9.12)

The taste buds are the receptors for taste sensation. They are present on the walls of the papilla.

The taste buds are oval-shaped structures containing

- receptor cells,
- supporting cells, and
- basal cells.

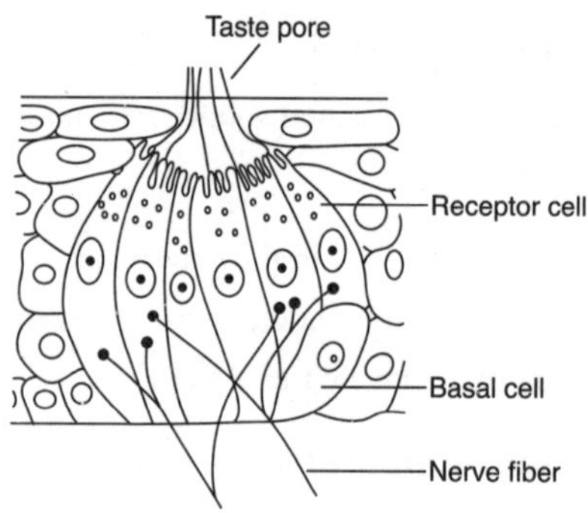

Fig. 9.12   Taste bud.

At the tip of taste bud, there is a taste pore. From the apical portion of receptor cells, hair-like projections come out of the taste pore. These are called the **microvilli**.

Fine sensory nerve fibers which arise from the receptor cells carry the taste sensations.

The basal cells form the receptor cells which are replaced periodically.

Nerve Supply to Tongue

The taste sensations from the anterior two-third of the tongue are carried by chorda tympani, branch of facial nerve. From posterior one-third, it is carried by glossopharyngeal nerve.

Taste Pathway (Fig. 9.13)

Nerve fibers from the anterior and posterior parts of the tongue end on gustatory portion of the nucleus of tractus solitarius (NTS) present in the medulla of brain.

The second-order neurons arising from NTS end in the ventral posteromedial (VPM) nucleus of the thalamus.

The third-order neurons arising from the thalamus end on the face area of the somatosensory cortex. (lower lateral part of postcentral gyrus deep in the lateral sulcus).

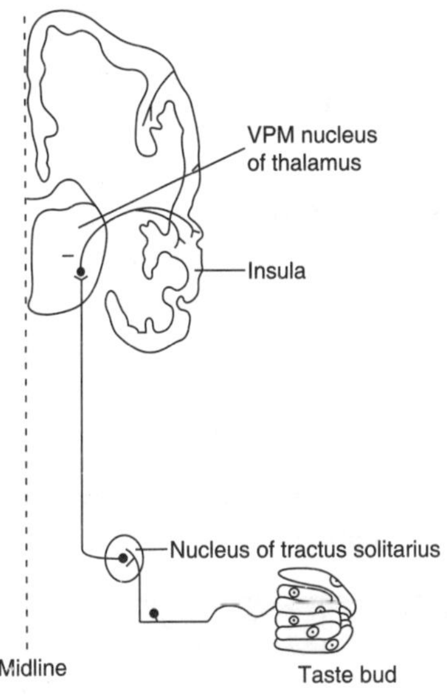

Fig. 9.13   Taste pathway.

Mechanism of Appreciation of Taste

The taste-producing substance dissolves in saliva and comes in contact with the villi through the taste pores present in the taste buds. This contact brings about changes in the receptors cells of the taste buds resulting in generation of the generator potential. This causes release of the neurotransmitter at the synapse between the receptor cell and the sensory nerve. The action potential is generated at the sensory neuron. Impulses from the receptor cells are carried to the foot of the postcentral gyrus in the parietal lobe of the cerebral cortex where different taste sensations are appreciated.

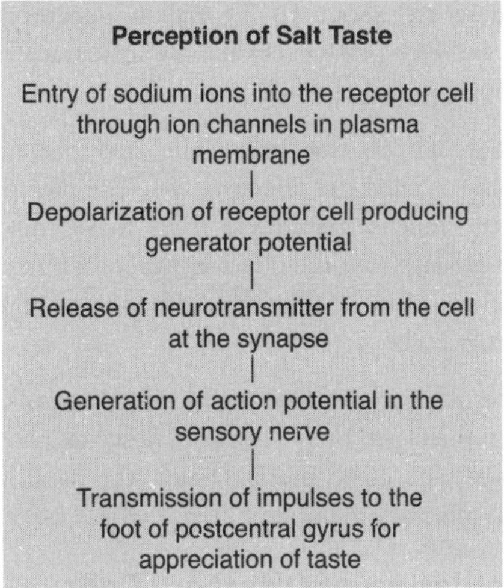

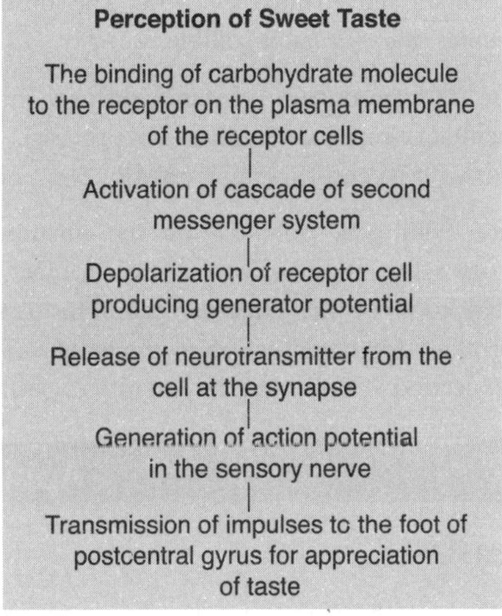

Each taste system is organized into specific coded pathway to the CNS.

The single taste receptor cell responds to more than one type of taste sensation to varying extent.

Appreciation of a specific taste sensation depends on the activation of a group of neurons from different receptor cell.

Smell (Olfaction)

The olfactory receptors are located in the yellowish pigmented olfactory mucus membrane of the nasal cavity.

The olfactory receptors are called the olfactory cells.

There are about 10–20 million olfactory cells. They are interspersed between the sustentacular cells (supporting epithelial cells).

They are bipolar cells. The dendrite has an expansion called the olfactory rod. The cilia project into the mucus membrane from these rods. The axons arising from the olfactory receptors pierce the cribriform plate of the ethmoid bone and enter the olfactory bulb.

The olfactory neurons are the only neurons known to be replenished by cell division. Mucus is produced by Bowman's gland present below the basal lamina of the olfactory membrane (Fig. 9.14).

Stimulation of Olfactory Cells

The smell of volatile substances can be appreciated when they are sniffed into the nostrils. The stimulating substances must be water soluble.

The odor-producing substance diffuses into the mucus that covers the cilia (hair-like process). Then it binds with receptor forming cAMP.

The membrane potential of the unstimulated olfactory cell is about –55 mV. The odorants cause depolarization of the olfactory cell. The olfactory receptors undergo adaptation to the extent of 50% in first second. Thereafter, they adapt very little and very slowly. Because of this mechanism, intensity of smell is high in the beginning but decreases thereafter.

Human olfactory system can recognize more than 10,000 different odors. This is possible by the presence of about 1000 different genes.

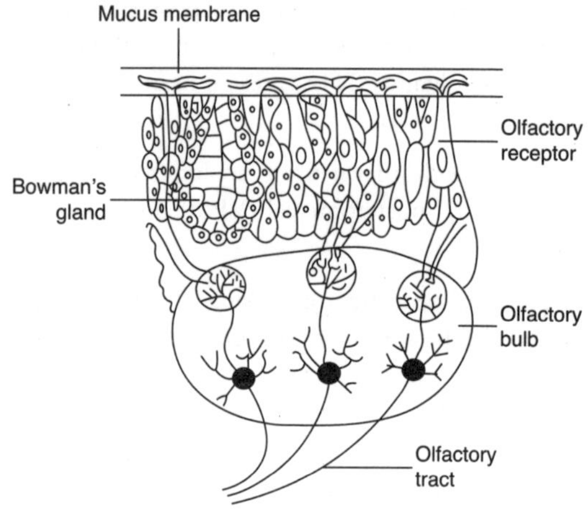

Fig. 9.14   Olfactory membrane.

Olfactory Pathway

The axons of the olfactory cells pierce the cribriform plate of the ethmoid bone and end in the olfactory bulb. (Olfactory bulb is an anterior outgrowth of brain tissue from the base of the brain.)

The short axons from the olfactory cells terminate in multiple globular structures within the olfactory bulb called **glomeruli**.

Applied Physiology

Ageusia

Absence of taste sensation

Hypogeusia

Decreased taste sensation

Dysgeusia

Disturbed taste sensation

Each glomerulus has dendrites from mitral cells and tufted cells. These cells in turn send axons through the olfactory tract to transmit olfactory sensations to the CNS.

The olfactory tract enters the brain at the anterior junction between the mesencephalon and the cerebrum.

The tract divides into two pathways: one passes medially to the medial olfactory area and the other laterally to the lateral olfactory area.

- **Medial olfactory area:** This consists of a group of nuclei located in the midbasal portions of the brain anterior to the hypothalamus.
- **Lateral olfactory area:** This is mainly composed of the prepyriform cortex, pyriform cortex, and cortical portion of the amygdaloid nuclei. From these areas, signals pass into almost all portions of the limbic system, especially to the hypothalamus.

The newer olfactory pathway pass through the thalamus, to the basomedial thalamic nucleus, and then to the lateral posterior quadrant of the orbitofrontal cortex.

Applied Physiology

Anosmia

Loss of sensation of smell.

Parosmia

Perverted smell sensation.

Pheromones

They are chemical substances produced by rodents and few mammals which can stimulate the sex drive in them. Thus pheromones play a major role in sexual and reproductive behavior of animals. Vomeronasal organs have receptors capable of identifying odors arising from pheromones.

Endocrinology

Endocrine and nervous systems are the two major regulatory systems of the body. The endocrine system consists of glands present in different parts of the body. They are called **endocrine glands** (Fig. 10.1) because they release their secretions directly into the bloodstream without the help of ducts (ductless glands).

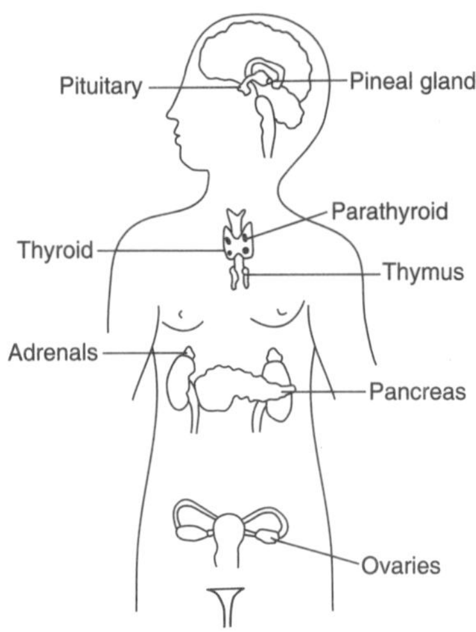

Fig. 10.1 Endocrine glands.

The endocrine glands are present scattered throughout the body. They are connected to each other and other organs of the body through vascular system. The chemicals secreted by the endocrine glands are called **hormones**.

Hormone

A hormone is a chemical substance secreted by the endocrine glands directly into the bloodstream. It regulates the function of a distant organ (target organ).

Types

1. **Classical hormones:** The hormones are liberated from the endocrine gland and carried by the blood or lymph. They reach the target cell and produce the desired effect. Examples include thyroid hormones and hormones of pancreas.
2. **Neurohormones:** These are secreted from the axon terminals and released into the circulation. Examples are hypothalamic-releasing hormones.
3. **Paracrine hormones:** These are the hormones which have effect on the adjacent cells.

For example, α and β cells of islets of Langerhans exert paracrine effect on each other.

4. **Autocrine hormones:** The cell regulates its own function. For example, platelet-activating factor from the endothelium acts on itself.

Chemistry

Chemically, hormones are of three types:

1. steroid hormones,
2. amines, and
3. proteins or peptides.

Steroid Hormones

These are synthesized from cholesterol. They have cyclopentanoperhydrophenanthrene ring. They are formed from smooth endoplasmic reticulum.

The different steroid hormones are cortisol, aldosterone, estrogens, progesterone, and testosterone.

Amines

These are derivatives of amino acid tyrosine. They are synthesized in the cell cytoplasm.

They include thyroid hormones and hormones of the adrenal medulla.

- Thyroid hormones are thyroxine and triiodothyronine.
- Adrenal medullary hormones are epinephrine and norepinephrine.

Protein (or Peptides)

They are water-soluble hormones and are carried in unbound form in the plasma. They are made up of chains of amino acids linked by peptide bonds. They are synthesized by rough endoplasmic reticulum.

Proteins (or peptide) hormones are

- anterior pituitary hormones;
- posterior pituitary hormones;
- insulin, glucagon, and parathormone.

Control of Hormone Secretion

Hormone secretion is regulated by its requirement. The regulation of hormonal secretion is brought about by feedback mechanisms, which are of two types:

1. negative feedback mechanism and
2. positive feedback mechanism.

Negative Feedback Mechanism

Increased levels of the hormone or its product inhibit the gland. This reduces the secretion of hormone from the gland.

Negative feedback becomes functional only when the target organ responds optimally to the hormone.

Positive Feedback Mechanism

Hormone secreted from a gland acts on the same gland to enhance synthesis and release of the hormone. Positive feedback mechanism regulates optimal hormone secretion.

For example, initial secretion of oxytocin further enhances its own secretion during parturition.

Hormone Receptors

Hormone receptors are modified proteins having specific binding sites for the respective hormone. Receptors are present on the surface or inside the cells.

The locations of receptors are as follows:

- **Cell membrane:** Protein, peptide, and catecholamine hormones have specific membrane receptors.
- **Cytoplasm:** Receptors for steroid hormones are usually found almost entirely in the cell cytoplasm.
- **Nucleus of the cell:** Receptors for the thyroid hormones are present in the nucleus.

The number of receptors in a cell is not a constant number. An increase in the concentration of hormones causes decrease in the number of receptors by inactivation or decreased production. This is called **downregulation** of receptors.

A decrease in the concentration of hormone triggers the formation of more receptors. This is called **upregulation** of receptors.

Hormonal Transport

Hormones after secretion enter the bloodstream and circulate in the plasma. They are carried either in free form or bound to the plasma. Usually the steroid hormones circulate in free form. Proteins and amines are transported bound to the globulins.

Mechanism of Action

Hormone regulates functioning of its target tissues by activating the receptors.

Hormone binds to the receptor to form a hormone–receptor complex. This complex alters the structure and function of the receptor.

Altered receptor produces the desired response by

- **Change in membrane permeability of the cell:** Hormones like epinephrine and norepinephrine secreted by the adrenal medulla act by this mechanism. They cause opening and closing of ion channels, thereby bringing about a change in the membrane permeability.

- **Activation of an intracellular enzyme:** Binding of hormone to its receptor activates an enzyme inside the cell membrane.

  For example, activation of adenylcyclase. This in turn catalyzes the formation of cAMP. It is called second messenger since it does not directly cause the effect.

- **Activation of genes:** Some hormones bind to the protein receptors inside the cell. The hormone–receptor complex binds to the proteins of DNA in the nucleus. This initiates transcription of genes to form mRNA.

Second Messenger System

Calcium ions, cyclic adenosine monophosphate (cAMP), cyclic guanosine monophosphate (cGMP), calmodulin, and products of membrane phospholipid breakdown are the various second messenger systems.

Cyclic AMP System

Cyclic AMP is the cyclic form of AMP. It is produced from ATP by action of adenyl cyclase.

The binding of hormones with receptors causes coupling of the receptors to a G-proton-stimulating adenyl cyclase. The stimulation of adenyl cyclase converts ATP into cAMP inside the cell. Cyclic AMP activates cAMP-dependent protein kinase.

Once cAMP is formed, it activates a cascade of enzymes which ultimately lead to phosphorylation of specific proteins in the cell. These proteins bring about the action through hormones.

Some hormones acting through cAMP second messenger system include ACTH, LH, and TSH.

Membrane Phospholipid Second Messenger System

Some hormones activate receptors that inactivate phospholipase C enzymes. This enzyme causes breakdown of some phospholipid in the cell membrane to inositol triphosphate (IP3) and diacylglycerol (DAG). IP3 activates calcium and causes second messenger effects. DAG activates enzyme protein kinase C which phosphorylates proteins.

Calcium–Calmodulin Second Messenger System

This system operates in response to the entry of calcium ions into the cell. Entry of calcium is by the opening of calcium channels caused by a change in membrane potential or action of hormone. On entry into the cell calcium binds to a protein called calmodulin. Calmodulin has four binding sites for calcium. Calmodulin changes its shape and initiates multiple effects inside the cell.

Hormonal Assay

It is the measurement of hormone concentration in the blood.

Since hormones are secreted in very minute quantities, it is difficult to measure them by conventional chemical methods. It is therefore measured by techniques called **radioimmunoassay** and **ELISA**.

Principle

Radioimmunoassay is based on competitive binding of hormone and radiolabeled hormone to a specific antibody. By estimating relative percentage of radiolabeled hormone bound to the antibody, the natural hormone concentration in the given sample can be calculated.

Hormonal Rhythm (Fig. 10.2)

Some of the endocrine glands exhibit a cyclic pattern of hormonal secretion (rhythm). These rhythms range from a few minutes to months. The rhythm having a 24-h cycle is termed **circadian rhythm**. Cortisol and growth hormone have circadian rhythm. Pulsatile rhythms occur over half an hour to 2-h period and appear as sudden bursts of secretion. Pulsatile rhythms with less than 24-h periodicity are termed **ultradian rhythms**. These rhythms denote normal functioning of the glands and are absent in disease conditions.

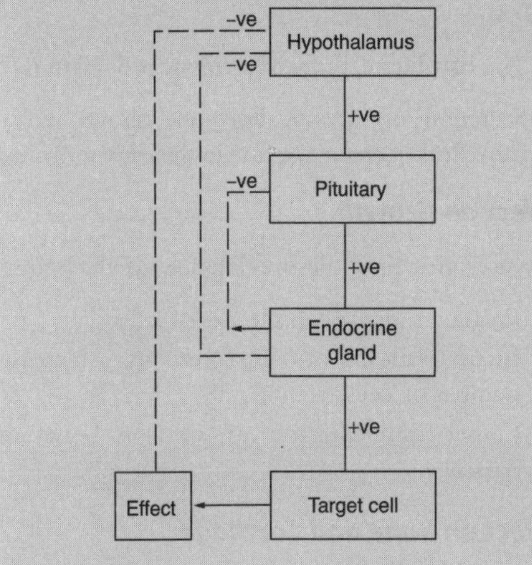

Fig. 10.2 General pattern of regulation of hormone secretion.

Hypothalamus

The hypothalamus secretes hypothalamic-releasing and -inhibiting factors which control the secretions of the pituitary gland. This control is brought about by hormonal and nervous mechanisms. The anterior pituitary is controlled by hormonal mechanism and posterior pituitary is controlled by nervous mechanism.

Hormones released by the hypothalamus are conducted through the hypothalamohypophysial portal system.

These are extensive capillary networks connecting the hypothalamus and anterior pituitary.

The hypothalamic hormones are secreted by the specialized cells in it. The nerve cells terminate in the median eminence and tuber cinereum of the pituitary stalk. Hormones secreted from these nerve terminals are immediately absorbed into the hypothalamohypophysial portal system and are carried to the sinuses of the anterior pituitary gland.

The anterior pituitary in turn secretes various hormones that act on other endocrine glands. These endocrine glands produce hormones which act on the target cells.

The hormones of the posterior pituitary are ADH and oxytocin.

They are synthesized in the hypothalamus and stored and released from the posterior pituitary.

Mechanism of Action

Hypothalamic-releasing hormones act on the anterior pituitary by binding to specific membrane receptors on the cells. Most of the hormones act by stimulating cAMP.

Important hypothalamic hormones are as under:

- **TRH (thyrotropin-releasing hormone):** It causes release of thyroid-stimulating hormone.

- **CRH (corticotropin-releasing hormone):** It causes release of ACTH.

- **GHRH (growth hormone–releasing hormone):** It causes release of growth hormone.

- **GHIH (growth hormone inhibitory hormone somatostatin):** It inhibits the release of growth hormone.

- **GnRH (gonadotropin-releasing hormone):** It causes release of two gonadotropic hormones, FSH and LH.

- **PIH (prolactin-inhibiting hormone):** It causes inhibition of prolactin secretion.

Pituitary Gland (Fig. 10.3)

This is also called the **hypophysis cerebri**. It is a small gland measuring 1 cm in diameter and weighing about 0.5–1 g. It is present at the base of brain and lies in the sella turcica of the sphenoid bone. It is connected to the hypothalamus by its stalk.

Pituitary gland is divided into two lobes:

1. anterior lobe (adenohypophysis) and
2. posterior lobe (neurohypophysis).

Pars intermedia is a small zone in between the anterior and posterior lobes of the pituitary. It secretes melanocyte-stimulating hormone.

The anterior pituitary originates from **Rathke's pouch,** which is an invagination of the pharyngeal epithelium. The cells of the anterior pituitary are therefore glandular in nature.

The posterior pituitary arises as an outgrowth of the hypothalamus. The posterior pituitary contains nerve cells.

The hormones secreted by the anterior pituitary are as follows:

- **Growth hormone (GH):** Growth hormone causes growth of the whole body by increasing protein synthesis and enhanced cell growth

- **Adrenocorticotropic hormone (ACTH):** ACTH controls secretion of the adrenocortical hormones, which in turn control carbohydrate, protein, and fat metabolism.

- **Thyroid-stimulating hormone (TSH):** TSH controls the rate of secretion of T_3 and T_4 hormones by the thyroid gland.

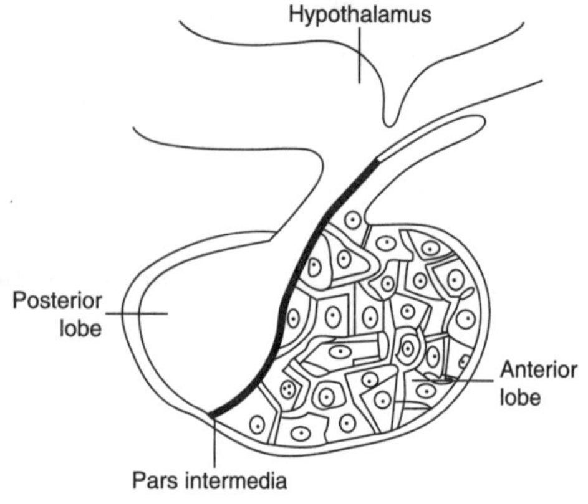

Fig. 10.3 Pituitary gland.

- **Prolactin:** Prolactin causes development of mammary gland and helps in milk production.

- **Follicle-stimulating hormone (FSH) and lutenizing hormone (LH):** FSH and LH control growth of ovaries and testes and thereby help in controlling reproductive activity. Hormones of the posterior pituitary are secreted in the hypothalamus and stored in the posterior pituitary.

The hormones of the posterior pituitary are

- **Antidiuretic hormone (vasopressin):** Antidiuretic hormone controls the amount of water in the body by regulating the urine output.

- **Oxytocin:** Oxytocin helps in expression of milk from breast. It also helps in delivery of the baby.

Growth Hormone (Somatotropin)

This is a small protein hormone containing 191 amino acids in a single chain. Its molecular weight is 22,000.

The half-life of growth hormone is 6–20 min.

Secretion of growth hormone shows diurnal rhythm. Peak secretion occurs in the early morning.

Effect on Growth

It causes growth of almost all tissues of the body.

- Promotes increase in the size of cells.
- Increases the rate of mitosis, resulting in increased number of cells.
- Causes differentiation of cells in bone and muscle.

Effect on Bone and Cartilage

Growth hormone stimulates bone growth.

- Increases the number of cells responsible for bone growth.
- Increases deposition of protein by chondrocytic and osteogenic cells.
- Causes growth of epiphysial cartilage.
- Delays fusion of epiphysis with the shaft.

Metabolic Effects

Effect on Protein Metabolism It increases the rate of protein synthesis in all the cells by

- enhancing amino acid transport through the cell membrane;

- increasing nuclear transcription of DNA to form mRNA;
- enhancing RNA translation to promote protein synthesis by ribosomes;
- decreasing the catabolism of protein and amino acids.

Effect on Carbohydrate Metabolism

- Decreases the use of glucose for energy; diminishes uptake of glucose by the cells and increases blood glucose concentration.
- Increases the secretion of insulin.

Effect on Fat Metabolism

- Increases mobilization of fats from adipose tissue.
- Increases free fatty acids in the blood.
- Enhances use of fatty acids for energy.
- Excess of growth hormone has a ketogenic effect.

Effect on Electrolyte Metabolism

- Causes rise in plasma phosphorous and fall in blood urea, nitrogen, and amino acid levels.
- Increases GI absorption of Ca^{++}.
- Reduces Na^+ and K^+ excretion.

Growth hormone is degraded in the liver and kidneys.

Regulation of Growth Hormone

The normal plasma concentration of growth hormone in adults is between 1.6 and 3 ng/mL. It is about 6 ng/mL in children and adolescents.

Growth hormone secretion increases during starvation, excitement, exercise, trauma, hypoglycemia, and sleep.

Hormones like testosterone and estrogens stimulate the secretion of growth hormone.

Secretion of growth hormone decrease with an increase in blood glucose level, cortisol, and free fatty acid levels.

Secretion of growth hormone is controlled by two factors produced in the hypothalamus. They are as follows:

1. **Growth hormone–releasing hormone:** It is a member of vasoactive intestinal peptide family. Its actions are mediated by cAMP. Dopamine stimulates release of GRH.
2. **Growth hormone–inhibiting hormone:** It is also called somatostatin. It is secreted in many areas of the body. It inhibits GH and TSH release, mediating through the GI-associated receptors.

Somatomedins

These are polypeptide growth factors secreted by the liver in response to stimulation by the growth hormone.

Effect of growth hormone on cartilage, protein metabolism, and general growth depends on its interaction with the somatomedins.

About four somatomedins have been isolated till now. The most important is somatomedin C. This is also called IGF-I (insulin-like growth factor I).

The pigmies of Africa and some congenital dwarfs have inability to synthesize IGF-I.

Insulin-like growth factors are multifunctional hormones that regulate cell growth, differentiation, and metabolism. They are proteins that resemble insulin in structure and function. IGFs are produced in many tissues and have autocrine and paracrine actions.

Applied Physiology

Altered growth hormone secretion results in gigantism.

Gigantism

This occurs due to an increased secretion of the growth hormone by acidophilic tumor or excessive stimulation of the acidophilic cells before puberty (before fusion of epiphysis).

There is excessive growth of long bones and the individual can grow to a height of about 8 ft.

Overstimulation of β-cells of the islets of Langerhans by growth hormone results in its destruction. This leads to **pituitary diabetes**.

Treatment

It is treated by surgical removal of tumor or irradiation of the gland.

Acromegaly

This is a condition in which the secretion of growth hormone is increased after puberty. Acromegaly means enlargement of periphery.

Clinical Features

- Excessive growth of mandible resulting in its protrusion (prognathism)
- Enlargement of frontal bone and facial sinuses producing frontal bossing
- Enlargement of hands and feet
- Bowing of the spine due to excessive growth of vertebrae (kyphosis)
- Excessive soft-tissue growth associated with organomegaly
- Thickening of the skin
- Individual has gorilla appearance

Dwarfism

This condition is due to reduced growth hormone production during childhood.

Clinical Features

- There is stunted growth. However, all physical parts of the body are proportional. Child aged 10 years may look like a child of 5 years.
- There is no mental retardation.
- They attain sexual maturity.

Treatment

Dwarfism can be treated by administration of human growth hormone.

Lorain Dwarf

This condition is characterized by the deficiency of somatomedin C. However, growth hormone secretion is normal. They are not responsive to growth hormone secreted by the body.

Lorain dwarfs have features of dwarfism but they do not respond to treatment with growth hormone.

Panhypopituitarism

The condition is due to a decreased secretion of all anterior pituitary hormones.

Panhypopituitary dwarfs do not attain puberty and do not develop sexual functions.

In adults, panhypopituitarism can occur due to destruction of the pituitary gland by tumors. The patient can develop thyroid, and gonadal and adrenocortical insufficiency.

Sheehan's Syndrome

This occurs in women during childbirth.

Excessive blood loss during delivery results in circulatory shock. Reduced blood flow causes infarction of adenohypophysis and hence pituitary insufficiency.

Physiology of Growth

Growth is a complex phenomenon which increases the size of different tissues and organs of the body.

Growth requires various hormones like growth hormone, thyroid hormone, androgens, estrogens, glucocorticoids, and insulin.

Growth is influenced by

- genetic factors and
- nutrition.

Growth of different parts of the body is not uniform. General growth occurs rapidly twice, one during infancy and second during puberty. Growth of lymphoid organs is more during childhood.

Neural growth occurs rapidly in the first two years of life. Gonadal growth occurs at puberty.

Posterior Pituitary

Posterior pituitary is an outgrowth of the floor of III ventricle. Posterior pituitary is mainly composed of glial cells called pituicytes. The pituicytes are only supporting cells.

Hormones of the posterior pituitary are synthesized in the cell bodies of the supraoptic and paraventricular nuclei of the hypothalamus. They are transported to the neurohypophysis by the axons of these cell bodies. The nerve endings of these cell bodies form bulbous knobs containing secretory granules. These secretory granules end on the surfaces of capillaries, thereby releasing secretions into circulation via the capillaries.

Two hormones of the posterior pituitary are

1. ADH (vasopressin) and
2. oxytocin.

ADH (Vasopressin)

Antidiuretic hormone is formed mainly in the supraoptic nuclei of the hypothalamus.

It is a polypeptide containing nine amino acids.

ADH and oxytocin are chemically similar. However, phenylalanine and arginine of ADH are replaced by leucine and isoleucine in oxytocin.

Actions

- Antidiuretic effect—ADH increases permeability of the distal convoluted tubule (DCT) and the collecting ducts to water, enhancing water reabsorption.

  ADH causes insertion of protein water channels in the principal cells of the collecting ducts. These water channels are called **aquaporins**.

  In the absence of ADH, DCT, and collecting tubules become impermeable to water. This prevents reabsorption of water and therefore produces dilute urine (diabetes insipidus).

- In high doses, ADH causes vasoconstriction and increases blood pressure.
- It causes contraction of mesangial cells present in the juxtaglomerular apparatus (JGA) and reduces the glomerular filtration rate (GFR).
- It acts on the JGA cells and inhibits renin secretion.
- It causes secretion of CRH and ACTH during stress.

Vasopressin Receptors   There are three kinds of vasopressin receptors V_{1A}, V_{1B}, and V_2.

V_{1A} and V_{1B} increase the intracellular calcium concentration. V_2 receptors increase cAMP levels.

Metabolism

ADH is rapidly inactivated in the liver and kidneys. It has a biological half life of 18 min.

Regulation

An increase in osmolarity of the blood causes increased ADH secretion.

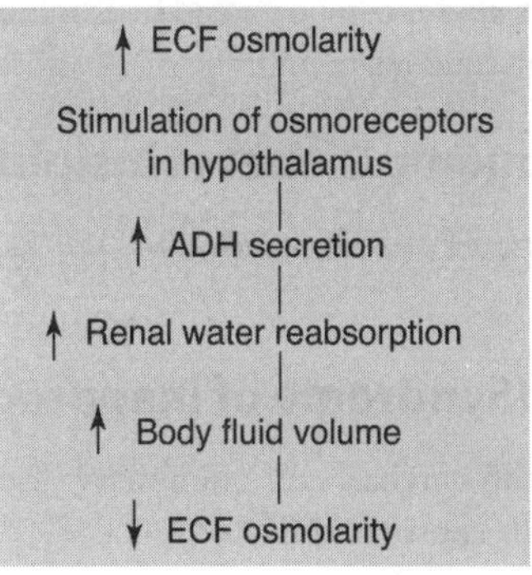

In the hypothalamus, there are modified receptors called the osmoreceptors. When the extracellular fluid (ECF) becomes too much concentrated, fluid moves out of the osmoreceptors by osmosis. This causes a decrease in the size of the osmoreceptors. This initiates nerve signals in the hypothalamus for ADH secretion.

When ECF becomes too dilute, water moves into the cell by osmosis causing decrease in the signals for ADH secretion.

Oxytocin

This is a polypeptide containing nine amino acids. It is formed primarily in the paraventricular nucleus of the hypothalamus and stored in the posterior pituitary.

Oxytocin circulates in the unbound form. It has a half-life of 3–5 min. Degradation occurs primarily in the liver and kidneys.

Actions

It acts mainly on

- uterus and
- breasts

On Uterus

Oxytocin causes contraction of smooth muscles of the pregnant uterus and relaxation of cervix.

In nonpregnant uterus, oxytocin facilitates sperm transport.

On Breast

It plays an important role in lactation. It causes contraction of myoepithelial cells that line the ducts of the breast, thus helping in milk ejection.

Milk Ejection Reflex (Milk Letdown Reflex)
This is a neuroendocrine reflex. Touch receptors are present in the breast around the nipple. Suckling the nipple stimulates these touch receptors. Impulses from the nipple reach the supraoptic and paraventricular nuclei through the somatic touch pathways. This causes secretion of oxytocin from the posterior pituitary. Oxytocin is then carried by blood to the breasts where it causes contraction of myoepithelial cells resulting in the ejection of milk.

Parturition (Delivery of the Baby)   Descent of the head of the baby at term causes stretch of the cervix. The impulses are carried to the hypothalamus.

Applied Physiology

Diabetes Insipidus

Diabetes insipidus develops due to deficiency of ADH. It is caused by disease of the supraoptic and paraventricular nuclei of the hypothalamus or the posterior pituitary gland.

The patient passes large quantity of dilute urine with reduced specific gravity (polyuria). It is associated with increased fluid intake (polydipsia). Unlike diabetes mellitus, the blood sugar levels are normal in diabetes insipidus.

Treatment

Diabetes insipidus can be treated by administration of desmopressin, an analogue of ADH having a longer half-life through mucous membrane of the nose.

Nephrogenic Diabetes Insipidus

In this type of diabetes insipidus, the kidneys are unable to respond to ADH. ADH production can be normal.

SIADH (Syndrome of Inappropriate Hypersecretion of ADH)

Patients with cerebral and pulmonary diseases tend to hypersecrete vasopressin. Pulmonary carcinoma and tuberculosis cause SIADH.

This results in the release of oxytocin from the posterior pituitary. Oxytocin acts on the gravid uterus to produce contraction of the uterus and relaxation of the cervix to deliver the baby. During labor, number of oxytocin receptors is increased.

This is an example of positive feedback mechanism.

Males also produce considerable amounts of oxytocin. But the exact role of oxytocin in males is unknown.

Other Actions

Oxytocin causes sodium retention and has an antidiuretic effect.

Thyroid (Fig. 10.4)

The thyroid gland is located in front of the larynx on either side and anterior to the trachea. It has two lobes connected by an isthmus.

It weighs 15–20 g in normal adult. This gland develops as an evagination of the floor of pharynx.

Thyroid gland has a rich blood supply. The rate of blood flow is 4–6 mL/g/min.

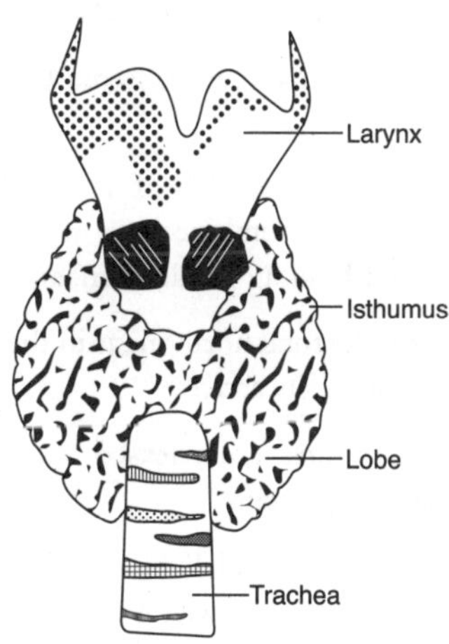

Fig. 10.4   Thyroid gland.

Histology (Fig. 10.5)

Thyroid gland is made up of multiple follicles (acini). Each follicle contains a single layer of cuboidal epithelium. It is filled with a clear, viscous material called colloid. The colloid contains thyroglobulin. The parafollicular cells are present in between the thyroid acini. The parafollicular cells secrete calcitonin.

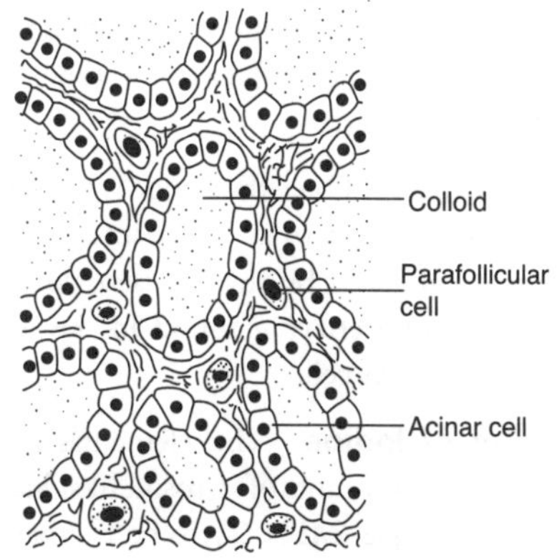

Fig. 10.5   Histology of thyroid glands.

Thyroid Hormones

Thyroid hormones are iodothyronines, i.e., compounds formed by coupling two iodinated tyrosine molecules with an ether linkage.

Thyroid hormones include

1. **Thyroxine (T_4):** It constitutes about 90% of the thyroid hormone.
2. **Triiodothyronine (T_3):** It constitutes about 9% of the thyroid hormone.
3. **Reverse T_3 (RT_3):** It constitutes only 1% of the thyroid hormone.
4. **Calcitonin:** It is secreted from the parafollicular cells.

Synthesis

Iodine is the most essential raw material for the synthesis of thyroid hormones. Ingested iodine

Applied Physiology

Synthetic oxytocin is used during delayed labor to induce uterine contractions.

It is used to prevent postpartum (after delivery) hemorrhage by producing contraction of the uterus.

is converted to iodide and absorbed by the gastrointestinal tract (GIT). Iodide enters the blood and is taken up by the thyroid gland by a process known as **iodide trapping**.

Iodide Trapping　Iodine is a trace element. Therefore, it is selectively trapped by the thyroid gland.

The basal membrane of the acinar cell has the ability to pump iodide by secondary active transport along with Na^+. By this method, concentration of iodide in the follicular cell is increased 30 times than its concentration in blood.

Oxidation of Iodide　Once the iodide is within the follicular cell, it is oxidized to an active intermediate. This reaction is catalyzed by thyroid peroxidase. It is a membrane-bound enzyme found in the apical portion of the follicular cell.

Organification of Iodine　The elemental iodine combines with third position of tyrosine residues to form monoiodotyrosine (MIT). Tyrosine is a part of the thyroglobulin molecule in the colloid. Addition of another iodine to this MIT at the fifth position of tyrosine results in the formation of diiodotyrosine (DIT).

Two DITs then condense to form T_4 (thyroxine). One MIT and one DIT condense to form T_3 (triiodothyronine). This is called **coupling reaction**. Thyroid peroxidase enzyme is involved in coupling reaction:

$$I_2 + Tyrosine = MIT$$

$$MIT + MIT = DIT$$

$$MIT + DIT = T_3$$

$$DIT + DIT = T_4.$$

Storage　The thyroid hormones remain attached to the thyroglobulin molecule and are stored in the colloid. Thyroid hormone stored in the gland is sufficient to meet the requirement of the body for 2–3 months.

Release　When the hormone is required, apical portion of the thyroid cells ingests small portion of colloid by endocytosis. The peptide bonds between iodinated tyrosine residue and thyroglobulin are broken down by proteases. Later, T_4, T_3, DIT_3, and MIT are released.

T_4 and T_3 are released into circulation. The remaining MIT and DIT are deiodinated. They are recycled for the synthesis of thyroid hormones.

Thyroglobulin

This is a glycoprotein molecule secreted into the follicles of thyroid gland. It is produced by the endoplasmic reticulum and the Golgi apparatus of thyroid acinar cells.

It has two subunits with a molecular weight of 6,60,000. It contains 123 tyrosine residues, of which only 4–8 are incorporated into the thyroid hormones. The thyroid hormones are formed within the thyroglobulin molecule and are bound to it until secretion.

During secretion, colloid is ingested by the thyroid cells. The peptide bonds are hydrolyzed; free T_4 and T_3 are released into the circulation.

Normal serum thyroglobulin is 6 ng/dL. It is increased in hyperthyroidism.

Secretion and Transport

The human thyroid gland secretes about 80 μg of T_4, 4 μg of T_3, and 2 μg of RT_3 each day.

The normal plasma T_4 is 8 μg/dL and T_3 is 0.15 μg/dL.

On entering the blood, 99% of T_4 and T_3 combine with proteins. They combine with thyroid-binding globulin, thyroid-binding prealbumin, and albumin.

Only 1% of the total hormone is in the free form and it is physiologically active.

Thyroid hormones are released slowly because they are bound to proteins.

Inside the tissue, T_3 and T_4 bind with intracellular proteins. They are used slowly over a period of days or weeks.

Pituitary secretion of TSH depends on free thyroid hormone levels in the blood.

Metabolism

T_3 and T_4 are deiodinated in the liver and kidney. One-third of circulating T_4 is converted to T_3. Forty-five percent is converted to reverse T_3.

Mechanism of Action

Thyroid hormones act at various sites including the nucleus, mitochondria, and plasma membrane.

Thyroid hormones enter the cells and bind to thyroid receptors in the nuclei. The hormone receptor complex then binds to DNA to form mRNA. Formation of mRNA and rRNA leads to the formation of a variety of proteins.

Proteins serve as structural and functional components of the cell and modify cell function.

Functions

Physiological Actions

1. **Calorigenic action:** Thyroid hormones increase the metabolism of almost all tissues of the body, exceptions being brain, testes, uterus, lymph nodes, spleen, and anterior pituitary.

   Thyroid hormones produced in excess can increase the BMR by 60–100%.

2. **General growth and development:** Thyroid hormones are essential for general growth. They stimulate the secretion of growth hormone. They also increase the synthesis of structural proteins.

3. **Metabolic actions:** Thyroid hormones have effects on various aspects of metabolism of carbohydrates, proteins, and lipids.

   (a) *Carbohydrate metabolism:* Thyroid hormones increase blood glucose level by
   - increasing the absorption of glucose from the gut;
   - increasing gluconeogenesis (formation of glucose from lipid and protein);
   - increasing insulin degradation;
   - increasing glycogenolysis (breakdown of glycogen);
   - causing rapid uptake of glucose by the cells.

   (b) *Lipid metabolism:* Lipid metabolism is enhanced by the thyroid hormones.
   - They increase the synthesis, mobilization, and degradation of lipids.
   - They decrease serum cholesterol level.

   (c) *Protein metabolism:* The thyroid hormones are essential for protein synthesis and growth. But excess thyroid hormones lead to protein catabolism (breakdown).

4. **Body weight:** An excess of thyroid hormones decreases the body weight due to increased catabolism.

5. **Effect on CVS:** Thyroid hormones
   - increase the heart rate;
   - increase the force of contraction;
   - systolic BP $\uparrow$ and diastolic BP $\downarrow$, but mean arterial pressure is unchanged;
   - cause vasodilatation.

6. **Action on CNS:**
   - Thyroid hormones have a marked effect on brain development.
   - They help in synaptic development and myelination.
   - They maintain normal reaction time of stretch reflex.

   Excess of thyroxine causes stimulation of CNS resulting in restlessness.

7. **Sleep:** Thyroid hormones maintain a normal sleep pattern. Sleep is disturbed in hyperthyroidism due to excessive stimulation of CNS. In hyperthyroidism, subject is exhausted but unable to sleep.

8. **Action on muscles:**
   - Thyroid hormones cause growth and maintenance of skeletal muscles.
   - They prevent muscle weakness.

9. **Effect on skin:** They maintain normal skin texture.

10. **Reproductive system:**
    - They maintain normal ovarian cycle in females.
    - They maintain spermatogenesis in males.
    - They maintain libido (sexual desire).

Other Functions

- Thyroid hormones stimulate erythropoiesis.

- They increase milk production.
- They exert permissive action on other hormones.
- They help in differentiation and maturation of cartilage.

Regulation

The specific feedback mechanisms operate through the anterior pituitary and the hypothalamus.

Thyroid function is mainly regulated by the pituitary TSH.

Feedback Regulation Increased level of thyroid hormones in the body decreases secretion of TSH from the anterior pituitary. It also has an effect on the hypothalamus to decrease the secretion of TRH. This is an example for negative feedback mechanism.

Thyroid-stimulating Hormone

It is also known as thyrotropin. Thyrotropin is a glycoprotein containing 211 amino acid residues, secreted by the anterior pituitary.

Its molecular weight is 28,000. The biological half-life of TSH is about 60 min. The secretion of TSH is pulsatile reaching a peak at midnight. The normal TSH secretion is 110 μg/day. The average plasma level is about 2μ units/mL.

Actions

- Increases the size and number of acinar cells.

- Increases the activity of iodide pump, which enhances the rate of iodide trapping.
- Increases iodination of tyrosine and coupling to form thyroid hormones.
- Increases proteolysis of thyroglobulin, releasing thyroid hormones into the blood.

The effect of TSH is brought about by the activation of second messenger cAMP system.

Thyroid Hormone-Releasing Hormone

This is secreted by the nerve endings in median eminence of the hypothalamus and transported to the anterior pituitary by the hypothalamohypophysial portal system.

TRH is a tripeptide amide. It acts on the anterior pituitary to increase the output of TSH.

TRH binds to the receptors present in the pituitary and activates phospholipase second messenger system.

Cold increases TRH and TSH secretion. Stress and anxiety decrease it.

Thyroid Function Tests

T_3, T_4 and TSH Levels Hormone levels are measured by radioimmunoassay. Serum T_3 and T_4 increase and serum TSH levels are reduced in hyperthyroidism.

The serum T_3 and T_4 decrease and serum TSH levels are increased in hypothyroidism.

Applied Physiology

Diseases of Thyroid Gland

The abnormalities of thyroid secretion can be due to either excess of thyroid hormones or deficiency of thyroid hormones.

Hypothyroidism

Deficiency of thyroid hormone secretion results in hypothyroidism.

There are two types of hypothyroidism:

- **Myxedema:** Hypothyroidism in adults
- **Cretinism:** Hypothyroidism in children

Myxedema   This condition develops due to hypothyroidism in adults. It is called myxedema due to the deposition of myxomatous tissue resulting in generalized edema.

Clinical Features

- Low BMR
- Thin and sparse hair
- Rough and dry skin
- Intolerance to cold
- Hoarse and slow voice
- Puffiness of face and increased body weight
- Mental sluggishness, delayed reaction times, and excessive sleep
- Nonpitting edema of feet due to deposition of mucopolysaccharides, protein hyaluronic acid, and choindroitin sulfate (myxomatous tissue)
- Decreased heart rate: reduced appetite
- Menstrual irregularity and infertility
- Low serum T_3–T_4 levels; increased TSH level

Treatment   Supplementation with hormone thyroxine

Cretinism   This is caused due to hypothyroidism during fetal life, infancy, and childhood.

Clinical Features

- The child will have stunted growth and mental retardation with idiotic appearance. The CNS manifestations are due to defective myelination
- Potbelly with umbilical hernia
- Enlarged and protruded tongue
- Failure of sexual development
- Low BMR; reduced appetite
- Dry, rough, and thick skin

Causes   Maternal iodine deficiency, fetal thyroid dysgenesis, and inborn errors of thyroid metabolism

Treatment   Supplementation with hormone thyroxine.

Goiter

It is a condition of enlargement of thyroid gland due to iodine deficiency.

- **Endemic goiter:** This disease occurs in people living in areas with deficiency of iodine in the food, e.g., Himalayan regions.

    Lack of iodine causes decreased production of T_3 and T_4. This causes increased secretion of TSH. TSH increases secretion of thyroglobulin. Accumulation of thyroglobulin causes enlargement of the gland.

- **Nonendemic goiter:** This disease occurs in persons whose iodine uptake is normal, but there is deficiency of enzymes involved in the synthesis of T_3 and T_4. Cabbage and turnip have goitrogenic effect.

Hyperthyroidism

Excess secretion of T_3 and T_4 leads to this condition.

The common form of hyperthyroidism is **Grave's disease**.

It is an autoimmune disease wherein antibodies are produced by B-lymphocytes. These antibodies activate thyroid receptors resulting in hyperthyroidism.

Clinical Features

- Exophthalmos (protrusion of the eyeball)
- Nervousness and fine tremors
- Increased cardiac output, systolic blood pressure, and increased resting pulse rate
- Intolerance to heat and excessive sweating
- Increased BMR
- Hyperglycemia and decreased cholesterol
- Weight loss, polyphagia, and diarrhea

Exophthalmos

It is the protrusion of eyeballs caused due to inflammation and edema of the retro-orbital structures.

Treatment

- Surgical removal of thyroid gland
- Use of antithyroid drugs
- Radioactive iodine therapy for destruction of the gland

Thyroiditis

This is an inflammation of the thyroid gland which causes progressive destruction and fibrosis of the gland.

Hashimoto's thyroiditis is an autoimmune disease caused due to the production of antibodies against thyroglobulin which ultimately destroys the gland.

Radioactive Iodine Uptake   Radiolabeled iodine is administered to the subject and uptake of iodine by the thyroid gland is evaluated.

This test helps to differentiate between normal, toxic nodule, thyroid cyst, and malignant nodule. Normal radioiodine uptake is 20–40%. In hyperthyroidism, there is increased uptake, and in hypothyroidism, there is decreased uptake of iodine.

Serum Protein-Bound Iodine (PBI)   Normal serum PBI is 4–8 μg/dL. Less than 3.5 μg/dL indicates hypothyroidism.

Sleeping Pulse Rate   Sleeping pulse rate is high in thyrotoxicosis.

Basal Metabolic Rate   Basal metabolic rate is high in hyperthyroidism (+100%).

BMR is low in hypothyroidism (–40%).

Other Investigations

- Serum cholesterol increased in hypothyroidism
- Serum creatinine increased in hyperthyroidism
- Radiography of the neck
- Thyroid gland biopsy
- Indirect laryngoscopy

Parathyroid Glands

There are four parathyroid glands. Two in the superior pole of the thyroid and two in the inferior pole.

Each parathyroid measures $3 \times 6 \times 2$ mm.

Total weight is 140 mg.

There are two types of cells in parathyroid gland:

1. chief cells and
2. oxyphil cells.

Chief cells contain Golgi apparatus, endoplasmic reticulum, and secretory granules. They secrete parathormone.

Oxyphil cells contain large number of mitochondria. Function of oxyphil cell is not known.

Parathormone

Parathormone (PTH) is a polypeptide hormone with molecular weight 9,500, containing 84 amino acid residues.

Normal plasma value is 10–55 pg/mL. Plasma half-life is 10 min.

Actions

Parathormone mainly acts on the bones, kidneys, and intestine. It indirectly acts on the nervous system, muscles, and other endocrine glands.

Bones It increases reabsorption of bone and mobilization of calcium from the bone.

It increases the activity of osteoclasts causing osteoclastic bone dissolution.

Kidneys Parathormone increases the reabsorption of calcium in the DCT.

It increases phosphate excretion in the urine by decreasing phosphate reabsorption in the proximal tubules.

It increases reabsorption of Mg^{++} and H^+ ions. It decreases reabsorption of Na^+, K^+, and amino acids.

Intestine Parathormone increases the synthesis of vitamin D. Calcium is absorbed from the GIT under the influence of vitamin D (1-25-dihydroxy cholecalciferol).

It enhances phosphate absorption from the intestine.

Parathormone therefore increases serum calcium level by

- increasing calcium mobilization from bones;
- increasing reabsorption in the kidney;
- increasing reabsorption from the intestine.

Synthesis

It is synthesized as preprohormone on the ribosomes. Later, it is cleaved to form prohormone and then to hormone containing 84 amino acids by the endoplasmic reticulum and Golgi apparatus. It is then packed in secretory granules in the cell cytoplasm.

Mechanism of Action

Three different receptor types have been identified. PTH activates the enzyme adenylate cyclase. This increases intracellular cAMP in the osteocytes, osteoclasts, and other target cells. Cyclic AMP is responsible for actions of the parathormone.

Regulation of Secretion

Parathormone secretion is regulated in negative feedback mechanism by action of ionized calcium on the parathyroid glands.

When plasma calcium is high, parathormone secretion is inhibited. Calcium is deposited in the bones. When plasma calcium becomes low, calcium is mobilized from the bones.

Applied Physiology

Hypoparathyroidism

The deficiency of parathormone occurs due to accidental removal of the parathyroid glands during thyroid surgery. Symptoms develop in 2–3 days. Decreased PTH causes decreased plasma Ca^{++} and increased plasma phosphate. Hypocalcemia leads to **tetany**.

Decreased serum calcium level in tetany leads to increased neuromuscular excitability. This leads to spasm of laryngeal and intestinal muscles. Involvement of the laryngeal muscles causes laryngeal stridor, airway obstruction, convulsions, and death.

Adduction of thumbs and extension of feet is termed **carpopedal spasm**.

In pseudohypoparathyroidism, secretion of PTH is normal, but there is a defect in receptors. Hence, the response to PTH is decreased.

Tests for Latent Tetany.

- **Chvostek's sign:** Tapping facial nerve causes contraction of facial muscles.
- **Trousseau's sign:** Occlusion of blood supply to upper limb causes flexion at wrist and thumb, and extension of fingers.

Hyperparathyroidism

This condition is due to tumor or hyperplasia of the parathyroid gland.

This leads to hypercalcemia, hypophosphatemia, demineralization of bones, hypercalciuria, and formation of renal stones.

It diminishes neuronal excitability, muscle weakness, and constipation.

Secondary Hyperparathyroidism

This occurs in conditions of chronic renal disease and rickets. The serum calcium is chronically low. Low calcium stimulates the parathyroid glands causing compensatory hypertrophy of the parathyroid and secondary hyperparathyroidism.

Decreased serum Mg^{++} also stimulates parathormone secretion.

Calcitriol (1,25-Dihydroxycholecalciferol)

It is an active form of vitamin D (D_3). It is formed by the action of UV radiation on 7-dehydrocholesterol present in the skin. Vitamin D_2 is available in the diet.

Synthesis

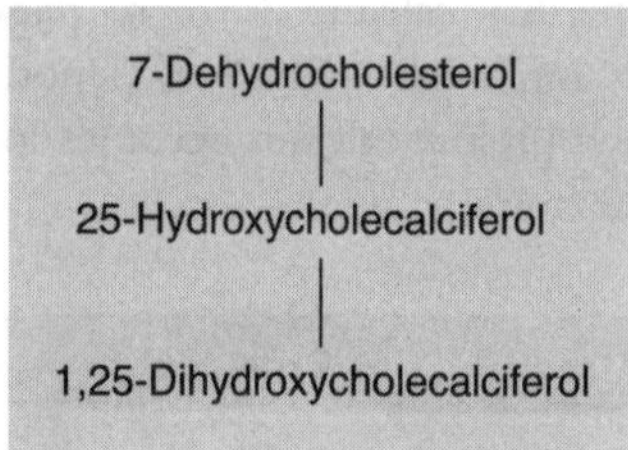

Functions

On GIT It stimulates the absorption of calcium from intestines by increasing the production of carrier protein for calcium.

It increases the intestinal absorption of phosphates as well as magnesium.

On Kidneys It increases the absorption of calcium and phosphate from the DCT.

On Bones It influences mineralization of bone. It increases synthetic activity of osteoblasts. It is

necessary for normal calcification. In large quantities, it causes the absorption of bone.

Calcitriol has a role in muscle function, development, and suppression. Serum calcitriol level increases in pregnancy.

Transport

Calcitriol is sparingly soluble in blood. Ninety-nine percent of calcitriol is transported in bound form with transcalciferin. Plasma half-life of calcitriol is 5–24 h.

Mechanism of Action

It acts through receptors in cytoplasm. The hormone–receptor complex causes synthesis of calcium-binding protein in the mucosa of the gastrointestinal tract.

A calcium-binding protein called calbindin facilitates the transport of calcium, magnesium, and phosphate. This is present in the intestinal mucosal epithelium. Synthesis of calbindin is regulated by calcitriol.

Regulation

Reduced levels of calcium or phosphate lead to increase in the formation of vitamin D_3 from vitamin D. Increased levels of calcium or phosphate lead to the formation of inactive forms of vitamin D_2 and vitamin D.

Calcitonin

Calcitonin is secreted by type C cells or parafollicular cells of the thyroid gland.

It is a polypeptide with 32 amino acids.

Molecular weight of calcitonin is about 3400.

Functions

- Promotes calcium deposition in the bones.
- Inhibits resorption of bone by the osteoclasts.
- Decreases serum calcium levels.

Mechanism of Action

It acts by stimulation of adenylate cyclase and increase in the levels of cAMP.

Regulation

High serum calcium levels stimulate calcitonin secretion.

Clinical Application

Used in the treatment of Paget's disease and senile osteoporosis.

Calcium Metabolism (Fig. 10.6)

Ionic calcium is important for physiological functions of the body. It is necessary for nerve conduction, excitability of the cell, muscle contraction, blood coagulation, and synaptic transmission.

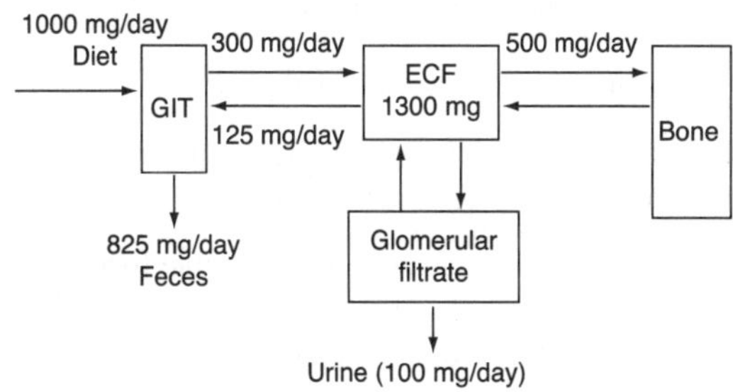

Fig. 10.6   Distribution and exchange of calcium in the body.

Source

Calcium is present in food and water. It is found in green leafy vegetables, milk, and dairy products.

Applied Physiology

Deficiency of vitamin D leads to **rickets** in children and **osteomalacia** in adults.

Rickets

Defective bone formation leads to frontal bossing, knock-knee, and rickety rosary (thickening and prominence of costochondral junction).

It can be corrected by exposure to sunlight and supplementation of vitamin D.

Osteomalacia

In this condition, bones become soft due to defective mineralization.

Hypervitaminosis D

It occurs due to excessive intake of vitamin D. This is characterized by nausea and vomiting.

In long-standing cases, it results in defective bone formation.

Osteoporosis

It occurs at old age and in postmenopausal females. The condition is due to loss of bone matrix. The bone looses calcium, becomes porous, and gets fractured easily.

Daily Intake

One thousand milligrams of calcium is consumed per day. About 300 mg is absorbed in upper part of small intestine. About 125 mg is secreted in the digestive juices. The net absorption is 175 mg/day.

Normal Serum Calcium Level
9–11 m/100 mL of blood

Calcium content of a normal adult is 1000 g.

Ninety-nine percent is present in the bones. One percent is in soft tissues and ECF.

About 50% of calcium is in diffusible form. This is ionic calcium and is biologically active. Decrease of ionic calcium results in tetany.

Absorption

Calcium is absorbed by both diffusion and carrier-mediated transport (with calbindin). Calcitriol increases GI absorption of calcium.

High levels of phosphate, and fat decrease calcium absorption; corticosteroids also inhibit calcium absorption.

Normal serum calcium levels are maintained by parathormone, calcitriol, and calcitonin. Regulation is by the action of hormones on the GI tract, kidneys, and bones.

Regulation of Calcium Ion Concentration

Exchangeable calcium salts in the bone are calcium phosphate compounds. They are loosely bound in the bone and are in reversible equilibrium with calcium and phosphate ions in ECF.

An increased calcium and phosphate level in ECF causes immediate formation of calcium phosphate.

Decrease in the concentration of calcium and phosphate causes immediate absorption of calcium phosphate.

Sudden increase in calcium ion concentration leads to decreased rate of parathormone secretion. There is increase in calcitonin secretion leading to deposition of calcium in bones.

Functions of Calcium Ions

- Needed for the formation of bone and teeth
- Maintains cell membrane integrity
- Helps in coagulation of blood
- Regulates neuromuscular excitability
- Needed for the contraction of muscle
- Facilitates the secretion of neurotransmitters and hormones

Phosphate Metabolism

Phosphate is a major intracellular ion. Intracellular levels are much greater than extracellular levels.

About 85% of plasma phosphate is in free form. Serum phosphate levels vary widely during the day. Phosphate enters the serum from GIT, bone, and soft tissue. It leaves the serum by renal excretion, and entry into bone and soft tissues.

Total amount of phosphate in the body is 500–800 g. It is mainly present in the skeleton (85–90%).

Plasma phosphate level is 3–5 mg/dL.

Phosphate is found in ATP, cAMP, ADP, and glucose-6-phosphate.

Regulation

Plasma phosphate is mainly controlled by parathormone.

Parathormone reduces tubular reabsorption of phosphate.

Applied Physiology

Hypophosphatemia

A severe decrease in phosphate levels leads to decreased nerve conduction and defective bone mineralization. In addition, it leads to hemolytic anemia due to reduced red cell ATP.

Endocrine Pancreas

The islets of Langerhans are microscopic nests of cells mainly concentrated in the tail portion of the pancreas.

There are 1–2 million islets in humans.

These islets contain four types of cells:

1. **Alpha cells:** 25%, secrete glucagon
2. **Beta cells:** 60%, secrete insulin
3. **Delta cells:** 10%, secrete somatostatin
4. **F cells:** 5%, secrete pancreatic polypeptide

Beta cells make up the large central mass of islets of Langerhans. They are surrounded by alpha, delta, and F cells.

Insulin

Insulin was isolated in the year 1922 by Banting and Best.

It is a polypeptide hormone with 51 amino acids having two chains.

A chain has 21 amino acids. B chain has 30 amino acids.

Molecular weight is 5808.

Secretion

It is secreted by rough endoplasmic reticulum of beta cells as preproinsulin.

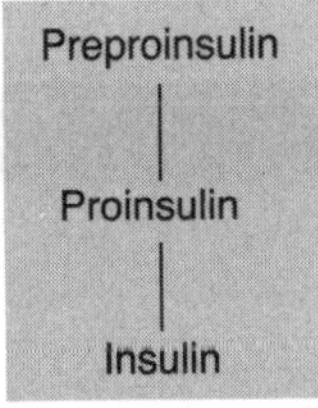

Insulin circulates in blood in unbound form.
Plasma half-life is 5 min.

Plasma Level

The plasma level of insulin is 20μ units/mL during fasting. It is 150μ units/mL after the consumption of food.

Mechanism of Action

Insulin binds to the insulin receptors which are present mainly in the liver, skeletal muscle, and adipose tissue.

The insulin receptors are large membrane proteins with two α and two β subunits. They are bound to each other by disulfide bridges. The insulin receptors are located on chromosome 19.

- Binding of insulin to α subunits brings about conformational change in β subunits.
- Conformational change in β subunits activates tyrosine kinase activity producing autophosphorylation of β subunits.
- This leads to phosphorylation of intracellular enzymes including a group of enzymes called insulin receptor substrates (IRS).
- IRS causes a variety of changes like activation or deactivation of target enzymes, translocation of GLUTs, and induction or suppression of genes.

In this way, insulin produces required effects on carbohydrate, fat, and protein metabolism.

Degradation

Insulin is cleared from circulation in 10–15 min. It is destroyed by insulin protease in the liver and kidney.

Actions

- **Rapid:** Increases transport of glucose, amino acids, and K^+ into insulin-sensitive cells.
- **Intermediate:** Stimulates protein synthesis; inhibits protein degradation.
- **Delayed:** Increases the formation of mRNA for lipogenic action.

Functions

Insulin has a wide range of activities that are broadly divided into two groups: metabolic functions and effect on growth.

Metabolic Functions

Carbohydrate Metabolism

- Helps in cellular uptake of glucose.
- Increases peripheral utilization of glucose.
- Prevents glycogenolysis and neoglucogenesis, and improves glycogen synthesis.

Insulin increases the activity of glucokinase enzyme. This enhances the utilization of glucose by catalyzing its phosphorylation. Increased utilization of glucose decreases its intracellular concentration. This leads to the entry of glucose by facilitated diffusion.

Glucose enters the cells by facilitated diffusion with the help of glucose transporters. In the intestine and kidneys it occurs by secondary transport with Na^+. In muscle and adipose tissue, insulin facilitates glucose entry into the cells by increasing the number of glucose transporters in the cell membrane.

Glucose Transporters

They are a family of closely related proteins having amino and carboxyl terminals inside the cell. They are different from sodium-dependent glucose transporters (SGLT-1 and SGLT-2). Seven GLUT transporters have been identified (GLUT 1–7).

Protein Metabolism

- Facilitates the transport of amino acids into cells.
- Increases mRNA translation.
- Increases protein synthesis.
- Prevents protein breakdown.

Hence, it is an anabolic hormone.

Lipid Metabolism

- Prevents lipolysis by inhibiting hormone-sensitive lipase.
- Decreases free fatty acid in the blood.

- Promotes the synthesis and storage of fats.

Ion Transport   Insulin increases K^+ transport into the cells.

Growth and Development   Insulin potentiates the action of growth hormone to promote growth.

Insulin and growth hormone act synergistically to promote growth.

Regulation

Factors Enhancing Insulin Release   Increased levels of glucose, amino acids, GI hormones, glucagon, and parasympathetic stimulation.

Factors Reducing Insulin Secretion   Increased secretion of somatostatin and sympathetic stimulation.

Control of insulin secretion is brought about by blood glucose concentration.

Insulin secretion increases as the concentration of blood glucose increases. This increases the transport of glucose into liver, muscles, and other cells, thereby reducing the blood glucose concentration toward normal.

Amino acids like arginine and lysine also stimulate insulin secretion.

Gastrin, secretin, cholecystokinin (CCK) and gastric inhibitory polypeptide (GIP) cause a moderate increase in insulin secretion.

Applied Physiology

Diabetes Mellitus

It is a condition caused due to the deficiency of insulin or decreased sensitivity of tissues to insulin. There is impaired carbohydrate, fat, and protein metabolism.

Types

1. **Type 1:** This is also called insulin-dependent diabetes mellitus (IDDM). It is caused by the lack of insulin secretion.
2. **Type 2:** This is also called noninsulin-dependent diabetes mellitus (NIDDM). It is caused by decreased sensitivity of tissues to insulin.

Symptoms

- Polyuria (increased urination)
- Polydipsia (increased fluid intake)
- Polyphagia (increased food intake)

- Weight loss
- Delayed wound healing

Polyuria   Increased blood glucose levels cause increased excretion of glucose in urine. This causes excessive excretion of water due to the osmotic effect of glucose.

Polydipsia   Increased excretion of urine leads to decreased body water. This causes sensation of thirst, resulting in increased water intake.

Polyphagia   There is reduced entry of glucose into glucostatic cells due to insulin lack. This suppresses the satiety center and stimulates the feeding center enhancing the desire to eat.

Treatment

- **IDDM**: Administration of insulin
- **NIDDM**: Diet and exercise (lifestyle modification); oral antidiabetic drugs; supplementation of insulin

Glucose Tolerance Test

This is a screening test for diabetes mellitus.

The individual is maintained on 3 days of balanced diet. He is advised to fast overnight. The patient is given 75 g of glucose orally and blood glucose levels are measured at periodic intervals. If the fasting glucose level is less than 115 mg/dL, 2 h level is <140 mg/dL, and none of the values exceed 200 mg/dL, the oral GTT is considered normal.

Control of Insulin Secretion

The serum insulin levels rise within 10 min after the ingestion of food. It reaches peak in 30–45 min. When stimulated, insulin is released in two phases: early phase due to the release of preformed insulin and late phase due to the release of newly formed insulin.

Insulin increases the uptake, storage, and utilization of glucose in almost all the tissues of the body. Muscles, adipose tissues, and liver utilize glucose under the influence of insulin.

Brain, RBC, kidney, and mucosa of small intestine are not dependent on insulin for the uptake and utilization of glucose.

Glucagon

This is a hormone secreted by the alpha cells of the islets of Langerhans. It is a polypeptide composed of 29 amino acids. Its molecular weight is 3485.

Glucagon is a hyperglycemic hormone. Physiological functions of glucagon are opposite to that of insulin.

Actions

- Causes glycogenolysis and gluconeogenesis. Therefore, it increases the blood glucose level.
- Increases the rate of amino acid uptake by the liver cells and converts them into glucose.
- Activates lipase which breaks down lipids into fatty acids.
- Stimulates the secretion of growth hormone, insulin, and pancreatic somatostatin.

Metabolism

It has a half-life of 5–10 min in circulation. It is degraded mainly in the liver.

Mechanism of Action

Glucagon activates adenylate cyclase in the liver cells. This causes formation of cyclic AMP. cAMP activates protein kinase, which in turn activates phosphorylase. Phosphorylase promotes the conversion of glycogen to glucose.

Regulation

Glucagon secretion is mainly controlled by the blood glucose concentration.

- Decrease in the blood glucose causes an increase in glucagon secretion.

- Increase in the blood glucose causes a decrease in glucagon secretion.
- Increased amino acids, severe exercise, CCK gastrin, and stress cause increased glucagon secretion.
- Increased glucose, free fatty acids, insulin, somatostatin, and GABA (gamma-aminobutyric acid) inhibit glucagon secretion.

Somatostatin

This is a polypeptide which functions both as a neurotransmitter and as a hormone. It is of two types: somatostatin 14 and somatostatin 28.

Functions

It functions as a neurotransmitter in various parts of the brain. It has an effect on the sensory input, locomotor activity, and cognitive function.

- In the hypothalamus, it acts as growth hormone–inhibiting hormone.
- In the pancreas, it inhibits the secretion of insulin and glucagon.
- It reduces GI motility and is an important inhibitory GI hormone.

Secretion

It is secreted by delta cells of islets of the Langerhans. It has a plasma half-life of 3 min.

Regulation

Increased blood glucose, amino acids, and fatty acids enhance somatostatin secretion.

Pancreatic Polypeptide

It is a polypeptide containing 36 amino acid residues. It is produced by F cells of the pancreas. It is closely related to polypeptide YY found in the intestine and neuropeptide Y found in the brain.

Secretion of pancreatic polypeptide is decreased by somatostatin and intravenous administration of glucose.

Pancreatic polypeptide slows the absorption of food but its exact function is still not known.

Adrenal Gland

Anatomy

There are two adrenal glands each weighing about 4 g.

They lie at the superior pole of both the kidneys.

It is a highly vascular gland receiving 6–7 mL of blood/g/min.

Adrenal gland consists of two parts:

1. **Adrenal cortex:** Occupies outer 80% of the gland. It secretes glucocorticoids, mineralo-corticoids, and sex steroids.
2. **Adrenal medulla:** Occupies inner 20% of the gland. It secretes epinephrine, norepinephrine, and dopamine.

Morphology

The adrenal cortex is composed of three relatively distinct layers:

1. **Zona glomerulosa** (outer 15–20%) secretes aldosterone.
2. **Zona fasciculata** (middle 50–55%) secretes cortisol, corticosterone, and small amounts of androgens.
3. **Zona reticularis** (inner 7–10%) secretes androgens and cortisol.

Chemistry

The adrenocortical hormones are steroid hormones derived from cholesterol.

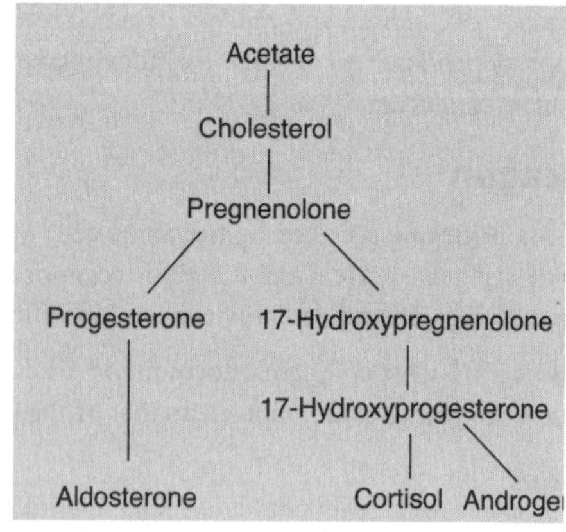

Important adrenocortical hormones are as under:

- **Mineralocorticoids:** Aldosterone and desoxycorticosterone
- **Glucocorticoids:** Cortisol and corticosterone

Mineralocorticoids

Aldosterone is the chief mineralocorticoid. It is secreted from the zona glomerulosa.

Mechanism of Action   It combines with receptors in the cytoplasm to form hormone–receptor complex. This complex induces portion of DNA to form mRNA. mRNA helps in the protein synthesis.

Transport and Secretion   Aldosterone combines loosely with the plasma proteins and about 50% of it is in free form.

It stays in circulation for around 30 min.

It is mainly degraded in the liver.

Actions

- Increase Na^+ and Cl^- absorption and decrease the absorption of K^+ and PO_4 in the renal tubules.
- Help in the regulation of body fluid volume.
- Help in the control of acid–base balance.

- Increase the reabsorption of Na^+ and Cl^- and secretion of K^+ ions in the sweat glands, salivary glands, and intestine.

Regulation of Aldosterone Secretion   Increased K^+ ion concentration in ECF increases aldosterone secretion.

Increased activity of renin–angiotensin system increases its secretion.

Increased Na^+ ion concentration in ECF marginally decreases its secretion.

Aldosterone Escape   Whenever aldosterone is increased, Na^+ ions are retained in the body. This causes osmotic absorption of water. Therefore, ECF volume increases. Increase in ECF leads to increase in arterial pressure, causing excretion of salt and water by pressure diuresis. This secondary increase in water and salt excretion by kidneys is called **aldosterone escape.**

Glucocorticoids

Cortisol   This is a C21 steroid produced mainly from the zona fasciculata.

It combines with cortisol-binding globulin.

Ninety-six percent of the cortisol is transported in bound form. Only 4% is transported in free form.

Applied Physiology

Aldosterone Excess

This is termed hyperaldosteronism.

It is of two types:

1. **Primary hyperaldosteronism (Conn's syndrome):** This occurs due to adenoma of zona glomerulosa. In this condition, there is K^+ depletion, Na^+ retention, weakness, hypertension, tetany, polyuria, and alkalosis.
2. **Secondary hyperaldosteronism:** This occurs due to the use of diuretics, nephrosis, cirrhosis of liver, and congestive cardiac failure. In this condition, circulating renin and angiotensin II levels are elevated.

Aldosterone Deficiency

Deficiency of aldosterone causes rise in K^+ ion concentration leading to cardiac toxicity. This results in reduced force of cardiac contraction and development of arrhythmias leading to heart failure.

Absence of aldosterone secretion causes death within 2 weeks. Without aldosterone, K^+ concentration in ECF increases. Na^+ and Cl^- concentration decreases. ECF volume and blood volume are greatly reduced. A person develops diminished cardiac output proceeding to a shock-like state followed by death.

It stays in circulation for 1–2 h.

It is degraded in the liver and conjugated to form glucuronides. It is excreted in the urine.

Mechanism of Action These hormones enter the cell and combine with receptors in the cytoplasm. Hormone–receptor complex induces portion of DNA to form mRNA. The mRNA causes protein formation. These proteins are responsible for actions of glucocorticoids.

Functions

- **On carbohydrate metabolism:** It stimulates gluconeogenesis by the liver. It decreases the rate of glucose utilization by the cells.

  Adrenal diabetes—The blood glucose increases as a result of increased gluconeogenesis and reduced glucose utilization by the cells. This condition is termed **adrenal diabetes**. This is moderately insulin sensitive.

- **On protein metabolism:** It reduces protein stores in all cells except the liver cells. This causes decreased protein synthesis.

  Cortisol enhances amino acid uptake by the liver cells. Hence, the liver proteins and plasma proteins are increased.

- **On fat metabolism:** It causes fatty acid mobilization from adipose tissue, increasing free fatty acids in plasma.

  It stimulates the absorption of lipids from the intestine.

  It causes redistribution of fats in the body.

- **Anti-inflammatory effect:** Cortisol inhibits all aspects of inflammation. It reduces leukocyte margination, chemotaxis, and phagocytosis of bacteria. Aggregation of monocytes is also inhibited.

  Cortisol inhibits the synthesis and release of chemical mediators of inflammation like prostaglandins and arachidonic acid.

- **Wound healing:** It prevents the development of fibroblasts and delays wound healing.

  It blocks the early stages of inflammation.

  If inflammation has already begun, it causes resolution of inflammation.

- **In stress:** Stress causes increase in ACTH secretion followed by secretion of cortisol.

Other Functions

- Cortisol has antiallergic effect.
- Decreases the number of eosinophils and lymphocytes in the blood.
- Causes demineralization of bone.
- Stimulates gastric secretion.
- Suppresses immune response by reducing circulating T-lymphocytes.

Regulation

Cortisol secretion is controlled by ACTH.

ACTH is secreted in irregular bursts throughout the day. Plasma cortisol rises and falls in response to these bursts. The plasma cortisol is high in the mornings (20 µg/dL) and very low (5 µg/dL) in the evenings.

Applied Physiology

Addison's Disease

This is caused due to failure of adrenal cortex to produce adrenocortical hormones. It is mostly caused by primary atrophy of adrenal cortex due to autoimmune disease, tuberculosis, and invasion by cancer.

Signs and Symptoms

- Loss of Na^+ and Cl^- ions through urine, leading to decreased ECF volume, hyponatremia, hyperkalemia, and mild acidosis
- Muscle weakness and depressed metabolic functions of the body
- Low blood glucose levels in spite of excess glucose in the body

- Highly susceptible to stress and infections
- Pigmentation of skin and mucus membrane

Addisonian Crisis

A person with Addison's disease succumbs to stress. This condition is called Addisonian crisis. They need extra amounts of glucocorticoids.

If the patient is not treated properly he/she dies of shock.

Cushing's Syndrome

It is a condition produced due to the excess secretion of glucocorticoids.

Causes

- Adrenocortical tumors
- Anterior pituitary tumors
- Ectopic ACTH-producing tumor
- Prolonged glucocorticoid therapy

    Cushing's syndrome caused due to tumors of anterior pituitary is called **Cushing's disease**.

Signs and Symptoms

- Fat collects in the abdominal wall, face, and upper back, producing buffalo hump and moon face.
- Skin and subcutaneous tissues are thin.
- Muscles are poorly developed.
- Wounds heal poorly; minor injuries cause bruises and ecchymoses, osteoporosis.
- There is insulin-resistant diabetes mellitus due to gluconeogenesis.
- There is salt and water retention, K^+ depletion, and weakness due to mineralocorticoid activity of cortisol.
- Protein depletion occurs due to its excessive catabolism.
- Hypertension develops due to increased deoxycorticosterone production.
- Reddish purple striae appear in the skin due to rupture of subdermal tissues.

Treatment

Treatment involves the removal of tumor in adrenal or pituitary gland. If removal of pituitary tumor is not possible then removal of both adrenals with supplementation of steroids.

Adrenogenital Syndrome

An adrenocortical tumor secretes excess amounts of androgens causing intense masculanizing effects. Females develop virile characteristics like growth of beard, deep voice, baldness, masculine distribution of hair, and growth of clitoris.

Prepubertal male has rapid development of sexual organs (precocious puberty).

In an adult male, it is difficult to diagnose the condition because the signs are obscured by normal virilizing characteristics of testosterone.

Cortisol-Binding Globulin

This is also called *transcortin*. It is an α-globulin that binds to cortisol. It is synthesized in the liver. CBG levels rise during pregnancy. It decreases during cirrhosis, nephrosis, and multiple myeloma.

ACTH

This is a single-chain polypeptide containing 39 amino acids. It is secreted by the anterior lobe of the pituitary gland. It is formed from a prohormone called pro-opiomelanocortin. Its plasma half-life is 10 min.

Actions

It stimulates the growth and secretion of zona fasciculata and zona reticularis of adrenal cortex. It controls the secretion of cortisol.

Mechanism of Action

ACTH acts through cAMP system. Cyclic AMP causes activation of protein kinase A. This causes conversion of cholesterol to pregnenolone.

Control

ACTH secretion is mainly controlled by CRH secreted by the hypothalamus. It increases blood steroids and decreases ACTH secretion.

Stress causes an increase in ACTH secretion.

ACTH is secreted in irregular bursts throughout the day. These bursts occur more frequently in the mornings. Therefore, secretion of cortisol is more in the mornings and less in the evenings.

Corticotropin-Releasing Factor

Corticotropin-releasing factor hormone (CRF) is secreted from the hypothalamus. It is a peptide with 41 amino acids. The cell bodies of neurons that secrete CRF are located in the paraventricular nucleus of the hypothalamus. CRF stimulates the secretion of ACTH.

Adrenal Medulla

Adrenal medulla is functionally related to the sympathetic system. It is a sympathetic ganglion in which the postganglionic neurons do not have axons and have become secretory cells.

It secretes the following hormones:

- epinephrine (adrenaline),
- norepinephrine (noradrenaline), and
- dopamine.

These hormones are not essential for life but they help to prepare the individual to deal with emergencies.

Ninety percent of the cells are epinephrine secreting type and 10% norepinephrine secreting type.

Synthesis

$$\text{Tyrosine} \xrightarrow{\text{Hydroxylation}} \text{DOPA}$$
$$\text{DOPA} \xrightarrow{\text{Decarboxylation}} \text{Dopamine}$$
$$\text{Dopamine} \xrightarrow{\text{Hydroxylation}} \text{Norepinephrine}.$$

Eighty percent of norepinephrine in the adrenal cortex is transformed to epinephrine:

$$\text{Norepinephrine} \xrightarrow{\text{Methylation}} \text{Epinephrine}.$$

The catecholamines have a half-life of 2 min in circulation.

The actions of epinephrine and norepinephrine are mediated through receptors.

There are two types of adrenergic receptors, α and β.

α receptors are of two types, α_1 and α_2.

β receptors are of three types, $\beta_1, \beta_2,$ and β_3.

Norepinephrine excites mainly α receptors.

Epinephrine excites both types of receptors equally.

Functions

- Norepinephrine causes constriction of all the blood vessels of the body.
- It causes inhibition of the GIT, reducing motility and secretion.
- It causes dilatation of pupils.
- Epinephrine causes dilatation of blood vessels in muscle and liver via β_2 receptors.

- Norepinephrine and epinephrine both increase the rate and force of contraction of the heart.
- They increase alertness, cause glycogenolysis, and also increase the metabolic activity of the body.

Regulation

The secretions from the adrenal medulla are influenced mainly through the nervous system. They increase in conditions of hypoglycemia, stress, anxiety, hemorrhage, exercise, and extremes of temperature.

Hemorrhage predominantly stimulates the epinephrine secretion.

Emotional stress and anger stimulate the norepinephrine secretion.

Pineal Gland

It forms a major part of the epithalamus. It weighs about 150 mg. It contains cells termed pinealocytes. It secretes the hormone melatonin.

Functions

- Controls reproductive function.
- Influences the function of other endocrine glands.
- Helps to maintain sleep-wakefulness cycle.
- Helps to maintain biological rhythms of the body.

Thymus

Thymus is present behind the upper part of the sternum. This gland processes the lymphocytes. These lymphocytes are called T-lymphocytes and they are responsible for cell-mediated immunity.

The endocrine role of the thymus gland is not clear. Thymus gland is known to interact with other endocrine glands.

Growth hormone promotes the growth of thymus. ACTH and glucocorticoids excess causes atrophy of thymus.

Thymus involutes at puberty possibly due to the effect of gonadal steroids.

Abnormal thymus function is implicated in the pathogenesis of autoimmune diseases like rheumatoid arthritis, hemolytic anemia, and myasthenia gravis.

Applied Physiology

Tumors of the adrenal medulla cause **pheochromocytoma**. In this condition, excess of catecholamines are produced. Symptoms of pheochromocytoma include hypertension, headache, anxiety, palpitations, and chest pain.

Reproductive System

The members of the same species are formed by the process of reproduction.

In unicellular organisms, reproduction occurs by division of the parent cell. It is an asexual type of reproduction.

In multicellular organisms, there is sexual type of reproduction. It occurs by the fusion of male and female gametes. Each of the male and female gametes has haploid number of chromosomes which fuse to form the fertilized egg or zygote.

Sexual reproduction is complex and needs specialized reproductive system.

Puberty

It is the period during which the increased endocrine and gametogenic functions of the gonads have acquired the capacity to reproduce.

Puberty occurs between the ages of 8 and 13 years in girls, and 9 and 14 years in boys.

The frequency and amplitude of pulsatile secretion of GnRH (gonadotropin-releasing hormone) increase at puberty. This causes increase in FSH (follicle-stimulating hormone) and LH (luteinizing hormone) secretion.

In males, FSH and LH stimulate Leydig cells to secrete testosterone.

In females, FSH and LH stimulate the production of estrogen and progesterone.

Changes Occurring at the Time of Puberty

Secondary Sexual Characters

In Boys

- Growth of the external genitalia
- Hypertrophy of the laryngeal mucosa and enlargement of the larynx causing a typical male voice

- Increased thickness of the skin, increased sebaceous secretion, and development of acne
- The pelvis becomes long, funnel shaped, and stronger
- Development of aggressive behavior and interest in opposite sex
- Increased muscular development
- Development of hair on face, axilla, and pubic region

In Girls

- Development of breasts
- Enlargement of the uterus, fallopian tube, ovaries, and vagina
- Onset of menstrual cycle
- Deposition of fat in the buttocks, thighs, and breast giving feminine appearance

- Growth of axillary and pubic hair
- Enlargement and widening of pelvis

Menarche   The onset of first menstruation is called menarche. It occurs at around 11–14 years of age.

Female Reproductive System

The female reproductive system has the following organs (Fig. 11.1):

- **Primary sex organ**

  Ovaries

- **Accessory sex organs**

  Fallopian tube

  Uterus

  Vagina

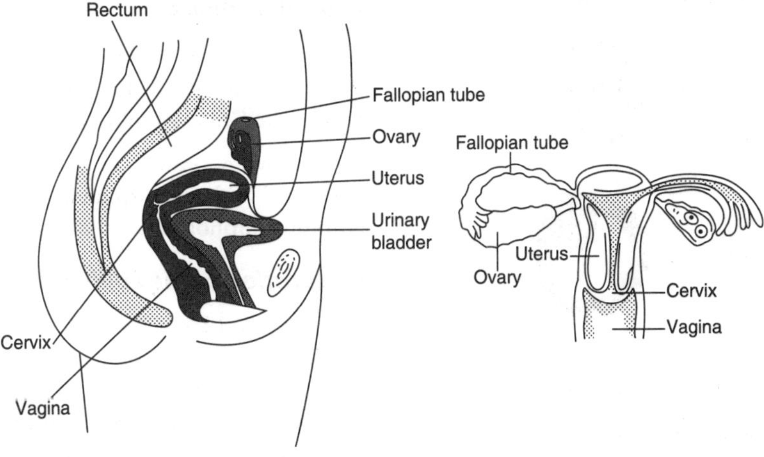

Fig. 11.1   Female reproductive organs.

Applied Physiology

Precocious Puberty

Onset of puberty at an early age is termed precocious puberty.

Delayed Puberty

If puberty does not occur before 18 years in females and 20 years in males, the condition is termed delayed puberty.

It can be caused due to conditions like hypopituitarism.

Development of Follicle (Fig. 11.2)

There are two ovaries each weighing 7–8 g. They produce female gametes. Each ovary is covered by tunica albuginea. Inside the tunica albuginea there are numerous follicles arranged in between the stroma.

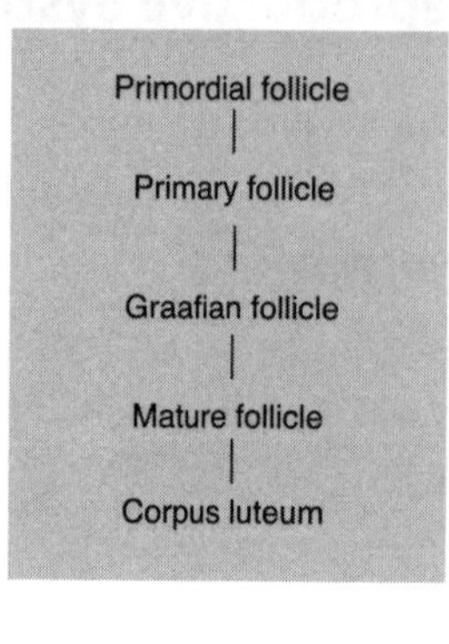

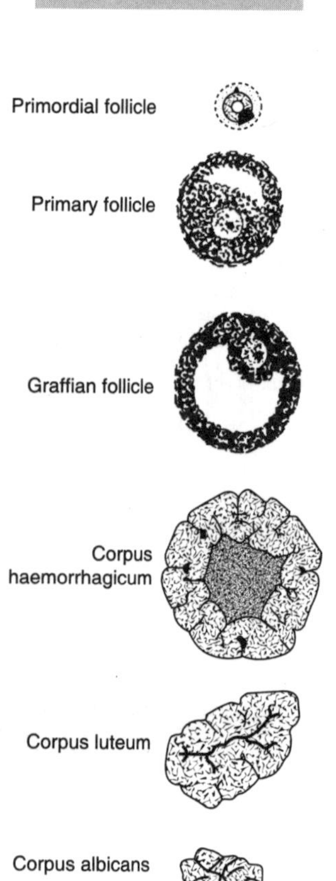

Fig. 11.2   Ovarian cycle.

Primordial Follicle

The primary oocyte (ovum) is surrounded by a single layer of spindle cells and is called a **primordial follicle**. At this stage the ovum is still immature. The primordial follicle is formed in the intrauterine life.

Primary Follicle

At the onset of ovarian cycle (at puberty) the follicles mature. The primordial follicle becomes a **primary follicle** due to the conversion of spindle cells into cuboidal epithelium. There is moderate enlargement of the ovum and growth of the additional layer of granulosa cells.

Approximately 6–12 follicles develop each month under the influence of FSH and LH. The rapid proliferation of granulosa cells forms multiple layers. The proliferation and differentiation of spindle cells form the theca interna and theca externa.

The theca interna secretes steroid hormones.

The theca externa transforms into vascular connective tissue capsule.

Graafian Follicle

The granulosa cells proliferate and secrete a fluid into the central cavity called the **antrum**. This follicle is termed the **Graafian follicle**.

The ovum present in the Graafian follicle is connected with its surrounding granulosa cells by **cumulus oophorus**.

Maturation of the Follicle (Fig. 11.3)

Out of the 6–12 follicles produced every month only one develops. The remaining follicles undergo atresia. The mature follicle secretes estrogen. Estrogen that is secreted exerts positive feedback to secrete more estrogen. Estrogen enhances FSH and LH receptors on theca cells.

At the time of ovulation the mature follicle attains the size of 1–1.5 cm.

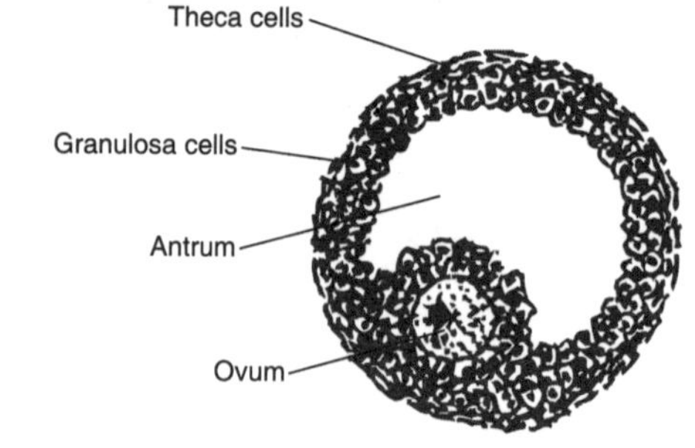

Fig. 11.3   Mature follicle.

Gametogenesis

The female gametes develop from the primordial germ cell (primitive sex cell) arising from the endoderm of the yolk sac. The mitotic proliferation of the primordial germ cell forms the **oogonia**. It later differentiates to form the **primary oocyte**.

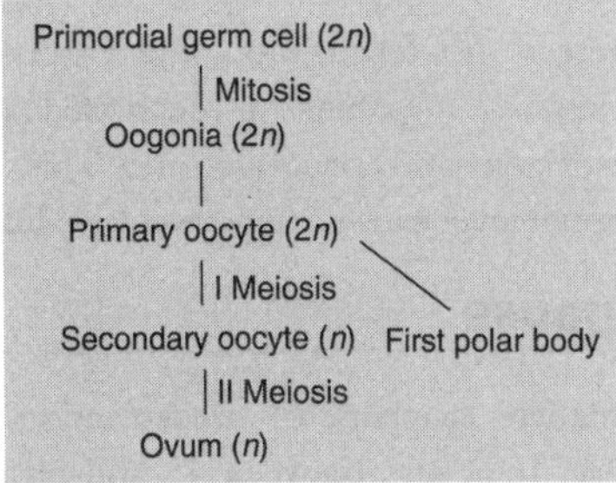

In the developing ovum, mitosis occurs till the fifth month of the intrauterine life. Later, mitosis stops and meiosis begins. This meiotic division is incomplete and stops at prophase.

Just before ovulation the first meiotic division is completed in the ova. One of the daughter cells receives most of the cytoplasm. This is termed the **secondary oocyte**, while the other cell called the **first polar body** disappears. After this the second meiotic division starts but it stops in metaphase and is completed only when the sperm enters the oocyte.

Menstruation

The periodic discharge of blood and cellular debris from the female genital tract is termed menstruation. The cyclical changes occurring from one menstruation to the next comprise a **menstrual cycle**.

The duration of the menstrual cycle is about 28 ± 4 days.

Phases

The menstrual cycle has three phases (Fig. 11.4):

1. proliferative phase,
2. secretory phase, and
3. menstrual phase.

Proliferative Phase (Follicular Phase)

The proliferative phase starts at the end of the menstrual phase. Its duration is about 10 days. At the beginning of this phase most of the endometrium has been desquamated. Later, the endometrium starts healing and then proliferates rapidly from fifth to fourteenth day of the menstrual cycle. This proliferation occurs under the influence of estrogen. There is growth of simple tubular glands and blood vessels. The endometrium increases in thickness to about 3–5 mm. The endometrial glands produce thick mucus. At the end of the proliferative phase ovulation occurs.

Secretory Phase (Luteal Phase)

The secretory phase lasts for about 14 days. It starts after ovulation and extends up to the next menstrual phase. The endometrium thickens up to 6 mm. The glands become bigger, tortuous, and filled with secretions. The stromal cells proliferate; spiral arteries become more coiled and dilated. This is caused due to the action of progesterone and estrogen on the uterine endometrium.

Menstrual Phase

The menstrual phase lasts for about 3–5 days.

If the ovum is not fertilized, the corpus luteum regresses from the 24th day of the cycle. This causes a decrease in the estrogen and progesterone levels. It results in shrinkage of the endometrium and coiling and spasm of the arteries leading to focal necrosis of the endometrium. The necrosed endometrium is shed along with blood and other secretions.

The normal quantity of blood loss during menstruation is about 50–60 mL.

The normal menstrual blood does not clot due to the release of fibrinolysin along with the necrotic endometrial material.

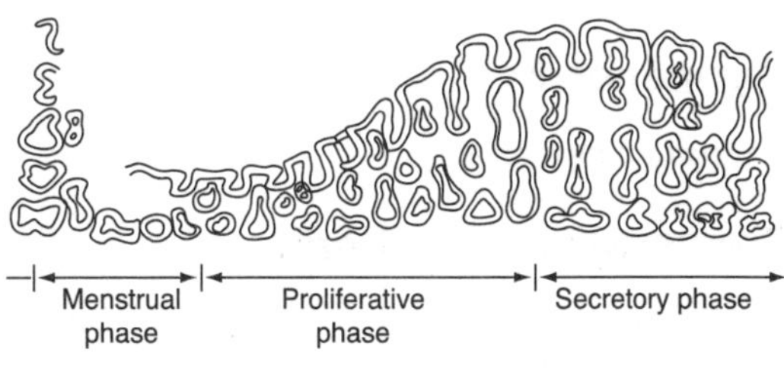

Fig. 11.4　Phases of menstrual cycle.

Ovarian Changes during Menstruation

During the proliferative phase, FSH from the anterior pituitary acts on the Graafian follicle of the ovary to produce estrogen. By the end of proliferative phase, LH is produced in large amounts. LH surge results in ovulation.

During the secretory phase, the ovary produces estrogen and progesterone.

During the menstrual phase, involution of the corpus luteum causes sudden decrease in the levels of estrogen and progesterone.

Hormonal Control of Menstruation

- GnRH from the hypothalamus increases gonadotropic secretion from the pituitary.
- Secretion of FSH causes development and maturation of the Graafian follicle.
- The granulosa cells of the developing follicles produce estrogen.
- An increased level of estrogen stimulates the pituitary glands to produce the LH surge.
- A rapid rise in LH secretion causes ovulation.

- The Graafian follicle after ovulation becomes the corpus luteum.
- The corpus luteum secretes progesterone and estrogen, which are responsible for secretory phase of the menstrual cycle.
- If there is fertilization, the corpus luteum continues to produce progesterone and becomes corpus luteum of pregnancy.
- If there is no fertilization, the corpus luteum degenerates. It results in decreased secretion of estrogen and progesterone. This reduced hormonal level causes menstrual bleeding.

Menopause

The permanent stoppage of menstruation is called menopause. It occurs between 45 and 50 years of age.

It is due to the depletion of functional follicles. Since follicles do not develop in response to LH and FSH secretion, the levels of estrogen and progesterone drop.

The symptoms associated with menopause are due to deficiency of estrogen. The vaginal epithelium atrophies and becomes dry. Bone loss is increased.

Applied Physiology

Amenorrhea

The absence of menstruation is called amenorrhea. Physiologically, it occurs during pregnancy.

Polymenorrhea

It is increased frequency of menstruation.

Menorrhagia

Menorrhagia is excessive bleeding during menstruation.

Dysmenorrhea

It is painful menstruation.

Premenstrual Syndrome

This is seen in the secretory phase of the menstrual cycle. The symptoms include irritability, depression, weight gain, breast tenderness, and headache. The symptoms subside during menstruation.

There is increased incidence of cardiovascular diseases.

Hot flashes due to peripheral vasodilatation and sweating are seen.

Ovulation

In women having a menstrual cycle of 28 days, ovulation occurs around the 14th day.

Just before ovulation, the outer wall of mature Graafian follicle protrudes to form the stigma. Rupture of the stigma releases viscous fluid containing the ovum into the abdominal cavity.

The ovum is surrounded by a number of granulosa cells forming the corona radiata.

The released ovum is ready for fertilization and is viable for 24 h.

Ovulation is a cyclical phenomenon. The cycle begins with bursts of GnRH secretion from the hypothalamus. GnRH secretion increases the release of FSH and LH. FSH acts on granulosa cells to produce estrogen. Estrogen and FSH increase the production of LH. LH surge in turn causes ovulation.

Corpus Luteum

After the extrusion of ovum, the remains of the Graafian follicle are together called the corpus luteum. Immediately after ovulation, it is filled with blood and therefore called corpus hemorrhagicum. Later, the granulosa cells and theca cells enlarge and get filled with lipid inclusions giving it a yellow appearance (luteinization).

The granulosa cells in the corpus luteum start forming large quantities of progesterone and small quantities of estrogens.

Theca cells form androgens, androstenedione, and testosterone. These are converted mainly to female hormones by granulosa cells.

In a normal female, the corpus luteum grows to about 1.5 cm in diameter in about 7–8 days after ovulation. If there is no pregnancy, it looses the secretory functions by about 12th day. The yellowish color is lost and it becomes corpus albicans. During the next few weeks it is replaced by fibrous tissue.

During pregnancy, the corpus luteum increases in size after fertilization. It is maintained by hCG (human chorionic gonadotropin) up to 90 days after fertilization. It is an important source of estrogen and progesterone.

Hormonal Regulation of Ovulation

The hormones regulating ovulation are

- GnRH,
- pituitary gonadotropins, and
- estrogens.

GnRH

GnRH is a 10 amino peptide secreted by neurons in the arcuate nucleus of the hypothalamus. Secretion from the arcuate nucleus is in turn controlled by the limbic system.

GnRH influences the secretion of FSH and LH from the anterior pituitary.

It is secreted intermittently, in pulses of 5–25 min every 1 h. This pulsatile release of GnRH causes intermittent output of LH secretion every 90 min.

Pituitary Gonadotropins

Pituitary gonadotropins like FSH and LH are secreted by the anterior pituitary gland. Secretion of these hormones begins at the age of 9–10 years and initiates menstruation by 11–14 years.

FSH   FSH is a small-molecular-weight glycoprotein with a molecular weight of 30,000.

The normal serum level of FSH is 5–30 million IU/mL.

Actions

- FSH causes the growth of primary follicles every month. It stimulates mitotic division of granulosa cells increasing their numbers and layers.
- It helps the theca interna to form estrogen.
- It helps in the formation of new FSH and LH receptors on the granulosa cells.

LH   The normal serum level of FSH is 5–25 million IU/mL.

Actions

- It is necessary for follicular growth and ovulation.

- LH secretion increases 10-fold before ovulation, causing secretion of follicular steroid hormones.
- It helps in the formation and maintenance of corpus luteum.
- It acts on granulosa cells and theca cells and converts them into progesterone-secreting cells. It also changes granulosa and theca cells into lutein cells after ovulation.
- It plays a role in the development of atretic follicles.

Estrogens

- Estrogens act synergistically with FSH to cause follicular development.
- They cause LH surge.
- They cause involution of the corpus luteum.

Physiology of Pregnancy

The normal duration of pregnancy in human beings is around 280 days. Pregnancy occurs when the ovum becomes fertilized. The fertilized ovum eventually develops into a full-term fetus.

Fertilization

Fertilization is the process of union of male and female gametes to form a zygote. It generally occurs at the outer end of the fallopian tube.

After the sexual act, the sperms travel toward the uterus and enter the fallopian tube. An ovum released from the mature Graafian follicle is taken up by the fimbrial end of the fallopian tube. The ovum meets the sperms in the fallopian tube. A single sperm enters the ovum to fertilize it.

The ovum survives in the genital tract for about 24 h and the sperm for 72 h.

Zygote

The fertilized ovum is called a zygote. The zygote has 46 chromosomes. It undergoes repeated division and forms a **morula**. The morula moves through the fallopian tube and gets implanted in the cavity of the uterus.

The morula touches the endometrium of the uterus to form a **blastocyst** by about fifth day after fertilization.

Applied Physiology

Detection of Ovulation

This is helpful in the diagnosis and treatment of infertility.

Tests to detect ovulation are as under:

1. **Basal body temperature (BBT) test:** In this test, the core body temperature (oral or rectal) should be recorded daily in the morning before the subject gets out of her bed (basal state). In the postovulatory phase, BBT increases by about 0.5°C due to increased secretion of the thermogenic hormone progesterone.
2. **Plasma progesterone levels:** By using the Elisa (enzyme-linked immunosorbent assay) technique, plasma progesterone is measured periodically throughout the menstrual cycle. A sharp increase in plasma progesterone indicates ovulation.
3. **Progesterone metabolites:** The estimation of urinary metabolites of progesterone gives an indication about ovulation.
4. **Endometrial biopsy:** The histological examination of the uterine endometrium in the second half of the menstrual cycle demonstrating secretory changes indicates that the ovulation has occurred.
5. **Fern test:** The cervical mucus is spread on a glass slide and observed. The absence of fern pattern in the endocervical mucus indicates ovulation.
6. **Ultrasonography:** This method is widely used in recent times. Size of Graafian follicle is measured daily; rupture of follicle and occurrence of ovulation can be detected.

The blastocyst looses its zona pellucida (membranous structure surrounding the ovum). A cavity is slowly formed inside the blastocyst.

The outer layers of the blastocyst form the trophoblasts. They are further divided into an outer **syncytiotrophoblast** and an inner **cytotrophoblast**.

The process of implantation is over by about 11 days.

Placenta

The trophoblastic cells begin to grow in the form of cords inside the endometrium of the uterus. These cords or processes are called the chorionic villi. The chorionic villi are surrounded by intervillous spaces which contain maternal blood. The fetal blood circulates through the chorionic villi. The maternal blood circulates through the intervillous space. Thus, the placenta connects the growing embryo with the mother.

Functions

- Provides nutrition to the growing embryo.
- Prevents entry of harmful substances into the fetus.
- Transfers waste products from the fetus to the maternal circulation.
- Secretes hormones like hCG, hCS, estrogen, progesterone, prostaglandins, and β-endorphins.

Placental Hormones

Human Chorionic Gonadotropin (hCG)   This is produced by the syncytiotrophoblast.

It is a glycoprotein hormone similar to LH. It is essential for the maintenance of corpus luteum in the early part of the pregnancy.

hCG production starts by 7 days after fertilization, reaches peak by 60 days, and decreases thereafter.

hCG is also necessary for the production of testosterone.

Human Chorionic Somatommotropin (hCS)
hCS is also called human placental lactogen secreted from the syncytiotrophoblast.

This hormone is responsible for the development of mammary glands and growth of the fetus.

Maternal Changes during Pregnancy

Body Weight

A woman puts on about 10–12 kg of weight during pregnancy. This is due to fetal weight, placental weight, fat deposition, and accumulation of fluid.

Blood

Erythropoiesis is increased during pregnancy. The bone marrow becomes hypercellular.

The concentration of plasma proteins is reduced.

The blood volume increases by 30% during the latter half of pregnancy. The ESR (erythrocyte sedimentation rate) increases.

Cardiovascular System

The blood volume and cardiac output increase by about 30%.

The systolic blood pressure is not altered significantly, but the diastolic blood pressure is reduced.

Respiratory System

The O_2 consumption increases by 20%. The tidal volume and respiratory rate increase to meet the demand for the excess supply of oxygen.

Central Nervous System

Excitement, irritability, and depression are commonly seen.

Gastrointestinal System

Morning sickness, nausea, and vomiting occur especially during the first three months of pregnancy.

Endocrine System

The anterior pituitary is depressed as hCG takes over the function.

The placenta secretes estrogen and progesterone.

Thyroid hormone secretion is increased.

Oxytocin, prolactin, and cortisol secretion increases.

Reproductive System

The uterus increases in weight and size. There is hypertrophy and hyperplasia of the myometrium.

The uterus weighs about 30 g in nulliparous woman. It increases to about 1 kg at term.

The mammary glands develop under the influence of estrogen and progesterone.

Pregnancy Tests

Immunological Test

This is the latest test based on the reaction between hCG and its antibody. The various immunological tests used are bioassay, immunoassay (antigen–antibody reaction), and radioimmunoassay. (Radiolabeled hCG is used.)

Principle

The urine of women is mixed with hCG antiserum. Later, hCG-coated latex particles are added to this mixture. Absence of agglutination is a positive pregnancy test.

Advantages

It is the most accurate test available, easier to perform and less expensive.

It gives result in 5–30 min.

Disadvantages

Proteinuria may give false-positive results.

Test becomes negative in later stages of the pregnancy.

Other Tests

- Aschheim–Zondek test
- Friedman test
- Galli-Mainini test

Parturition

This is the process of delivery of the baby.

Factors Initiating Parturition

They are broadly divided into two categories:

1. hormonal factors and
2. mechanical factors.

Hormonal Factors

(a) Fetal hormones
(b) Maternal hormones

Role of Fetal Hormones   Increase of fetal CRH (corticotropin-releasing hormone) causes increased ACTH secretion.

This increases the fetal androgens.

The fetal androgens are converted to estrogens.

Estrogen increases the secretion of prostaglandins.

Prostaglandins enhance uterine contractions, which helps in the delivery of the baby.

Role of Maternal Hormones

Estrogen/Progesterone Ratio   Progesterone has an inhibitory effect on uterine contractility. Estrogen has stimulatory effect. Throughout pregnancy, both estrogen and progesterone are secreted. But from seventh month onward, estrogen content increases and progesterone level decreases. This alteration in estrogen progesterone ratio favors increased contractility of the uterus.

Effect of Oxytocin   Oxytocin increases uterine contractions by causing direct stimulation of uterine smooth muscle and also by the formation of prostaglandins.

As pregnancy approaches full term there is

- increase in sensitivity of the uterus to circulating oxytocin;
- increase in the rate of oxytocin secretion.

Relaxin   This hormone produced by the corpus luteum of pregnancy relaxes the pelvic joints and softens uterine cervix helping in easy delivery of the baby.

Mechanical Factors

Stretch of Uterine Muscle   This increases uterine contractility. Intermittent stretch of smooth muscle caused by the movement of fetus also causes uterine contraction.

Stretch of Cervix   This increases uterine contractions. Stretching of nerves in the cervix causes reflex contraction of the uterine muscles by release of oxytocin (neuroendocrine reflex).

Braxton Hick's Contractions   These are weak and slow contractions of the uterus occurring throughout the pregnancy. Toward the end of pregnancy, these contractions become very strong resulting in dilatation of the cervix and expulsion of the baby through the birth canal.

Labor

The process of birth of the baby is termed labor. Labor is due to a mechanism of positive feedback. The uterine contractions stimulate stronger uterine contractions subsequently resulting in birth of the baby. The contraction of the abdominal muscles facilitates labor.

The process of parturition occurs in three stages (Fig. 11.5).

First Stage

- It involves dilatation of cervix and opening of the vaginal canal.
- This stage lasts for 8–24 h in primigravida (first pregnancy).

Second Stage

- Membranes rupture and fetal head descends down the birth canal and the baby is delivered.
- This lasts for about 20–30 min in primigravida.

Third Stage

- It involves expulsion of placenta.
- It occurs 10–15 min after the delivery of the baby.
- During this stage, about 350 mL of blood is lost from the mother.

Involution of Uterus

The uterus starts decreasing in size. By 4–5 weeks after the delivery of the child it reaches the prepregnant state. This process of involution is facilitated by lactation.

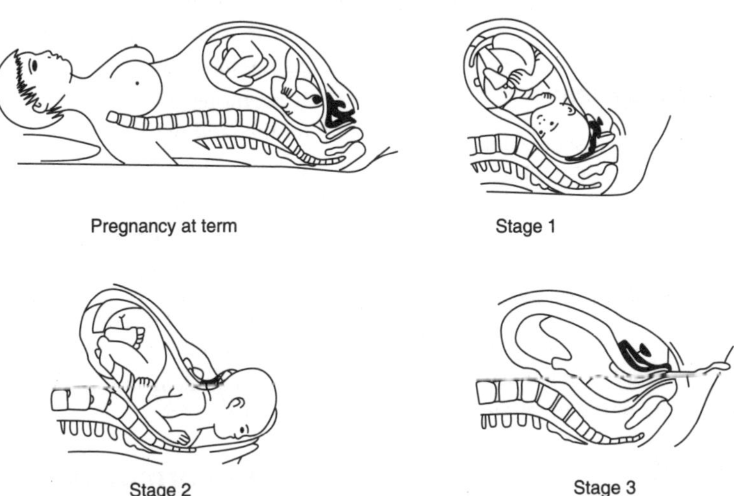

Fig. 11.5   Stages of labor.

Applied Physiology

If the uterine contractions are not strong enough, it can be enhanced by giving *synthetic oxytocin*.

If there is no improvement, *forceps delivery* is done.

If the pelvic canal is small and there is obstruction to childbirth (labor) or if the uterine contractions do not become strong, *caesarian section* operation is performed.

Loss of more than 500 mL of blood during placental delivery is termed *postpartum hemorrhage*.

Lactation

Lactation is the process of synthesis, secretion, and ejection of milk by the mammary glands.

Mother's milk has the ideal composition suitable for the infant.

Hormonal Control

- Estrogen causes development of the duct system of breast and collection of fat tissue.
- Progesterone helps in the development of alveoli of the breast.
- Prolactin helps in the formation of milk.
- Oxytocin causes ejection of milk.

Development of Breasts

The breasts begin to develop at puberty under the influence of estrogen. During pregnancy, estrogen and progesterone help in further development of the breasts.

Growth of the Ductal System

Throughout pregnancy, there is significant growth of the ductal system and stroma of the breasts. A large amount of fat is stored in the stroma. These changes occur due to the influence of estrogen.

Development of the Alveolar System

The lobules and alveoli develop under the influence of progesterone. The secretory characteristics develop in these alveoli due to the action of progesterone.

Formation of Milk

Prolactin, an anterior pituitary hormone, is responsible for the production of milk. During pregnancy there is no milk production because of the inhibitory effect of estrogen and progesterone on prolactin.

Once the baby is delivered and placenta is expelled, levels of these two hormones diminish and, therefore, lactogenic effect of prolactin is seen.

The influence of prolactin in the formation of milk is aided by growth hormone, cortisol, parathyroid hormone, and insulin.

Each time the mother nurses the child, prolactin level rises and causes the secretion of milk.

Expulsion of Milk

Milk secreted by the mammary gland is ejected out from the alveoli into the ducts. This is called letdown of milk.

Milk Ejection Reflex

When the baby suckles the nipple, the sensory impulses travel through the somatic nerves from the nipples to the hypothalamus, which causes secretion of oxytocin. Oxytocin is carried in the blood to the breast causing contraction of the myoepithelial cells resulting in expulsion of milk.

The average milk production in humans is about 500–800 mL/day.

Breastfeeding is very important for both the mother and the child.

Advantages of breastfeeding are as under:

- The baby gets sterile, easily digestible, nutritive, and inexpensive food which is delivered at the right temperature.
- It promotes an emotional bonding between the mother and the child.
- Women who breastfeed their babies are less likely to suffer from breast cancer.
- It is a form of contraception.
- It provides immunity to the child.

In nursing mothers, the ovarian cycle and ovulation do not occur till the mother stops nursing the child. This is because of the inhibition of secretion of FSH and LH.

Ovarian Hormones

The ovarian hormones are estrogens and progesterone.

Estrogens

They are secreted from

- granulosa and theca cells of the ovary,
- corpus luteum,
- placenta during pregnancy, and
- adrenal cortex.

Three main estrogens present in humans are

- 17-β-estradiol

- estrone, and
- estriol.

The 17-β-estradiol is the most potent form of estrogen. It is produced primarily in granulosa and luteal cells.

Estriol is less potent when compared to 17-β-estradiol. It is produced by ovaries during pregnancy. In nonpregnant women it is produced in the liver.

Estrone is the least potent of all the estrogens. Most of the estrone is produced from peripheral conversion of estradiol.

Biosynthesis

All the three forms of estrogens are C18 steroids. They are formed from cholesterol which is derived from acetate or drawn from the plasma pool.

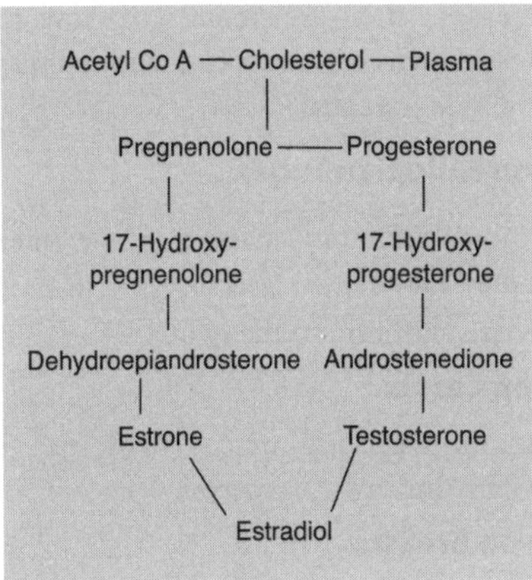

Transport and Secretion

Estrogen is transported in the blood mainly bound to the plasma albumin (60%) and specific estrogen-binding globulin called the **gonadal-binding globulin** (38%). This binding is loose and is released into the tissues in about 30 min. Only 2% of the circulating estradiol is in free form.

Daily Secretion

In the early follicular phase, daily estradiol secretion is 30 μg/day. It peaks to 380 μg/day before ovulation. It is around 250 μg/day in the midluteal phase.

Mechanism of Action

The estrogens penetrate the cell membrane of the target cells and combine with the cytosol receptor in the cytoplasm. The hormone–receptor complex enters the nucleus and gets attached to the DNA molecules. This stimulates DNA to produce mRNA facilitating protein synthesis.

The action of DNA also stimulates mitosis, resulting in hypertrophy and hyperplasia of the target organs.

Metabolism

The estrogens are degraded in the liver to inactive metabolites. They are later excreted through urine.

Functions

Action on Uterus and External Genital Organs

- Increases the size of the female reproductive organs.
- Helps to convert vaginal epithelium into stratified squamous epithelium.
- Causes acidification of vagina, thus preventing infections.
- Causes development of endometrial glands.

Action on Breasts

- Causes enlargement of breasts and pigmentation of areola during puberty.
- Causes development of stromal tissue and ductal system of breasts during pregnancy.
- Causes fat deposition in the breasts.

Action on Skeleton

- Causes rapid growth of bones at puberty and early union of epiphysis with shaft of long bones.
- It is responsible for the feminine shape: narrow shoulders, broad hips, converging thighs, and diverging arms.
- Its action leads to the skin becoming smooth and soft with increased fat deposition in subcutaneous tissues.
- Lowers plasma cholesterol, thereby preventing atherosclerosis, coronary heart disease, and hypertension.
- Increases body protein.
- Increases basal metabolic rate.
- Causes sodium and water retention by kidneys.
- Inhibits the formation of acne and blackheads.

- Causes typical female behavior and is responsible for increased libido.

Synthetic Estrogens

Uses

- Synthetic estrogens are used as oral contraceptives.
- They are used in the treatment of post menopausal syndrome, e.g., ethinyl estradiol and diethylstilbestrol.

Progesterone

This is a C21 steroid, secreted by

- corpus luteum,
- placenta during pregnancy, and
- zona reticularis of the adrenal cortex.

Biosynthesis

The chief precursor of progesterone is cholesterol.

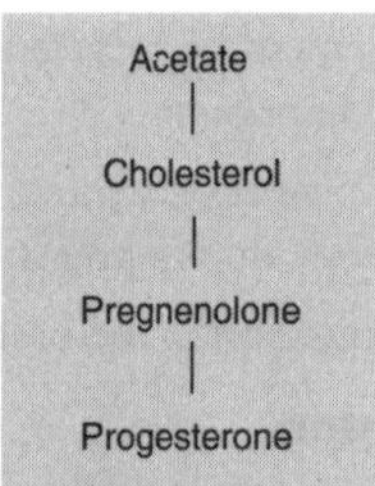

Transport and Secretion

It is mainly transported bound to albumin (80%). Eighteen percent is bound to steroid-binding globulin. Only 2% is in free form.

Plasma Progesterone

- **In women**

  0.9 ng/mL in follicular phase

  18 ng/mL in luteal phase

- **In men**

  0.3 ng/mL

It is mainly degraded in the liver into pregnanediol and excreted in urine.

Mechanism of Action

Like other steroids, its action is brought about by action on DNA to initiate the synthesis of new mRNA.

Metabolism

Progesterone is degraded in the liver to inactive metabolites. They are later excreted in the urine.

Functions

Effect on Uterus

- Promotes secretory changes in the uterine endometrium and, therefore, prepares the uterus for implantation of the fertilized ovum.
- Decreases the frequency and intensity of uterine contractions.
- Has antiestrogenic effect on myometrial cells.
- Decreases the excitability of myometrium and sensitivity to oxytocin, and increases the membrane potential.

Effect on Fallopian Tubes

- Promotes secretory changes in the mucosa of fallopian tubes.
- Provides nutrition to the ovum.

Effect on Cervix

- Makes the cervical mucus thick and thereby prevents the entry of sperms.

Action on Breasts

- Causes development of the alveoli of the breasts and makes them secretory in nature.

Effect on Electrolyte Balance

- Reduces the total body water and sodium since it blocks the effect of aldosterone.

Effect on Body Temperature

- Raises the body temperature. Therefore the basal body temperature is raised after ovulation.

Effect on Respiration

- Stimulates respiration causing a decrease in alveolar PCO_2.

Relaxin

This is a polypeptide hormone secreted by the corpus luteum, uterus, placenta, mammary glands, and prostate (in men).

It has an α and β chain connected by two disulfide bridges.

Functions

- Relaxes the pubic symphysis during pregnancy.
- Softens and dilates the cervix, thus facilitating the delivery.
- Inhibits uterine contractions.
- Plays a role in the development of mammary glands.
- In males, it is found in semen, and helps in sperm motility and penetration.

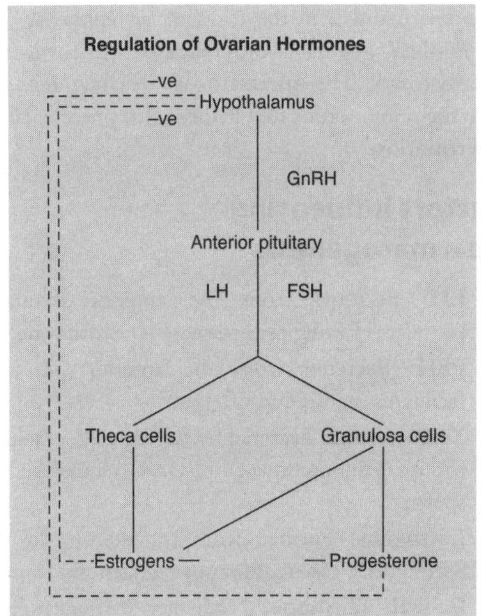

Male Reproductive System (Fig. 11.6)

The reproductive functions of the male have three components:

1. spermatogenesis (formation of sperms),
2. male sexual act, and
3. regulation of male reproductive functions by various hormones.

The primary sex organ of the male is **testis**.

The accessory sex organs are epididymis, vas deferens, seminal vesicles, prostate, and penis.

Physiological Anatomy

The testis is made up of loops of convoluted seminiferous tubules in which sperms are formed. There are up to 900 seminiferous tubules in each testis. The average length of each tubule is around 0.5 m.

The testis also contains the interstitial cells of Leydig and Sertoli cells.

The seminiferous tubules open into the epididymis, which is a coiled tube about 6 m in length.

From the head of the epididymis, the sperm enters the vas deferens.

The vas deferens enlarges to form the ampulla before it enters the body of the prostate gland. The seminal vesicles located on either side of the prostate gland empty their secretions into the prostatic end of the ampulla.

The contents of both the ampulla and the seminal vesicle pass into the ejaculatory duct and empty into the internal urethra. The prostatic ducts also empty into the internal urethra.

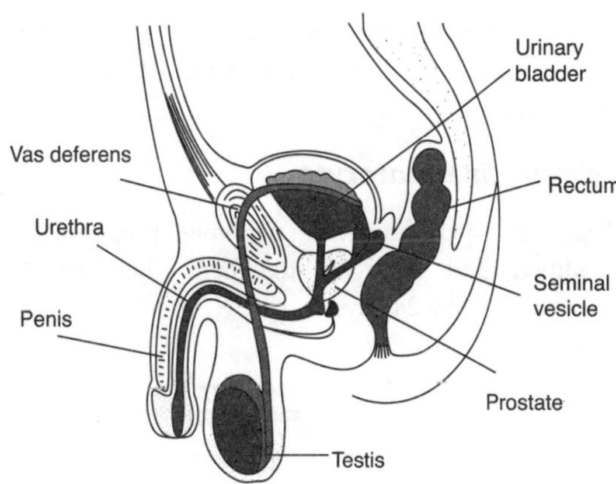

Fig. 11.6   Male reproductive system.

Spermatogenesis

Spermatogenesis is the process of formation of sperms in the seminiferous tubules (Fig. 11.7). It begins at around 13 years of age and continues throughout life.

Stages

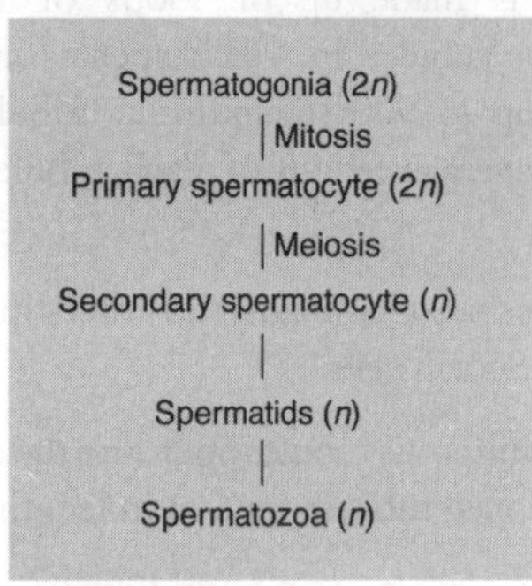

Spermatogonia

The seminiferous tubules contain large number of germinal epithelial cells, spermatogonia. They continually proliferate and a portion of them differentiates to form the sperm.

The primordial spermatogonia which is present near the basement membrane of the germinal epithelium is called **type A spermatogonia**. These type A spermatogonia divide four times to form 16 cells called **type B spermatogonia**.

The spermatogonia penetrate the blood testis barrier and become enveloped within the folds of sertoli cells.

Primary Spermatocyte

Type B spermatogonia become progressively modified and enlarged to form the primary spermatocyte by 24 days.

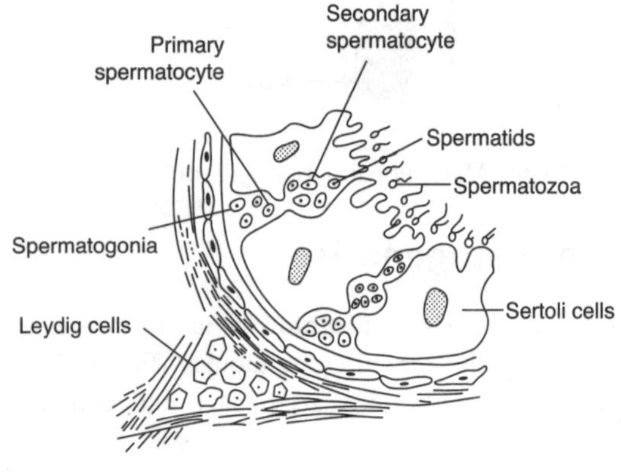

Fig. 11.7   Section of seminiferous tubule.

Secondary Spermatocyte

At the end of 24 days, each primary spermatocyte divides to form two secondary spermatocytes. This division occurs by meiosis.

I Meiotic Division The primary spermatocyte divides into two secondary spermatocytes, each containing 23 chromosomes with two chromatids.

II Meiotic Division Within 2–3 days, a second meiotic division occurs forming two daughter spermatids with 23 chromosomes each.

Spermiogenesis

It is the conversion of spermatids into spermatozoa. The spermatid is in the form of an epithelial cell. It is then gradually differentiated to form the spermatozoa. The spermatozoa are then released into the seminiferous tubule through a process called **spermiation**.

Factors Influencing Spermatogenesis

- **LH:** Secreted from the anterior pituitary, stimulates Leydig cells to secrete testosterone.
- **FSH:** Secreted from the anterior pituitary, facilitates maturation of sperm.
- **Testosterone:** Secreted by Leydig cells, essential for growth, multiplication, and maturation of sperm.
- **Estrogens:** Formed from testosterone in the Sertoli cells, essential for spermiogenesis.
- **Growth hormone:** Necessary for controlling metabolic functions of testis, promotes division of spermatogonia.
- **Temperature:** 32°C is ideal for spermatogenesis.
- **Exposure to X-rays:** Repeated exposure to X-rays reduces spermatogenesis.

Capacitation of Sperm

The movement of sperm is sluggish inside the male genital tract. The sperms move vigorously when they enter the female genital tract and develop an ability to fertilize the ovum.

The movement of sperm inside the female genital tract is assisted by cervical and uterine movements and sucking effect of the uterus.

Sperm

The sperms are elongated cells measuring about 55–65 μ. They are motile, moving at the rate of 1–4 mm/min. After production, they are stored in the epididymis and are viable for a month.

The sperm has a head, middle piece, and tail (Fig. 11.8).

Head

It is 4–5 μ long and contains the nucleus. The anterior portion of the head is covered by acrosomal cap. The acrosomal cap contains hyaluronidase, mucopolysaccharide, and acid phosphatase enzymes.

Middle Piece

This is made up of the axial filament surrounded by the mitochondria. The mitochondria provide energy for the movement of sperm.

Tail

The tail causes the movement of sperm.

Nutrition for the sperm is provided by Sertoli cells and the fluid in the seminiferous tubule.

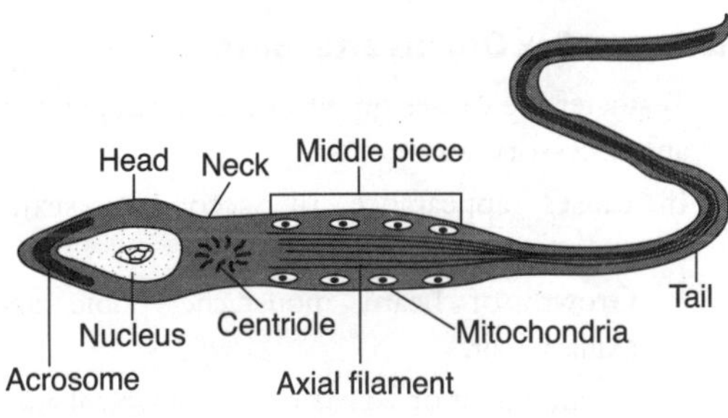

Fig. 11.8   Structure of sperm.

Sertoli Cells

These are special cells present in the seminiferous tubules. They are large cells with abundant cytoplasm.

Functions

- Form a blood–testis barrier.
- Provide nutrition to sperms.
- Destroy defective sperms.
- Produce inhibin, Mullerian regression factor, estradiol, and androgen-binding protein.

Semen

Semen is the fluid ejaculated from the male genital tract during orgasm.

Normal sperm count is 60–120 million/mL.

pH is 7.4 –7.5.

Contents

Normal volume is 2–6 mL per ejaculation.

It contains the following:

- sperms and fluid from vas deferens—10%;
- seminal fluid—60%;
- prostatic fluid—30%.

Semen contains fructose which is necessary to provide nutrition to the sperms.

It also contains prostaglandins, phospholipids, citric acid, spermin, and clotting enzyme.

Functions

- Provides bulk to the sperm.
- Maintains alkaline environment.
- Provides nutrition to sperms.

Applied Physiology

Oligospermia

Sperm count less than 20 million/mL is termed oligospermia.

Azoospermia

Absence of sperms is termed azoospermia.

Male Sex Hormones

Androgens are male sex hormones secreted by the testis.

They include testosterone, dihydrotestosterone, and androstenedione.

Zona reticularis of the suprarenal cortex produces androstenedione and dehydroepiandrosterone.

Testosterone

It is the most powerful male sex hormone.

It is formed by interstitial cells of Leydig present in between the seminiferous tubules. Interstitial cells constitute 20% of the adult testicular mass.

The activity of Leydig cells begins at seventh week of fetal life. The Leydig cells are normally stimulated by hCG secreted by the placenta. These Leydig cells go into quiescence after the birth of the child because hCG is no longer available. But at the time of puberty, they again get activated due to LH secretion and continue to function till death.

Chemistry

Testosterone is a C19 steroid hormone. It is synthesized from either cholesterol or acetyl coenzyme A.

Secretion

The rate of testosterone secretion is 4–9 mg/day in normal adult male. A small amount of testosterone is also secreted in females by ovaries and adrenal glands.

Transport

Almost 98% of testosterone is transported either loosely bound to the **plasma albumin** (33%) or tightly bound to the **testosterone-binding globulin** (65%). It circulates in blood for 1 h. About 2% of testosterone circulates in free form.

Plasma testosterone level in adult male is 525 ng/dL.

In the target tissues, testosterone is converted to dihydrotestosterone.

Degradation and Excretion

Testosterone is converted to androsterone and dehydroepiandrosterone and is conjugated in the liver. These are excreted into the gut either through bile or through urine.

Functions

- Helps in the development of male sex organs, secondary sex characteristics, and sex behavior.
- Acts as an anabolic hormone.

Action on Sex Organs in the Fetus

- Testosterone is produced at around seventh week of intrauterine life. Before 7 weeks of intrauterine life fetus has both **Wolffian** and **Mullerian** ducts. Male sex chromosomes cause the genital ridge to secrete testosterone. This causes disappearance of Mullerian duct system and development of male accessory sex organs. Absence of testosterone causes development of Mullerian duct into accessory female sex organs.
- Testosterone helps in the descent of testis into the scrotum during the last trimester of pregnancy.
- The exposure of hypothalamus and other parts of the brain to testosterone in the male fetus determines the sexual behavior in adult life.

Action on Sex Organs after Birth

- Testosterone causes growth of external genitalia and accessory sex organs.
- It causes appearance of secondary sexual characteristics such as

  Growth of beard, moustache, pubic, and axillary hair.

  Enlargement of larynx causing a typical adult male voice.

  Increased thickness of the skin.

  Increased sebaceous secretion which causes acne.

- It is necessary for spermatogenesis and sperm motility.
- It is responsible for aggressive behavior.

Anabolic Effect

- Testosterone increases the synthesis and decreases the breakdown of proteins.
- It causes linear growth of skeleton and muscle tissue.

Other Effects

- Testosterone increases basal metabolic rate (BMR).
- It increases RBC production.

Regulation

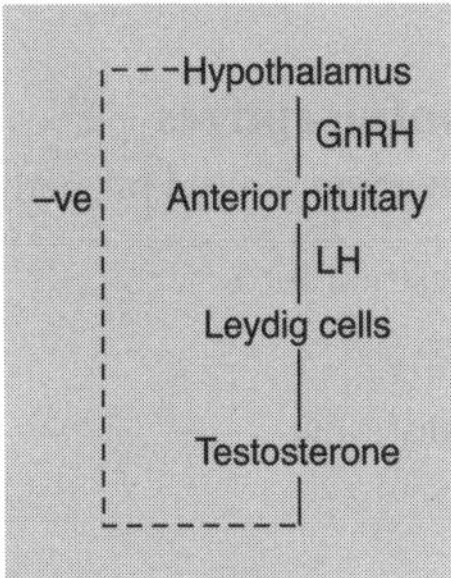

Inhibin

This is produced by Sertoli cells in males and the granulosa cells in females.

It is a glycoprotein. Its molecular weight is 10,000–30,000.

Function

It helps in the regulation of spermatogenesis by

- causing inhibition of FSH secretion by acting directly on the anterior pituitary;
- acting on the hypothalamus to inhibit secretion of GnRH.

Contraceptive Methods

India is the second most populated country in the world next to China, and by 2035 it is likely to become the most populated country. With only 2.4% of the world's land area, we support 16% of the world's population. In order to check the growing population, it is necessary to follow family planning methods. They mainly involve various methods of contraception.

Contraception in Males

- **Temporary methods:**
  Barrier methods
  Hormonal methods
- **Permanent method:**
  Vasectomy

Applied Physiology

Cryptorchidism

The failure of testis to descend into the scrotum is called cryptorchidism. The testis develops in the abdominal cavity and migrates into the scrotum during fetal development under the influence of testosterone. Approximately 10% of the newborn babies can have undescended testis but they later descend by the age of 1 year.

Treatment

- Administration of gonadotropic hormones
- Surgery to mobilize the testis and bring it down to the scrotum as early as possible

Treatment should be done as early as possible, otherwise high temperature in the abdominal cavity can damage spermatogenic epithelium causing sterility. The testis located in the abdominal cavity may develop malignancy.

Anabolic Steroids

These are synthetic substances having anabolic effects.

They are banned in sports since they are known to enhance performance. Examples include nandrolone and stanozolol.

Contraception in Females

- **Temporary methods:**

  Barrier methods

  Intrauterine devices

  Hormonal methods

  Postconceptional methods

- **Permanent method:**

  Tubectomy

Temporary Methods

Barrier Methods

(a) **Physical methods:**

Condom

- This is the most widely used male contraceptive method.

- Its advantages are that it is easily available, safe, inexpensive, easy to use, prevents sexually transmitted diseases, and has no side effects.

- The disadvantage is that incorrect use leads to tear of condom.

Diaphragm

- This is a rubber cup to be inserted into the vagina of the female before intercourse. It is not used because of difficult technique in using it.

(b) **Chemical methods:**

- Foams, creams, jellies, and suppositories are available in the market. All these contain spermicides. For example, polyurethrene foam sponge, which is saturated with spermicide nonoxynol-9.

Intrauterine Contraceptive Devices   These are small inert substances inserted into the cavity of uterus. The use of IUCD was known to ancient Arabs. They used to insert small stones into the uterus of camels.

- **First-generation IUCD:** Lippe's loop. It is made of polyethylene.

- **Second-generation IUCD:** Copper T. Copper is used since it has antifertility effect.

- **Third-generation IUCD:** Progestasert. This is a device filled with progesterone. This device releases the progesterone slowly.

Mechanism of Action   They act as foreign bodies in the uterine cavities, thereby preventing fertilization and implantation.

Advantages Simple, insertion takes few minutes, inexpensive, and no systemic side effects.

Disadvantages Excessive menstrual bleeding, pain, pelvic infection, uterine perforation, and ectopic pregnancy.

Hormonal Contraceptives   They are the most effective contraceptives if used properly.

They are classified into

- oral pills and

- depot preparations.

Oral Pills

1. **Combined pill:** This pill contains synthetic estrogen and progesterone. Pill is given orally for 21 days beginning from fifth day of last menstrual cycle.

2. **Progesterone-only pill:** This is called mini pill. It contains only progesterone and is not as effective as the combined pill.

3. **Postcoital pill:** It contains high doses of estrogens. It is used daily for 5 days after the sexual act.

4. **Once-a-month pill:** It is not commonly used due to high bleeding and high failure rate.

Mechanism of Action

- Prevent ovulation.

- Prevent implantation of ovum.

- Restrict the entry of sperm by altering the character of cervical mucus.

Disadvantages

- Increased risk of myocardial infarction, thrombosis, increased risk of cancer cervix, weight gain, migraine, and liver disorders.

5. **Male pill:** It is still in the trial stage. Gossypol tried as a male contraceptive is toxic and may result in permanent azoospermia.

Depot Preparations

1. **Injectable contraceptives:**
    - DMPA (depot medroxyprogesterone acetate)

- NET-EN (norethisterone enantate)

This is not widely used because the injections are painful. Women may have irregular cycles and sometimes it may even lead to permanent amenorrhea.

2. **Subdermal implants**: This needs surgical procedure and is still in trial stage. It can provide long-term reversible contraception.

Postconceptional Methods

- **Menstrual regulation**: This is aspiration of uterine contents 6–14 days after missed periods.

- **Medical termination of pregnancy (abortion):** This is termination of pregnancy before 28 weeks of gestation.

Permanent Methods

Male Sterilization—Vasectomy   In this procedure, the vas deferens is clamped and cut and the cut ends are ligated. It is a very safe procedure but not widely practised probably due to male ego or fear of decreased sexual vigor.

Precaution   The person undergoing vasectomy is not immediately sterile. A minimum of 30 ejaculations are required for all the remaining sperms to be washed off.

Female Sterilization—Tubectomy   This is done by identifying the fallopian tubes and ligating them. Later, the ligated ends are cut and sutured.

Biological Methods

Abstinence   Avoiding sexual intercourse.

Coitus Interruptus   This method was practised during olden days. In this method, the male withdraws from the act just before ejaculation. Failure rate is very high since a small change in the timing of withdrawal can cause problems.

Safe Period (Rhythm Method)   This is based on the fact that ovulation occurs between 12th and 16th day in menstrual cycle of the duration of 28 days. The couple is advised to avoid intercourse from 8th to 22nd day of menstrual cycle. Its disadvantages are high failure rate and cannot be practised in women having irregular menstrual cycle.

Question Bank

1. General Physiology

Long Essay

1. Give the normal value of total body water? Classify its various compartments giving the normal values. Explain the methods of measurement of various compartments.

Short Essay

1. Explain the structure and functions of the following cellular components:
   (a) Cell membrane
   (b) Nucleus
   (c) Mitochondria
   (d) Golgi apparatus
   (e) Endoplasmic reticulum
   (f) Lysosomes
2. Explain the different types of intercellular connection. What are its functions?
3. Describe the phases of mitotic cell division.
4. What are the types of RNA? Add a note on their functions.
5. Describe the proteins that help in transport across the cell membrane.
6. Describe different mechanisms of passive transport across the cell membrane.
7. Describe different mechanisms of active transport across the cell membrane.
8. Explain the distribution of fluid in various compartments of the body.
9. Describe the methods of measurement of different fluid compartments of the body.

2. Blood

Long Essay

1. Name the plasma proteins. Explain their chemical nature. Add a note on their functions.
2. What is erythropoiesis? Describe the stages and factors influencing it.
3. What is anemia? Describe the types of anemia. Give the blood picture in each of them.
4. Explain the structure, synthesis, functions, and breakdown of hemoglobin.
5. Classify leukocytes. Describe their morphology. Add a note on their functions.
6. Describe the various stages of leukopoiesis.
7. What is immunity? Explain its types.
8. Describe the mechanism of cellular immunity.

9. Explain intrinsic and extrinsic mechanisms of blood clotting.
10. Name the blood group systems. Explain the basis for its classification. Add a note on its clinical importance.

Short Essay

1. List the functions of blood.
2. What is polycythemia? Explain its different types.
3. Describe any two abnormal types of hemoglobin.
4. Explain the absorption, storage, and functions of iron in the body.
5. Explain the role of lymphocytes in immunity.
6. What are immunoglobulins? What are their functions?
7. Discuss the changes that occur during phagocytosis.
8. Explain the formation, composition, and functions of lymph.
9. What is reticuloendothelial (monocyte-macrophage) system? Outline its functions.
10. Explain the functions of platelets.
11. Explain the mechanism of hemostasis.
12. Give a brief account of hemophilia.
13. Explain in brief the thrombocytopenic purpura.
14. Name the clotting factors. Explain the properties of factor VIII.
15. Name any *four* anticoagulants. Explain the mechanism of action of any *one* of them.
16. Explain the consequences of mismatched blood transfusion.

Short Answer

1. Name the plasma proteins.
2. What is albumin–globulin ratio? What is its clinical importance?
3. Give an account of blood picture in pernicious anemia.
4. Give an account of blood picture in iron-deficiency anemia.
5. What are reticulocytes? How are they demonstrated in the blood film?
6. What are the structural and functional differences between adult and fetal hemoglobin?
7. What is the normal ESR? Mention factors that influence it.
8. Give the normal value for MCV, MCH, MCHC, and color index.
9. What is normal PCV? When is it altered?
10. Mention the causes for leukocytosis and leukopenia.
11. What is a plasma cell? What is its function?
12. What is active and passive immunity?
13. Name any *four* anticoagulants.
14. What is Landsteiner's law?
15. What is cross-matching? What are its types?
16. What is erythroblastosis fetalis?
17. How is blood stored in blood banks?

3.   Nerve–Muscle Physiology

Long Essay

1. Describe the structure of neuromuscular junction (NMJ) with the help of a diagram and explain the mechanism of transmission of nerve impulse across it.
2. Describe the molecular basis for muscle contraction.

3. Discuss excitation–contraction coupling in a skeletal muscle.

Short Essay

1. What is resting membrane potential? Explain its ionic basis.
2. Describe an action potential recorded from a nerve fiber. Explain its ionic basis.
3. What are the types of action potentials?
4. Classify nerve fibers based on velocity and diameter. Explain the factors influencing the velocity of nerve impulse.
5. Explain the properties of nerve fibers.
6. Describe the transmission of impulse in myelinated and unmyelinated nerve fibers.
7. Explain the types of nerve injuries.
8. Describe Wallerian degeneration.
9. Explain the changes during regeneration of a damaged nerve.
10. List the types of neuroglia. Explain their structure and functions.
11. Describe the structure of neuromuscular junction.
12. Explain the transmission of impulse across neuromuscular junction.
13. What is myasthenia gravis? Explain its pathophysiology and clinical features. Add a note on its management.
14. List the neuromuscular blocking agents. Explain their mechanism of action.
15. Describe the structure of sarcomere.
16. Name the muscle proteins. Explain their chemical nature.
17. Define refractory period for an excitable tissue. Explain how it differs in cardiac and skeletal muscles.
18. Describe the sarcotubular system. What is its function?
19. Discuss the molecular basis of muscle contractions.
20. Define chronaxie and rheobase. Draw a strength–duration curve explaining its importance.
21. Discuss the properties of skeletal muscle.
22. Define fatigue. What is the site of fatigue? What are the causes for it?
23. What is beneficial effect? Explain the molecular basis for it.
24. What is rigor mortis? Describe the biochemical and physical changes associated with it. What is its medicolegal importance?
25. Explain denervation hypersensitivity.
26. Explain the molecular basis for smooth muscle contraction.
27. Explain the cardiovascular and respiratory changes during exercise.

Short Answer

1. Describe the structure of a neuron.
2. Give the classification of neurons.
3. What is myelinogenesis?
4. Define a nerve impulse. What is saltatory conduction?
5. What is orthodromic and antidromic conduction?
6. What is compound action potential?
7. What is a nerve growth factor?
8. What is all-or-none law? How does it vary in different excitable tissues?
9. What is end-plate potential?
10. What is miniature end-plate potential?
11. What is Lambert–Eaton syndrome?
12. Give the classification of muscle fibers.

13. Name the muscle proteins.
14. Draw a labeled diagram of sarcomere.
15. Define latent period in a skeletal muscle. What are the factors influencing its duration?
16. Define the terms (a) resting length, (b) equilibrium length, and (c) optimal length.
17. What is "active tension" and "passive tension" in a muscle?
18. Define Starling's law of muscle contraction.
19. What is all-or-none law in an excitable tissue?
20. What is isometric and isotonic contraction?
21. Define motor unit.
22. Explain the terms temporal, spatial, and quantal summation.
23. Define the terms treppe, clonus, and tetanus.
24. List the differences between red and white muscles.
25. Define the terms (a) hypotonia, (b) hypertonia, and (c) atonia. Mention one condition of their occurrence.
26. Define muscle tone. What is its clinical importance?
27. What are the types of smooth muscles?
28. What is oxygen debt?

4. Cardiovascular System

Long Essay

1. Explain the properties of cardiac muscle.
2. Define cardiac cycle. Explain with the help of a diagram the mechanical and pressure changes during cardiac cycle.
3. Draw a labeled diagram showing the innervations of heart. Describe the regulation of heart rate.
4. Define blood pressure. Give its normal value. Explain short-term and long-term mechanisms of its regulation.
5. Define cardiac output and cardiac index. Give its normal values. Describe the factors regulating cardiac output.
6. What is shock? What are its types? Discuss the cardiovascular compensatory changes that occur during shock.

Short Essay

1. Describe the conducting system of heart.
2. Explain origin and spread of cardiac impulse.
3. Discuss briefly the pacemaker potential.
4. Explain cardiac muscle action potential.
5. Define Starling's law. Explain its molecular basis and clinical importance.
6. Explain all-or-none law and staircase phenomenon.
7. List the differences between first and second heart sounds.
8. Define pulse. Describe a normal arterial pulse tracing.
9. Describe the waves in a normal jugular venous pulse.
10. Explain sinoaortic mechanism.
11. Explain the factors influencing blood pressure.
12. Explain the intermediate-term regulation of blood pressure.
13. Define cardiac output. Explain one method to measure it.
14. Explain the factors influencing venous return.
15. Draw a normal ECG. Explain the cause for different waves.

16. Describe the circulatory changes during muscular exercise.
17. Explain the factors influencing coronary circulation.
18. Describe the changes during irreversible shock.
19. Explain triple response.
20. Explain fetal circulation. Add a note on changes at births.

Short Answer

1. What is pulmonary and systemic circulation?
2. What is AV nodal delay? What is its clinical significance?
3. Define refractory period in a cardiac muscle. What is its importance?
4. What is staircase phenomenon? What is the molecular basis for it?
5. What is echocardiography?
6. How are different heart sounds produced?
7. What is pulse deficit?
8. What is Marey's law? Mention one condition that is an exception to this.
9. Explain briefly bainbridge reflex.
10. What is Cushing's reaction?
11. What are Korotkoff's sounds? How are they produced?
12. What is auscultatory gap?
13. Mention four factors influencing the cardiac output.
14. Draw a labeled diagram of ECG.
15. What is PR interval? What is its significance?
16. Mention two ECG changes in myocardial infraction.
17. What are artificial pacemakers? When are they used?
18. Mention the role of thoracic pump in venous return.
19. What is autoregulation? Mention three theories that explain it.
20. What is heart block? What is the ECG change in first-degree heart block.
21. What are (a) resistance vessels and (b) capacitance vessels?
22. List the factors influencing cerebral circulation.
23. Mention four methods of measuring cardiac output.

5. Respiratory System

Long Essay

1. Describe the mechanics of breathing.
2. Name the respiratory centers. Explain the neural regulation of respiration.
3. Discuss the transport of carbon dioxide in the blood.
4. Explain oxygen transport in the blood. Add a note on oxygen dissociation curve.
5. Classify hypoxia. Describe them with suitable examples.

Short Essay

1. Explain the structure and functions of respiratory membrane.
2. Explain the functions of lungs.
3. Draw a spirogram indicating various lung volumes and capacities.
4. Define lung volumes and give their normal values.
5. Define lung capacities and give their normal values.
6. What is timed vital capacity? How is it measured? Give its clinical importance.
7. What is dead space? What are its types? How is it measured?

8. Explain the chemical nature and the role of surfactant in pulmonary function.
9. What is ventilation–perfusion ratio? Explain its significance.
10. Explain the intrapleural and intrapulmonary pressure changes during different phases of respiration.
11. Give an account of Hering–Breuer reflex.
12. Define lung compliance. Mention the factors affecting it. How does it vary in health and disease?
13. Discuss the chemical regulation of respiration. Discuss the cause, consequence, and management of respiratory distress syndrome.
14. Explain briefly Hamburger's (chloride shift) phenomenon.
15. Classify hypoxia. Explain any two of them.
16. Explain the types of periodic breathing.
17. Name the methods of artificial respiration. Explain any one of them.
18. Discuss the changes that occur during acclimatization to high altitude.
19. What is decompression sickness? Add a note on its management.
20. What are the nonrespiratory functions of lungs?

Short Answer

1. List the functions of nasal cavity.
2. Name the muscles of respiration.
3. Define the following giving their normal values: (a) inspiratory reserve volume and (b) vital capacity.
4. Define the following giving their normal values: (a) inspiratory capacity and (b) expiratory reserve volume.
5. Define the following giving their normal values: (a) tidal volume and (b) total lung capacity.
6. Define the following giving their normal values: (a) residual volume and (b) functional residual capacity.
7. What is hyaline membrane disease?
8. Name the respiratory centers.
9. Draw an oxygen dissociation curve. List the factors influencing it.
10. What is P50?
11. What is Bohr and Haldane effect?
12. Give the normal partial pressures of oxygen and carbon dioxide in the arterial and venous blood.
13. List the types of hypoxia.
14. What is cyanosis? What are its types?
15. What is asphyxia? When is it produced?
16. Define the terms (a) dyspnea, (b) apnea, and (c) orthopnea.
17. Explain mouth-to-mouth breathing.
18. Write briefly about oxygen therapy in clinical practice.
19. Explain the Drinker's method of artificial respiration.

6.   Gastrointestinal System

Long Essay

1. What is the composition of saliva? What are its functions?
2. Describe the phases of gastric secretion. Give suitable experimental evidences to prove it.
3. Describe the phases of pancreatic secretion.

Short Essay

1. Name the phases of deglutition. Explain any one of them.
2. Explain the movements of stomach. Mention the factors influencing gastric emptying.

3. Explain the movements of small intestine.
4. Describe briefly the defecation reflex.
5. Explain the mechanism of salivary secretion.
6. Describe the functions of saliva.
7. Explain the composition and functions of gastric juice.
8. Explain the gastric function tests.
9. Explain the mechanism of secretion of HCl in the stomach.
10. What is the normal gastric emptying time? Explain the factors that alter it?
11. What is jaundice? What are its types?
12. Give the composition and functions of pancreatic juice.
13. Explain liver function tests.
14. Give the composition and function of succus entericus.
15. Explain the chemistry, action, and regulation of secretion of gastrin.
16. Explain the chemistry, action, and regulation of secretion of secretin.

Short Answer

1. What is antiperistalsis?
2. What is Pavlov's pouch? What is its importance?
3. What is sham feeding?
4. Explain the movements of large intestine.
5. Name any four gastrointestinal hormones.
6. List four important functions of saliva.
7. List four functions of stomach.
8. Give the composition of gastric juice.
9. Name the different cell types of gastric mucosa. Mention their functions.
10. Enumerate the functions of HCl present in gastric juice.
11. What is Heidenhain's pouch? What is its importance?
12. What is achlorhydria? What is its effect?
13. List any four functions of bile.
14. List four functions of liver.
15. What is enterohepatic circulation?
16. Name the bile salts and bile pigments.
17. Explain the functions of colon.

7. Excretory System

Long Essay

1. Describe the mechanism of urine formation.
2. Draw a labeled diagram showing nerve supply to the urinary bladder. Explain the mechanism of micturition. What is a neurogenic bladder?
3. Describe the role of countercurrent multiplier and exchange system in concentrating urine.

Short Essay

1. Describe the structure of a nephron.
2. Describe the functions of proximal convoluted tubules of the kidney.
3. Explain the structure of juxtaglomerular apparatus. What are its functions?
4. Explain the theories of autoregulation.
5. What is GFR? What is its normal value? How is it measured?

6. What is effective filtration pressure in the kidney? List the factors influencing it.
7. What is the normal renal blood flow? How is it measured?
8. Define renal clearance. Explain standard and maximal urea clearance.
9. Describe the renal tubular handling of sodium.
10. Describe the reabsorption of water in renal tubules.
11. Describe the glucose reabsorption in the kidney. Give the normal value for renal threshold and tubular maximum for glucose.
12. Explain the mechanism of bicarbonate absorption.
13. Explain the nerve supply to urinary bladder. Add a note on micturition reflex.
14. Write briefly about artificial kidney.
15. Explain renal function tests.

Short Answer

1. Draw a labeled diagram of a nephron.
2. List the functions of kidney.
3. What are the peculiarities of renal circulation?
4. List the factors influencing GFR.
5. What is PAH clearance? What is its clinical application?
6. Mention the components of filtration membrane.
7. What is filtration fraction? What is its normal value?
8. What is renal glycosuria?
9. What is tubuloglomerular feedback?
10. Mention substances secreted and reabsorbed in the distal convoluted tubule of the kidney.
11. How do you distinguish between diabetes mellitus and diabetes insipidus by examination of urine?
12. What is automatic urinary bladder?
13. What is atonic bladder?
14. What is cystometrogram?
15. What is renal failure? What are its types?
16. Enumerate the pathological constituents of urine.

Skin and Body Temperature Regulation

Short Essay

1. What is the normal body temperature? Describe the role of hypothalamus in its regulation.
2. What are the physiological changes that occur in the body when exposed to high temperature?
3. What are the physiological changes that occur when the body is exposed to low temperature?
4. What is fever? Describe the mechanism of its causation.
5. Explain the mechanisms for heat loss and gain by the body.

8.   Central Nervous System

Long Essay

1. Explain the mechanism of synaptic transmission. Explain briefly the properties of synapses.
2. Classify sensory receptors. Explain the properties of receptors.
3. Describe with the help of a diagram the pathway for pain sensation. Explain the basis of phantom limb.
4. Describe the origin, course, and termination of the pyramidal tract with the help of a labeled diagram. Add a note on hemiplegia.

5. Describe the immediate and delayed effects of complete transection of spinal cord.
6. List the nuclei of hypothalamus. Explain the functions of hypothalamus.
7. List the nuclei and describe the connections and functions of thalamus.
8. Name the nuclei of basal ganglia. Describe the functions of basal ganglia with relevant connections. Add a note on Parkinsonism.
9. What are the functional divisions of the cerebellum? Describe their functions with relevant connections. Explain the signs of cerebellar dysfunction.

Short Essay

1. Explain the structure of a synapse. What are its types?
2. Explain EPSP and IPSP. Add a note on its ionic basis.
3. Explain presynaptic inhibition.
4. Explain postsynaptic inhibition.
5. Explain Renshaw cell inhibition.
6. Explain a reflex arc with the help of a diagram.
7. What is conditioned reflex? Explain it with an example.
8. Explain the structure and functions of muscle spindle.
9. Write the neural circuit for reciprocal innervation. Explain its functional importance.
10. What is referred pain? Explain the theories of referred pain.
11. Briefly outline the role of endogenous pain-inhibiting system?
12. List the differences between upper and lower motor neuron lesion.
13. Explain the sensory and motor changes in a hemisection of the spinal cord.
14. Draw a diagram showing Brodmann cortical areas. Mention functions corresponding to these areas.
15. What is EEG? What are its normal waves? List the changes of EEG during sleep.
16. What are the different types of memory? Explain briefly the mechanism of formation of long-term memory.
17. What is REM sleep? List the features associated with it.
18. What is reticular activating system? What are its functions?
19. Describe the formation, circulation, and functions of cerebrospinal fluid. Add a note on hydrocephalus.
20. Describe the structure and functions of vestibular apparatus.
21. Explain the types and physiological basis for memory.
22. Explain the mechanism for speech. What is dyslexia?
23. Compare and contrast the actions of sympathetic and parasympathetic divisions on different systems.

Short Answer

1. Explain the division of nervous system.
2. Explain habituation and sensitization.
3. Name different types of synapses.
4. Name excitatory and inhibitory neurotransmitters.
5. What are neurotrophins and neuromodulators?
6. What is withdrawal reflex?
7. What is inverse stretch reflex?
8. What is crossed extensor response?
9. What is axon reflex?
10. What is stereognosis?
11. List the ascending tracts. Indicate the sensations carried by them.

12. List the descending tracts.
13. List the features of Brown Sequard syndrome.
14. List the clinical features of upper motor neuron lesion.
15. List the clinical features of lower motor neuron lesion.
16. What is Babinski's sign? Explain the physiological basis for it.
17. What is hemiplegia? List the clinical features of this condition.
18. List the features of facial palsy.
19. What is decerebrate rigidity? What is its practical application?
20. List the clinical manifestations of the lesion of basal ganglia.
21. List the functions of limbic system.
22. Explain the features of NREM sleep.
23. Discuss the disorders of sleep.
24. Explain the structure and functions of blood–brain barrier.
25. What is lumbar puncture? What is its clinical importance?
26. What is aphasia? What are its types?

9. Special Senses

Long Essay

1. Trace the visual pathway. Explain the effects of lesion at six levels in its course.

Short essay

1. Explain the formation, drainage, and functions of aqueous humor. What is glaucoma?
2. Name the errors of refraction. Explain its corrections with the help of a diagram.
3. Explain direct and indirect light reflex with their pathways. What is Argyll Robertson pupil?
4. Trace the pathway for accommodation reflex. Explain the changes during accommodation.
5. How is visual acuity tested?
6. Explain rhodopsin cycle.
7. Explain Young–Helmholtz theory of color vision. Name the defects of color vision.
8. What is color-blindness? How are they classified?
9. What are the contents and functions of middle ear? Explain the tympanic reflex.
10. Explain the mechanism of appreciation of sound.
11. Trace the auditory pathway with a neat, labeled diagram.
12. Explain the tests for hearing.
13. Trace the taste pathway.
14. Trace the olfactory pathway. What is anosmia?

Short Answer

1. What are the functions of iris?
2. List the functions of lacrimal secretion.
3. Name the functions of rods and cones.
4. Draw a labeled diagram of cone.
5. Explain the basis of visual acuity.
6. What is Argyll Robertson pupil?
7. Discuss the location and types of visual cortex.
8. What is macular sparing?
9. Mention extraocular muscles and movements produced by them.
10. What is squint? What are its types?

11. Explain the structure of rods and cones.
12. What is nyctalopia?
13. What are the changes during dark adaptation?
14. Mention the changes during light adaptation.
15. List the primary colors of vision.
16. Mention the disorders of color vision.
17. Explain the tests for color vision.
18. Draw a labeled diagram of the organ of Corti.
19. Explain traveling wave theory of hearing.
20. What is cochlear microphonic and endolymphatic potential?
21. What are the types of deafness?
22. Explain briefly audiometry.
23. Name auditory cortical areas.
24. Explain Rinne's test.
25. What is Weber's test? What is its clinical importance?
26. Name the primary taste sensations.
27. Draw a diagram of a taste bud.
28. Explain the mechanism for appreciation of taste.
29. Explain the terms (a) ageusia, (b) hypogeusia, and (c) dysgeusia.
30. Name four different types of taste sensations.
31. Draw a diagram of otolith organs.
32. What are pheromones?

10. Endocrinology

Long Essay

1. Name the anterior pituitary hormones. Describe the secretion, regulation, and functions of growth hormone.
2. Describe the steps involved in the synthesis of thyroid hormones. Explain its physiological functions. Add a note on cretinism.
3. What is the normal serum calcium level? Describe the hormonal regulation of serum calcium. What is tetany?
4. What is the normal blood sugar level? How is it regulated? Add a note on diabetes mellitus.
5. Enumerate the adrenal cortical hormones. Describe briefly the functions of glucocorticoids.

Short Essay

1. Classify hormones. Explain the mechanism of action of hormones.
2. Explain negative and positive feedback mechanism of hormonal regulation.
3. Explain briefly radioimmunoassay (RIA).
4. Describe the hypothalamohypophysial axis.
5. Explain the role of hypothalamus as an endocrine gland.
6. Name the posterior pituitary hormones. Explain their actions.
7. Describe the milk ejection reflex.
8. What are the functions of oxytocin?
9. What are the functions of antidiuretic hormone?
10. What are the differences between pituitary dwarf and thyroid dwarf?
11. What are second messengers? Explain the mechanism of action of any one of them.
12. Describe the iodide trapping mechanism in thyroid gland. How is it inhibited?

13. Enumerate the actions of thyroxin.
14. What are clinical features of cretinism? How are they produced?
15. Explain the clinical features of myxedema. Add a note on its management.
16. What is tetany? What are its clinical features?
17. Name the hyperglycemic hormones. Give the mechanism of action of any one of them.
18. Explain the symptoms of diabetes mellitus. Add a note on its management.
19. Discuss the actions, metabolism, and regulation of secretion of glucagon.
20. Explain the anti-inflammatory effect of cortisol.
21. What is Cushing's syndrome? What are its clinical features?
22. Explain the cause and features of Addison's disease.
23. Compare and contrast the actions of epinephrine and norepinephrine.

Short Answer

1. Name the stimulating and inhibitory hormones of hypothalamus.
2. What is panhypopituitarism?
3. What is hormonal rhythm?
4. Name the clinical conditions associated with altered secretion of growth hormone.
5. Name the hormones secreted by anterior pituitary.
6. What is pituitary diabetes?
7. Name the diabetogenic hormones.
8. Mention two examples of neuroendocrine reflex.
9. What is the difference between diabetes mellitus and diabetes insipidus?
10. What are somatomedins? Where are they secreted?
11. What are somatostatins? Where are they secreted?
12. List important tests for the assessment of thyroid functions.
13. Explain the tests to detect latent tetany.
14. What is rickets? Mention its clinical features.
15. What is permissive action of hormones? Give an example.
16. Name the hormones secreted by pancreas.
17. Name the cell layer and hormones secreted by adrenal cortex.
18. List the functions of aldosterone.
19. What is aldosterone escape?
20. What is Addisonian crisis?
21. What is adrenogenital syndrome?
22. List the functions of pineal gland.

11. Reproductive System

Long Essay

1. Describe the hormonal, uterine, ovarian, and vaginal changes during different phases of menstrual cycle.

Short Essay

1. Explain gametogenesis in female.
2. List the secondary sexual characters in males and females.
3. What is ovulation? Explain its hormonal control.
4. Write briefly about corpus luteum.
5. Explain the tests to detect ovulation.

6. Describe the immunological test for pregnancy.
7. Describe briefly fetoplacental unit.
8. Discuss physiological changes during pregnancy.
9. Explain the contraceptive methods in females.
10. Explain the mechanism of action of oral contraceptive pill.
11. Briefly describe the functions of placenta.
12. Discuss the hormonal control of lactation.
13. Explain the stages of spermatogenesis. Add a note on the factors influencing it.
14. Describe the actisons of testosterone.
15. Explain the methods of contraception in males.

Short Answer

1. Mention the primary organ of sex in males and females.
2. Define menarche and menopause.
3. List the functions of estrogen.
4. List the functions of progesterone.
5. List the hormones of placenta.
6. Explain the role of oxytocin during parturition.
7. List the functions of FSH.
8. Mention the functions of LH.
9. Define the terms (a) amenorrhea, (b) menorrhagia, and (c) polymenorrhea.
10. List the methods of contraception in females.
11. Give an account of source and action of inhibin.
12. Give an account of actions of relaxin.
13. List contraceptive methods in males.
14. List the functions of Sertoli cells.
15. What is cryptorchidism?

Multiple Choice Questions

1. General Physiology

1. The movement of particles from the region of higher concentration to the region of lower concentration is termed

   (a) Diffusion
   (b) Osmosis
   (c) Endocytosis
   (d) Pinocytosis

2. The movement of solvent from the region of higher concentration to the region of lower concentration through semipermeable membrane is

   (a) Diffusion
   (b) Osmosis
   (c) Endocytosis
   (d) Pinocytosis

3. The powerhouse of the cell is

   (a) Centriole
   (b) Centrosome
   (c) Mitochondria
   (d) Lysosomes

4. The structure in the cell that helps in digestion of bacteria is

   (a) Centriole
   (b) Centrosome
   (c) Mitochondria
   (d) Lysosomes

5. The system of fibers maintaining the structure of the cell is

   (a) Actin
   (b) Myosin
   (c) Cytoskeleton
   (d) Troponin

6. The part of the cell that monitors the steps of cell division is

   (a) Ribosome
   (b) Centrosome
   (c) Mitochondria
   (d) Lysosomes

7. The type of intercellular connection through which the molecules move easily is

   (a) Desmosomes
   (b) Gap junction
   (c) Tight junction
   (d) Ion channels

8. Each chromosome is made up of a giant molecule of

   (a) Gene
   (b) Chromatin
   (c) DNA
   (d) RNA

9. The ultimate units carrying hereditary characters are

   (a) Gene
   (b) Chromatin
   (c) DNA
   (d) RNA

10. Germ cell is a

   (a) Haploid cell
   (b) Diploid cell
   (c) Zygote
   (d) Mature cell

11. **The number of lipid layers present in the cell membrane is**

    (a) One
    (b) Two
    (c) Three
    (d) Four

12. **Ribosomes are present on**

    (a) Centriole
    (b) Endoplasmic reticulum
    (c) Nucleus
    (d) Lysosomes

13. **Granular endoplasmic reticulum forms**

    (a) Proteins
    (b) Lipids
    (c) Carbohydrates
    (d) Steroids

14. **Smooth endoplasmic reticulum forms**

    (a) Proteins
    (b) Lipids
    (c) Carbohydrates
    (d) Vitamins

15. **The processing of protein and formation of secretory granules is done by**

    (a) Ribosomes
    (b) Centrosome
    (c) Golgi apparatus
    (d) Cytoskeleton

16. **The type of cell division in which the chromosomal number gets reduced to half is**

    (a) Mitosis
    (b) Meiosis
    (c) Prophase
    (d) Telophase

17. **The cell division in which the chromosomal number remains the same is**

    (a) Mitosis
    (b) Meiosis
    (c) Prophase
    (d) Telophase

18. **Release of contents of vesicles outside the cell with the membrane kept intact is termed**

    (a) Phagocytosis
    (b) Pinocytosis
    (c) Exocytosis
    (d) Endocytosis

19. **The other name for "cell eating" is**

    (a) Phagocytosis
    (b) Pinocytosis
    (c) Exocytosis
    (d) Endocytosis

20. **Cell drinking is also known as**

    (a) Phagocytosis
    (b) Pinocytosis
    (c) Exocytosis
    (d) Endocytosis

21. **The form of transport that requires the expenditure of energy is**

    (a) Diffusion
    (b) Osmosis
    (c) Active transport
    (d) Facilitated diffusion

22. **The movement of a substance along its concentration gradient with the help of carrier protein is**

    (a) Diffusion
    (b) Osmosis
    (c) Countertransport
    (d) Facilitated diffusion

23. **Transport of sodium and glucose is an example of**

    (a) Antiport
    (b) Symport
    (c) Uniport
    (d) Diffusion

24. **Transport of sodium and hydrogen ions is an example of**

    (a) Antiport
    (b) Symport
    (c) Uniport
    (d) Diffusion

25. **The second messenger systems are the following *except***

    (a) cAMP
    (b) cGMP
    (c) Calmodulin
    (d) GABA

26. **Maintenance of constancy of the internal environment is**

    (a) Hemostatic
    (b) Homeostasis
    (c) Hypoxia
    (d) Hypercapnia

27. **The type of cellular connection for the tissue to function as syncytium is**

    (a) Desmosomes
    (b) Gap junctions
    (c) Tight junction
    (d) Hemidesmosomes

28. **The phases of meiotic cell division are the following** *except*

    (a) Prophase
    (b) Anaphase
    (c) Telophase
    (d) Interphase

29. **The chromosomal number in a normal human being is**

    (a) 23
    (b) 44
    (c) 46
    (d) 48

30. **The process of formation of mRNA is**

    (a) Translation
    (b) Transcription
    (c) Duplication
    (d) Cell division

2. Blood

1. **The fluid component of plasma present in the blood constitutes about**

    (a) 40%
    (b) 55%
    (c) 75%
    (d) 90%

2. **The total volume of blood present in an adult human is around**

    (a) 3 L
    (b) 5 L
    (c) 8 L
    (d) 10 L

3. **Normal plasma protein value is**

    (a) 2 g/dL
    (b) 2–4 g/dL
    (c) 6–8 g/dL
    (d) 8–10 g/dL

4. **Most of the plasma proteins are synthesized by**

    (a) Liver
    (b) Kidney
    (c) Spleen
    (d) Pancreas

5. **The most abundant plasma protein present in the blood is**

    (a) Albumin
    (b) Globulin
    (c) Fibrinogen
    (d) Prothrombin

6. **Normal RBC diameter is**

    (a) $3.8\ \mu$
    (b) $5.4\ \mu$
    (c) $7.2\ \mu$
    (d) $8.6\ \mu$

7. **Erythropoiesis normally occurs in the adult in**

    (a) Liver
    (b) Yolk sac
    (c) Spleen
    (d) Bone marrow

8. **The process of erythropoiesis takes**

    (a) 7 min
    (b) 7 h
    (c) 7 days
    (d) 7 weeks

9. **Normal RBC count in males is**

    (a) 5–5.5 lakh cells/mm^3
    (b) 1.4–4 million cells/mm^3
    (c) 4–11 million cells/mm^3
    (d) 5–5.5 million cells/mm^3

10. **The most common type of anemia found in our country is**

    (a) Thalassemia
    (b) Aplastic anemia
    (c) Vitamin B_{12} deficiency anemia
    (d) Iron-deficiency anemia

11. Erythropoietin is mainly produced in

(a) Kidneys
(b) Bone marrow
(c) Spleen
(d) Lungs

12. Increase in RBC count is called

(a) Anemia
(b) Leukocytosis
(c) Polycythemia
(d) Leukemia

13. The granulocytes include all *except*

(a) Neutrophils
(b) Lymphocytes
(c) Basophils
(d) Eosinophils

14. Normal WBC count in adults is

(a) $400–1100$ cells/mm^3
(b) $4000–11000$ cells/mm^3
(c) $4–11$ lakh cells/mm^3
(d) $4–11$ million cells/mm^3

15. The percentage of neutrophil is

(a) $10–15$
(b) $40–45$
(c) $60–65$
(d) $90–95$

16. The diameter of an eosinophil is

(a) $2–4\,\mu$
(b) $4–6\,\mu$
(c) $7.2\,\mu$
(d) $10–14\,\mu$

17. The least numerous of WBCs are

(a) Neutrophils
(b) Monocytes
(c) Eosinophils
(d) Basophils

18. The largest WBC is

(a) Neutrophil
(b) Monocyte
(c) Eosinophil
(d) Basophil

19. The antiallergic cell is

(a) Neutrophil
(b) Monocyte

(c) Eosinophil
(d) Basophil

20. Phagocytic cell is

(a) Neutrophil
(b) RBC
(c) Platelet
(d) Astrocyte

21. Cell-mediated immunity is produced by

(a) T-lymphocytes
(b) B-lymphocytes
(c) Eosinophils
(d) Basophils

22. Increase in WBC count is termed

(a) Leukocytosis
(b) Leukopenia
(c) Leukopoiesis
(d) Leukocytes

23. The type of WBC increased in tuberculosis is

(a) Neutrophils
(b) Lymphocytes
(c) Basophils
(d) Eosinophils

24. Normal size of platelet is

(a) $1–1.5\,\mu$
(b) $2–4\,\mu$
(c) $4–6\,\mu$
(d) $7–8\,\mu$

25. Platelets are formed from

(a) Early normoblasts
(b) Myelocytes
(c) Megakaryocytes
(d) Proerythroblasts

26. Purpura is caused due to the deficiency of

(a) RBCs
(b) WBCs
(c) Clotting factors
(d) Platelets

27. The most important ion required for clotting is

(a) Mg^{++}
(b) Ca^{++}
(c) Na^{+}
(d) K^{+}

28. Fibrinogen is converted into fibrin by

(a) Thrombin
(b) Prothrombin
(c) Prothrombin activator
(d) Calcium

29. Clotting time is prolonged in all *except*

(a) Hemophilia
(b) Thrombocytopenia
(c) Vitamin K deficiency
(d) Afibrinogenemia

30. Normal bleeding time is

(a) 2–4 s
(b) 4–8 s
(c) 2–4 min
(d) 4–8 min

31. Normal clotting time by capillary tube method is

(a) 1–4 s
(b) 3–8 s
(c) 1–4 min
(d) 3–8 min

32. Blood group antigens are present on

(a) RBCs
(b) WBCs
(c) Platelets
(d) Hemoglobin

33. Individual with O blood group has

(a) A antigen
(b) B antigen
(c) Both AB antigens
(d) No antigen

34. Blood groups were discovered by

(a) William Harvey
(b) Louis Pasteur
(c) Duffy
(d) Karl Landsteiner

35. Erythroblastosis fetalis can occur when Rh+ child is born to

(a) Rh– mother
(b) Rh+ mother
(c) Rh+ mother and Rh– father
(d) Rh– mother and Rh– father

36. Indications of blood transfusion include all *except*

(a) Major surgeries
(b) Severe burns
(c) Severe anemia
(d) Cardiac failure due to MI

37. Kernicterus is caused due to accumulation of bilirubin in

(a) Liver
(b) Spleen
(c) Kidneys
(d) Brain

38. Heparin is released by

(a) Neutrophils
(b) Basophils
(c) Lymphocytes
(d) Eosinophils

39. Histamine is released by

(a) Neutrophils
(b) Monocytes
(c) Eosinophils
(d) Basophils

40. The percentage of eosinophil is around

(a) 0–1
(b) 1–4
(c) 10–14
(d) 25–30

41. The percentage of monocyte is around

(a) 0–1
(b) 1–4
(c) 2–8
(d) 20–30

42. ESR decreases in

(a) Infections
(b) Tuberculosis
(c) Rheumatoid arthritis
(d) Polycythemia

43. Hemoglobin mainly contains

(a) Copper
(b) Magnesium
(c) Iron
(d) Nickel

44. **Hemophilia is caused due to the deficiency of clotting factor**

    (a) VII
    (b) VIII
    (c) XI
    (d) X

45. **The anticoagulants include the following *except***

    (a) Heparin
    (b) EDTA
    (c) Vitamin K
    (d) Trisodium citrate

46. **Life span of an RBC is**

    (a) 100 days
    (b) 102 days
    (c) 120 days
    (d) 135 days

47. **The percentage of neutrophils present is**

    (a) 0–1
    (b) 1–4
    (c) 25–30
    (d) 60–65

48. **The normal plasma volume is**

    (a) 1–1.5 L
    (b) 3–3.5 L
    (c) 5–6 L
    (d) 7–8 L

49. **The percentage of basophils present is**

    (a) 0–1
    (b) 1–4
    (c) 10–14
    (d) 25–30

50. **The percentage of Lymphocytes present is**

    (a) 0–1
    (b) 1–4
    (c) 10–14
    (d) 25–30

51. **Specific gravity of whole blood is**

    (a) 1010–1015
    (b) 1030–1035
    (c) 1055–1060
    (d) 1075–1080

52. **Normal albumin–globulin ratio is**

    (a) 1:2.3
    (b) 1:1.7
    (c) 1.7:1
    (d) 2.3:1

53. **The molecular weight of albumin is**

    (a) 22,000
    (b) 44,000
    (c) 66,000
    (d) 88,000

54. **The main function of albumin is maintenance of**

    (a) Heart rate
    (b) Colloid osmotic pressure
    (c) Body temperature
    (d) Blood flow

55. **The most abundant cells present in blood are**

    (a) RBCs
    (b) WBCs
    (c) Platelets
    (d) Natural killer cells

56. **Surface area of an RBC is**

    (a) $85\ \mu^2$
    (b) $102\ \mu^2$
    (c) $135\ \mu^2$
    (d) $185\ \mu^2$

57. **Normal RBC count in infants is**

    (a) $2\text{–}3\ \text{million/mm}^3$
    (b) $3\text{–}4\ \text{million/mm}^3$
    (c) $6\text{–}7\ \text{million/mm}^3$
    (d) $10\text{–}12\ \text{million/mm}^3$

58. **Volume of normal RBC is**

    (a) $87\ \mu^3$
    (b) $104\ \mu^3$
    (c) $127\ \mu^3$
    (d) $135\ \mu^3$

59. **RBC mainly contains**

    (a) Carbohydrates
    (b) Lipids
    (c) Hb
    (d) Electrolytes

60. Metabolic needs of an RBC are met by

(a) Fatty acids
(b) Amino acids
(c) Glucose
(d) Cholesterol

61. Red bone marrow is found in

(a) Cranial bones
(b) Vertebrae
(c) Pelvic bones
(d) All the above

62. All of the following facilitate erythropoiesis
except

(a) Erythropoietin
(b) Estrogens
(c) Vitamin B_{12}
(d) Folic acid

63. Increase in RBC count above 8 million cells/mm^3 is termed

(a) Anemia
(b) Leukopenia
(c) Leukocytosis
(d) Polycythemia

64. The polypeptide chains present in HbA are

(a) $\alpha_2 \beta_2$
(b) $\alpha_2 \delta_2$
(c) $\alpha_2 \gamma_2$
(d) $\beta_2 \delta_2$

65. The polypeptide chains present in HbA$_2$ are

(a) $\alpha_2 \beta_2$
(b) $\alpha_2 \delta_2$
(c) $\alpha_2 \gamma_2$
(d) $\beta_2 \delta_2$

66. The polypeptide chains present in HbF are

(a) $\alpha_2 \beta_2$
(b) $\alpha_2 \delta_2$
(c) $\alpha_2 \gamma_2$
(d) $\beta_2 \delta_2$

67. Under normal conditions, one molecule of Hb carries

(a) 1.34 mL of O_2
(b) 1.72 mL of O_2
(c) 2.34 mL of O_2
(d) 2.72 mL of O_2

68. Oxidation of ferrous iron to ferric iron forms

(a) Carboxyhemoglobin
(b) Oxyhemoglobin
(c) Methemoglobin
(d) Sulphemoglobin

69. In a Hb molecule, 1 molecule of globin combines with

(a) 2 heme molecules
(b) 4 heme molecules
(c) 6 heme molecules
(d) 8 heme molecules

70. HbS is an abnormal hemoglobin in which glutamic acid is replaced by

(a) Leucine
(b) Isoleucine
(c) Methionine
(d) Valine

71. During breakdown of Hb, heme is broken down into iron and

(a) Stercobilinogen
(b) Urobilinogen
(c) Biliverdin
(d) Bilirubin

72. Abnormal condition caused due to decreased production of alpha and beta chains of Hb is called

(a) Sickle cell anemia
(b) Thalassemia
(c) Hereditary spherocytosis
(d) Iron-deficiency anemia

73. Normal amount of iron present in the body is

(a) 10–20 mg
(b) 1–2 g
(c) 3–5 g
(d) 10–20 g

74. The rate at which red cells settle down is termed

(a) ESR
(b) Fragility
(c) Specific gravity
(d) PCV

75. Normal color index is

(a) 0.1–0.3
(b) 0.45–0.6
(c) 0.85–1.15
(d) 1.15–1.65

76. Normal MCH is

(a) 28–32 pg
(b) 42–46 pg
(c) 87–93 pg
(d) 125–132 pg

77. The relative percentage of Hb in a single RBC is called

(a) CI
(b) MCH
(c) MCHC
(d) MCV

78. Life span of neutrophils in blood is

(a) 6–7 h
(b) 6–7 days
(c) 6–7 months
(d) 6–7 weeks

79. The multilobed leukocyte is

(a) Monocyte
(b) Small lymphocyte
(c) Neutrophil
(d) Large lymphocyte

80. Kidney-shaped nucleus is present in

(a) Monocyte
(b) Basophil
(c) Neutrophil
(d) Eosinophil

81. The size of monocyte is around

(a) 6–8 μ
(b) 8–10 μ
(c) 10–12 μ
(d) 12–18 μ

82. The size of a small lymphocyte is around

(a) 7 μ
(b) 11 μ
(c) 13 μ
(d) 18 μ

83. The process of squeezing of neutrophils through pores of blood vessels is termed

(a) Margination
(b) Chemotaxis
(c) Diapedesis
(d) Phagocytosis

84. Parasitic infestations produce increase in

(a) Neutrophils
(b) Eosinophils
(c) Basophils
(d) Lymphocytes

85. Most abundant immunoglobulin present in the body is

(a) IgG
(b) IgA
(c) IgM
(d) IgE

86. Immunoglobulin secreted in saliva, tears, and milk is

(a) IgG
(b) IgA
(c) IgM
(d) IgE

87. ABO antibodies are formed by

(a) IgG
(b) IgA
(c) IgM
(d) IgE

88. HIV virus causes destruction of

(a) Helper T cells
(b) Cytotoxic T cells
(c) Suppressor T cells
(d) Memory T cells

89. All the following are autoimmune diseases *except*

(a) Myasthenia gravis
(b) Rheumatoid arthritis
(c) Grave's disease
(d) Typhoid

90. Immunoglobulins are produced by

(a) Neutrophils
(b) Basophils

   (c) Eosinophils

   (d) Lymphocytes

91. The normal platelet count is

   (a) 150–400 cells/mm^3

   (b) 1.5–4 thousand cells/mm^3

   (c) 1.5–4 lakh cells/mm^3

   (d) 1.5–4 million cells/mm^3

92. Deficiency of platelets is termed as

   (a) Anemia

   (b) Leukopenia

   (c) Thrombocytopenia

   (d) Polycythemia

93. Vitamin K deficiency reduces the formation of all clotting factors *except*

   (a) Factor V

   (b) Factor VII

   (c) Factor IX

   (d) Factor X

94. Normal prothrombin time is

   (a) 1–4 s

   (b) 2–4 s

   (c) 2–8 s

   (d) 11–16 s

95. Bleeding time is prolonged in

   (a) Afibrinogenemia

   (b) Hemophilia

   (c) Chrismas disease

   (d) Purpura

96. A person is said to be Rh+ if he has

   (a) D antigen

   (b) d antigen

   (c) E antigen

   (d) e antigen

97. Blood is stored at

   (a) –80 °C

   (b) 2–4 °C

   (c) Room temperature

   (d) 42 °C

98. All are hazards of mismatched blood transfusion *except*

   (a) Shock

   (b) Renal failure

   (c) Jaundice

   (d) Iron overload

99. A group individual has

   (a) α-agglutinin

   (b) β-agglutinin

   (c) α- and β-agglutinin

   (d) No agglutinin

100. Anticoagulation within the body is brought about by all of the following *except*

   (a) Prostacyclin

   (b) Anti thrombin III

   (c) EDTA

   (d) Thrombomodulin

101. Excessive increase in the number of WBCs is termed

   (a) Leukocytosis

   (b) Leukopoiesis

   (c) Leukopenia

   (d) Leukemia

102. Dead neutrophils, necrotic tissue, dead bacteria all combine to form

   (a) Pus

   (b) Lymph

   (c) Serum

   (d) Plasma

103. Mean corpuscular volume is reduced in

   (a) Vitamin B$_{12}$ deficiency anemia

   (b) Folic acid deficiency anemia

   (c) Iron deficiency anemia

   (d) Aplastic anemia

104. Packed cell volume is increased in

   (a) Pregnancy

   (b) Anemia

   (c) Polycythemia

   (d) Overhydration

3. Nerve–Muscle Physiology

1. The structural and functional unit of nervous system is

   (a) Neuroglia

   (b) Nephron

   (c) Neuron

   (d) Renshaw's cell

2. **The following factors influence the velocity of the nerve impulse *except***

   (a) Myelination
   (b) Diameter
   (c) Temperature
   (d) Size of the cell body

3. **Resting membrane potential in a motor nerve is**

   (a) $-90\ mV$
   (b) $-70\ mV$
   (c) $70\ mV$
   (d) $90\ mV$

4. **Resting membrane potential is produced by the following *except***

   (a) Greater permeability of the membrane to potassium ions
   (b) Presence of large, nondiffusible, negatively charged proteins within the cell
   (c) Efflux of chloride ions
   (d) Action of sodium–potassium ATPase pump

5. **The following features are true for a local response *except***

   (a) It is graded
   (b) It is nonpropagated
   (c) It has a long latent period
   (d) It decays exponentially

6. **Depolarization in a motor nerve action potential is due to**

   (a) Entry of potassium ion
   (b) Entry of sodium ion
   (c) Exit of potassium ion
   (d) Entry of calcium ion

7. **Repolarization in a motor nerve is due to**

   (a) Influx of chloride ion
   (b) Efflux of potassium ion
   (c) Efflux of calcium ion
   (d) Influx of sodium ion

8. **Hyperpolarization in a motor nerve is due to**

   (a) Influx of chloride ion
   (b) Continued efflux of potassium ion
   (c) Efflux of calcium ion
   (d) Influx of sodium ion

9. **Depolarization in an excitable tissue**

   (a) Increases its excitability
   (b) Decreases its excitability
   (c) Keeps the excitability unchanged
   (d) Makes it functionless

10. **Hyperpolarization in an excitable tissue**

    (a) Increases its excitability
    (b) Decreases its excitability
    (c) Keeps the excitability unchanged
    (d) Makes it functionless

11. **Saltatory conduction**

    (a) Increases the velocity of nerve impulse
    (b) Decreases the velocity of nerve impulse
    (c) Has no influence on the velocity of nerve impulse
    (d) Alters the direction of nerve impulse

12. **Myelin sheath for the peripheral nerve is formed by**

    (a) Schwann cells
    (b) Microglia
    (c) Oligodendroglia
    (d) Astrocytes

13. **The following are the glial cells *except***

    (a) Pyramidal cells
    (b) Microglia
    (c) Oligodendroglia
    (d) Astrocytes

14. **The myelin sheath for the neuron of the CNS is formed by**

    (a) Schwann cells
    (b) Microglia
    (c) Oligodendroglia
    (d) Astrocytes

15. **Neurotransmitter is released at the neuromuscular junction due to**

    (a) Entry of calcium
    (b) Entry of sodium
    (c) Entry of potassium
    (d) Exit of calcium

16. **The neurotransmitter at neuromuscular junction is**

    (a) Acetylcholine
    (b) Epinephrine
    (c) Dopamine
    (d) GABA

17. **Neurotransmitter at the neuromuscular junction is broken down by**

    (a) Cholinesterase
    (b) Acetylcholine synthetase
    (c) Phosphodiesterase
    (d) Decarboxylase

18. **Myasthenia gravis is produced due to**

    (a) Defective production of acetylcholine
    (b) Excessive destruction of acetylcholine
    (c) Delayed breakdown of acetylcholine
    (d) Destruction of acetylcholine receptors

19. **Myasthenia gravis is treated effectively by using**

    (a) Acetylcholine receptor blockers
    (b) Acetylcholinesterase
    (c) Acetylcholinesterase inhibitors
    (d) L-dopa precursor of dopamine

20. **Compound action potential is produced by**

    (a) A single motor nerve
    (b) A group of nerve fibers
    (c) A myelinated nerve fiber
    (d) An unmyelinated nerve fiber

21. **Structural and functional unit of the muscle is**

    (a) Sarcomere
    (b) Sarcotubular system
    (c) Sarcoplasmic reticulum
    (d) Sarcolemma

22. **The voluntary muscle in the following is**

    (a) Biceps
    (b) Multiunit smooth muscle
    (c) Visceral smooth muscle
    (d) Cardiac muscle

23. **Resting membrane potential in a cardiac muscle is**

    (a) –80 to –90 mV
    (b) –70 mV
    (c) 70 mV
    (d) 80 to 90 mV

24. **The following are the properties of skeletal muscle *except***

    (a) Excitability
    (b) Autorhythmicity

    (c) Conductivity
    (d) Contractility

25. **Starlings' law states that**

    (a) Force of contraction of muscle is directly proportional to initial length of the muscle
    (b) Force of contraction is not related to initial length
    (c) Force of contraction is indirectly proportional to the initial length
    (d) Force of contraction is proportional to initial length within physiological limits

26. **In isotonic contraction**

    (a) Length of the muscle increases
    (b) Tone of the muscle changes
    (c) Tone remains the same
    (d) Length remains the same

27. **In isometric contraction**

    (a) Length of the muscle changes
    (b) Tone of the muscle decreases
    (c) Tone remains the same
    (d) Length remains the same

28. **Lifting a weight of 2 kg from the ground is an example of**

    (a) Isotonic contraction
    (b) Isometric contraction
    (c) Clonus
    (d) Fatigue

29. **The muscle fails to respond to second stimuli of any magnitude if it is in**

    (a) Isotonic contraction
    (b) Isometric contraction
    (c) Relative refractory period
    (d) Absolute refractory period

30. **The muscle responds to second stimuli of a greater magnitude if it is in**

    (a) Isotonic contraction
    (b) Isometric contraction
    (c) Relative refractory period
    (d) Absolute refractory period

31. **Pushing the wall is an example of**

    (a) Isotonic contraction
    (b) Isometric contraction
    (c) Relative refractory period
    (d) Absolute refractory period

32. All-or-none law is applicable to the following *except*

(a) A motor nerve fiber

(b) A single skeletal muscle fiber

(c) Entire cardiac muscle

(d) A bundle of skeletal muscle fibers

33. Chronaxie is

(a) Minimum strength of current given indefinitely to excite a tissue

(b) Minimum time required to excite with twice the rheobasic strength of current

(c) Minimum time needed to excite with rheobasic strength of current

(d) Maximum strength of current to excite the tissue

34. Rheobase is

(a) Minimum strength of current given indefinitely to excite a tissue

(b) Minimum time required to excite a tissue

(c) Maximum time needed to excite a tissue with maximum strength of current

(d) Maximum strength of current given indefinitely to excite a tissue

35. Utilization time is

(a) Minimum strength of current given indefinitely to excite a tissue

(b) Minimum time required to excite a tissue with twice the rheobasic strength of current

(c) Minimum time needed to excite a tissue with rheobasic strength of current

(d) Maximum strength of current to excite a tissue

36. The electrical changes occurring at the anode of the recording electrode is

(a) Catelectrotonic potential

(b) Anelectrotonic potential

(c) Action potential

(d) Receptor potential

37. The electrical changes occurring at the cathode of the recording electrode is

(a) Catelectrotonic potential

(b) Anelectrotonic potential

(c) Action potential

(d) Receptor potential

38. End-plate potential has the following characteristics *except*

(a) It is graded

(b) It is nonpropagated

(c) It has no latency

(d) It is propagated

39. Transmission of impulse away from the cell body is termed

(a) Orthodromic conduction

(b) Antidromic conduction

(c) Saltatory conduction

(d) Axoplasmic flow

40. Transport of substances from the cell body to the nerve terminal occurs by

(a) Orthodromic conduction

(b) Antidromic conduction

(c) Saltatory conduction

(d) Axoplasmic flow

41. Transmission of impulse toward the cell body is termed

(a) Orthodromic conduction

(b) Antidromic conduction

(c) Saltatory conduction

(d) Axoplasmic flow

42. Denervation hypersensitivity is true in the following conditions *except*

(a) Occurs in denervated muscle

(b) Due to increased Ach receptors

(c) Results in rigidity of the muscle

(d) Responds to circulating acetylcholine

43. The following are the contractile proteins *except*

(a) Actin

(b) Myosin

(c) Troponin

(d) Myoglobin

44. A threshold stimulus produces

(a) Action potential

(b) Local response

(c) Impulse

(d) Tetanus

45. A subthreshold stimulus produces

(a) Action potential

(b) Local response
(c) Receptor potential
(d) No response

46. **Action potential in a motor nerve has the following phases** *except*

(a) Depolarization
(b) Repolarization
(c) Hyperpolarization
(d) Plateau

47. **Responding property of the excitable tissue are the following** *except*

(a) Excitability
(b) Conductivity
(c) Contractility
(d) Rigor mortis

48. **The property of the motor nerve is**

(a) Conductivity
(b) Contractility
(c) Autorhythmicity
(d) Clonus

49. **Following are the properties of motor nerve** *except*

(a) Excitability
(b) Conductivity
(c) All-or-none law
(d) Tetanus

50. **The components of the neuromuscular junction are the following** *except*

(a) Prejunctional terminal
(b) Synaptic cleft
(c) Motor end plate
(d) Gap junction

51. **The period in which a second stimulus of greater intensity produces a response is termed**

(a) Latent period
(b) Relative refractory period
(c) Absolute refractory period
(d) Contraction period

52. **The period during which a second stimulus of greater intensity does not produce a response is termed**

(a) Latent period
(b) Relative refractory period

(c) Absolute refractory period
(d) Contraction period

53. **Thin filaments of muscles are made up of the following proteins** *except*

(a) Actin
(b) Myosin
(c) Troponin
(d) Tropomyosin

54. **The following statement is not true for skeletal muscle**

(a) It can be tetanized
(b) It obeys all-or-none law
(c) It can be fatigued
(d) It shows autorhythmicity

55. **The following statement is not true for smooth muscle**

(a) It is voluntary
(b) It can contract with external stimuli
(c) It is nonstriated
(d) It is supplied by autonomic nervous system

56. **The following statement is not true for cardiac muscle**

(a) It is involuntary
(b) It can be tetanized
(c) It exhibits autorhythmicity
(d) It obeys all-or-none law

57. **The action potential in a cardiac muscle is different from that of skeletal muscle by the presence of phase**

(a) Depolarization
(b) Repolarization
(c) Hyperpolarization
(d) Plateau

58. **Smooth muscle does not restore original length immediately after relaxation due to the presence of**

(a) Actin and myosin filaments
(b) Presence of Latch bridges
(c) Absence of sarcotubular system
(d) Absence of striation

59. **The potential developed at the postjunctional membrane in a neuromuscular junction is**

(a) Receptor potential
(b) Pacemaker potential

(c) End-plate potential

(d) Action potential

60. End-plate potential has the following characters *except*

(a) It is an all-or-none response

(b) It is a graded response

(c) It is a nonpropagated response

(d) It has no latency

61. Miniature end-plate potential is produced due to

(a) Stimulation of presynaptic terminal

(b) Release of small quantity of acetylcholine at rest

(c) Activation of postjunctional membrane

(d) Alteration in permeability of motor end-plate to calcium

62. Troponin has the binding sites for the following *except*

(a) Actin

(b) Tropomyosin

(c) Calcium ions

(d) Myosin

63. The sarcotubular system consists of the following structures *except*

(a) Sarcoplasmic reticulum

(b) T-tubules

(c) Terminal cistern

(d) Ribosomes

64. The theory that explains the basis of muscle contraction is

(a) Sliding filament theory

(b) Traveling wave theory

(c) Myogenic theory

(d) Metabolite theory

65. Causes for fatigue are the following *except*

(a) Accumulation of metabolic end products

(b) Exhaustion of neurotransmitter

(c) Depletion of ATP

(d) Decreased temperature

66. The site of fatigue in an intact animal is

(a) Neuromuscular junction

(b) Synapse

(c) Spinal cord

(d) Medulla

67. A state of sustained contraction is

(a) Tetanus

(b) Clonus

(c) Treppe

(d) Fatigue

68. Incomplete tetanus is called

(a) Clonus

(b) Tetanus

(c) Tetany

(d) Treppe

69. Following are the features of red muscle *except*

(a) Has a short latency

(b) Responds slowly

(c) They are postural muscles

(d) They are the muscles of the back

70. The character of white muscle is

(a) It has a short latency

(b) It has a long latency

(c) They respond slowly

(d) They are postural muscles

71. The calcium-binding protein which acts as second messenger is

(a) Calmodulin

(b) cAMP

(c) cGMP

(d) Adenosine

72. Recording of electrical activities of the muscle is

(a) EEG

(b) EMG

(c) EOG

(d) ECG

4. Cardiovascular System

1. Human heart has

(a) Four chambers

(b) Three chambers

(c) Two chambers

(d) One chamber

2. **The layers of the heart are the following except**

(a) Epicardium
(b) Myocardium
(c) Pericardium
(d) Endocardium

3. **In pulmonary circulation, the blood is pumped from**

(a) Right atrium
(b) Right ventricle
(c) Left atrium
(d) Left ventricle

4. **In systemic circulation, the blood is pumped from**

(a) Right atrium
(b) Right ventricle
(c) Left atrium
(d) Left ventricle

5. **In pulmonary circulation blood reaches**

(a) Right atrium
(b) Right ventricle
(c) Left atrium
(d) Left ventricle

6. **In systemic circulation, the blood reaches**

(a) Right atrium
(b) Right ventricle
(c) Left atrium
(d) Left ventricle

7. **The atrioventricular opening on the right side is guarded by**

(a) Tricuspid valve
(b) Mitral valve
(c) Semilunar valve
(d) None of the above

8. **The atrioventricular opening on the left side is guarded by**

(a) Tricuspid valve
(b) Mitral valve
(c) Semilunar valve
(d) None of the above

9. **The opening of aorta is guarded by**

(a) Tricuspid valve
(b) Mitral valve
(c) Semilunar valve

(d) None of the above

10. **The opening of pulmonary artery is guarded by**

(a) Tricuspid valve
(b) Mitral valve
(c) Semilunar valve
(d) None of the above

11. **________ are called resistance vessels.**

(a) Arteriole
(b) Veins and venules
(c) Capillaries
(d) Large-sized arteries

12. **________ are called capacitance vessels.**

(a) Arteriole
(b) Veins and venules
(c) Capillaries
(d) Large-sized arteries

13. **________ are called exchange vessels.**

(a) Arteriole
(b) Veins and venules
(c) Capillaries
(d) Large-sized arteries

14. **Following are the properties of cardiac muscle except**

(a) Excitability
(b) Conductivity
(c) Autorhythmicity
(d) Irradiation

15. **The cause for depolarization in ventricular muscle action potential is**

(a) Entry of sodium ions
(b) Exit of potassium ions
(c) Entry of calcium ions
(d) Entry of chloride ions

16. **The cause for repolarization in ventricular muscle action potential is**

(a) Entry of sodium ions
(b) Exit of potassium ions
(c) Entry of calcium ions
(d) Entry of chloride ions

17. **Cause for sustained depolarization (plateau) in ventricular muscle action potential is**

(a) Entry of sodium ions

(b) Exit of potassium ions
(c) Entry of calcium ions
(d) Entry of chloride ions

18. The pacemaker of the human heart is

(a) SA node
(b) AV node
(c) Sinus venosus
(d) Bundle of His

19. Conducting system of the heart has the following parts *except*

(a) SA node
(b) AV node
(c) Mossy fibers
(d) Purkinje fibers

20. Velocity of conduction of cardiac impulse is fastest in

(a) Internodal fibers
(b) SA node
(c) Purkinje fibers
(d) Ventricular muscle

21. Long absolute refractory period in a cardiac muscle is useful as

(a) It cannot be tetanized
(b) It improves efficiency
(c) It decreases excitability
(d) It prolongs contraction

22. All-or-none law in a cardiac muscle is applicable to

(a) Single muscle fiber
(b) Both the atria
(c) One ventricle
(d) One atrium

23. Following is not an event in the ventricular systole

(a) Isometric contraction phase
(b) Diastasis
(c) Maximum ejection phase
(d) Reduced ejection phase

24. Following is an event in the ventricular diastole

(a) Isometric contraction phase
(b) Rapid-filling phase
(c) Maximum ejection phase
(d) Reduced ejection phase

25. Following are the events in ventricular diastole *except*

(a) Isovolumetric relaxation phase
(b) First rapid-filling phase
(c) Diastasis
(d) Rapid ejection phase

26. First heart sound is produced due to closure of

(a) Semilunar valves
(b) Mitral valve
(c) Tricuspid valve
(d) Both mitral and tricuspid valves

27. Second heart sound is produced due to the closure of

(a) Semilunar valves
(b) Mitral valve
(c) Tricuspid valve
(d) Atrioventricular valves

28. The heart sound that corresponds with carotid artery pulsation is

(a) First sound
(b) Second sound
(c) Third sound
(d) Fourth sound

29. Stimulation of sympathetic nerve to the heart results in

(a) Increased heart rate
(b) Decrease in the heart rate
(c) Vasodilatation
(d) No change in the heart rate

30. Stimulation of parasympathetic nerve to the heart results in

(a) Increased heart rate
(b) Decrease in the heart rate
(c) Vasoconstriction
(d) No change in the heart rate

31. First heart sound is heard best in

(a) Mitral area
(b) Aortic area
(c) Pulmonary area
(d) All the above areas

32. Second heart sound is heard best in

(a) Mitral area
(b) Tricuspid area

   (c) Pulmonary area
   (d) All the above areas

33. In human heart, right vagus supplies

   (a) SA node
   (b) AV node
   (c) Ventricular musculature
   (d) Purkinje fibers

34. In human heart, left vagus supplies

   (a) Ventricular musculature
   (b) AV node
   (c) SA node
   (d) Purkinje fibers

35. First-degree heart block is detected by

   (a) Increased PR interval
   (b) Inverted T wave
   (c) Elevated ST segment
   (d) Inverted P wave

36. Myocardial infarction is diagnosed by

   (a) Increased PR interval
   (b) Inverted T wave
   (c) Depressed ST segment
   (d) Inverted P wave

37. P wave in ECG is produced due to

   (a) Atrial depolarization
   (b) Ventricular depolarization
   (c) Atrial repolarization
   (d) Ventricular repolarization

38. QRS complex in ECG is produced due to

   (a) Atrial depolarization
   (b) Ventricular depolarization
   (c) Atrial repolarization
   (d) Ventricular repolarization

39. T wave in ECG is produced due to

   (a) Atrial depolarization
   (b) Ventricular depolarization
   (c) Atrial repolarization
   (d) Ventricular repolarization

40. Normal heart rate in humans is

   (a) 40–60 beats/min
   (b) Less than 60 beats/min
   (c) 72–80 beats/min
   (d) More than 90 beats/min

41. Normal systolic blood pressure is

   (a) Less than 90 mm Hg
   (b) 60–90 mm Hg
   (c) 60–160 mm Hg
   (d) 100–140 mm Hg

42. Normal diastolic blood pressure is

   (a) Less than 90 mm Hg
   (b) 60–90 mm Hg
   (c) 60–160 mm Hg
   (d) 100–140 mm Hg

43. Blood pressure depends on the following *except*

   (a) Stroke volume
   (b) Heart rate
   (c) Peripheral resistance
   (d) End systolic volume

44. Marey's law states that

   (a) Heart rate varies directly as blood pressure
   (b) Heart rate varies inversely as blood pressure
   (c) Heart rate and blood pressure do not have any relationship
   (d) Heart rate varies directly as the cardiac output

45. Koratkoff sound is produced due to

   (a) Turbulence to the flow of blood
   (b) Laminar flow of blood
   (c) Closure of AV valves
   (d) Closure of semilunar valve

46. Stimulation of baroreceptor results in

   (a) Increased respiratory rate
   (b) Inhibition of vasomotor center
   (c) Increased heart rate
   (d) Increased peripheral resistance

47. Stimulation of chemoreceptor results in

   (a) Stimulation of vagal nuclei
   (b) Stimulation of vasomotor center
   (c) Decreased heart rate
   (d) Decreased peripheral resistance

48. Normal cardiac output is

   (a) 5–6 mL/min
   (b) 70–80 mL/min
   (c) 5–6 L/min
   (d) 20–30 L/min

49. Normal stroke volume is

(a) 5–6 mL/beat
(b) 70–80 mL/beat
(c) 5–6 L/beat
(d) 20–30 L/beat

50. Cardiac output is measured by the following methods *except*

(a) Dye dilution method
(b) Thermodilution method
(c) Fick's principle
(d) Inulin clearance

51. Ischemia of vasomotor center results in

(a) Decreased heart rate
(b) Decreased blood pressure
(c) Decreased peripheral resistance
(d) Reduced cardiac output

52. Following are not the mechanisms of intermediate-term regulation of blood pressure

(a) Stress relaxation
(b) Fluid shift mechanism
(c) Sinoaortic mechanism
(d) Renin–angiotensin mechanism

53. The mechanism for long-term regulation of blood pressure is

(a) Renin–angiotensin–aldosterone mechanism
(b) Stress relaxation
(c) Fluid shift mechanism
(d) Sinoaortic mechanism

54. Stretch of great vein results in increased heart rate. This relationship is explained by

(a) Bainbrige reflex
(b) Marey's law
(c) Starling's law
(d) Laplace law

55. Stretch of great vein results in

(a) Increased heart rate
(b) Decreased heart rate
(c) Decreased cardiac output
(d) Decreased blood pressure

56. Stimulation of right atrial stretch receptors causes

(a) Increased heart rate

(b) Decreased heart rate
(c) Decreased cardiac output
(d) Decreased blood pressure

57. Stimulation of left atrial stretch receptors causes

(a) Decreased heart rate
(b) Increased heart rate
(c) Increased blood pressure
(d) Increased cardiac output

58. Alteration of heart rate in different phases of respiration is

(a) Tachycardia
(b) Bradycardia
(c) Sinus arrhythmia
(d) Fibrillation

59. Collapsing pulse is pathologically seen in

(a) Exercise
(b) Emotions
(c) Aortic regurgitation
(d) Shock

60. Rolling back of blood in aorta at the beginning of ventricular diastole causes _______ in arterial pulse.

(a) Dicrotic notch
(b) Dicrotic wave
(c) a-wave
(d) c-wave

61. Following are the positive waves in jugular venous pulse *except*

(a) c-wave
(b) a-wave
(c) x-wave
(d) v-wave

62. Dicrotic wave in the arterial pulse tracing is due to

(a) Sudden closure of AV valves
(b) Sudden closure of semilunar valves
(c) Sudden rush of blood
(d) Opening of AV valves

63. Increased intracranial pressure reflexly increases blood pressure acting through vasomotor center. This reflex is

(a) Cushing's reflex
(b) Marey's reflex

   (c) Bainbridge reflex
   (d) Stretch reflex

64. **Increase of blood pressure without a demonstrable cause is**

   (a) Primary hypertension
   (b) Secondary hypertension
   (c) Hypotension
   (d) Orthostatic hypotension

65. **Increase of blood pressure with a demonstrable cause is**

   (a) Primary hypertension
   (b) Secondary hypertension
   (c) Hypotension
   (d) Orthostatic hypotension

66. **Venous return depends on the following factors** *except*

   (a) Respiratory pump
   (b) Muscle pump
   (c) Gravity
   (d) Blood pressure

67. **The law which states greater the preload greater the force of contraction is**

   (a) Starling's law
   (b) Laplace law
   (c) Bell–Magendie law
   (d) Marey's law

68. **The condition of circulatory failure is termed**

   (a) Shock
   (b) Bradycardia
   (c) Tachycardia
   (d) Coma

69. **Excessive bleeding and sudden loss of fluid results in**

   (a) Hypovolemic shock
   (b) Cardiogenic shock
   (c) Septicemic shock
   (d) Anaphylactic shock

70. **The type of shock seen immediately after myocardial infarction is**

   (a) Hypovolemic shock
   (b) Cardiogenic shock
   (c) Septicemic shock
   (d) Anaphylactic shock

71. **The shock produced due to hypersensitivity reaction is**

   (a) Hypovolemic shock
   (b) Cardiogenic shock
   (c) Septicemic shock
   (d) Anaphylactic shock

72. **The shock produced due to uncontrolled and fulminant infection is**

   (a) Hypovolemic shock
   (b) Cardiogenic shock
   (c) Septicemic shock
   (d) Anaphylactic shock

73. **Following are the properties of cardiac muscle** *except*

   (a) Fatigue
   (b) Excitability
   (c) Conductivity
   (d) Contractility

74. **Staircase phenomenon in a cardiac muscle is due to the following** *except*

   (a) Accumulation of calcium ions
   (b) Increased temperature
   (c) Decreased viscosity
   (d) Increased permeability to sodium

75. **All-or-none law is applicable to**

   (a) Single cardiac muscle fiber
   (b) Entire cardiac muscle
   (c) A group of skeletal muscle fibers
   (d) A bundle of nerve fibers

76. **Entire phase of cardiac contraction is in absolute refractory period. Hence, cardiac muscle**

   (a) Can be tetanized
   (b) Cannot be tetanized
   (c) Can be excited
   (d) Cannot be excited

77. **During moderate exercise, the following changes are seen** *except*

   (a) Increased heart rate
   (b) Decreased peripheral resistance
   (c) Increased systolic blood pressure
   (d) Decreased cardiac output

78. **Following are the internodal pathway (conducting system of the heart)** *except*

(a) Wenckebach
(b) Thorel
(c) Bachman
(d) Burdach

79. Irreversible shock results in the following changes *except*

(a) Acidosis
(b) Vasodilation
(c) Toxemia
(d) Increased BP

80. General principle in the management of shock is

(a) Maintenance of fluid and electrolyte balance
(b) Correction of alkalosis
(c) Increasing the cardiac output
(d) Maintenance of oxygen supply

81. Increase in heart rate is termed

(a) Shock
(b) Bradycardia
(c) Tachycardia
(d) Coma

82. Decrease in heart rate is called

(a) Shock
(b) Bradycardia
(c) Tachycardia
(d) Coma

5. Respiratory System

1. The normal respiratory rate is

(a) 6–8 cycles/min
(b) 12–16 cycles/min
(c) 30–40 cycles/min
(d) 72 cycles/min

2. The thickness of respiratory membrane is

(a) $0.6\ \mu$
(b) $2.5\ \mu$
(c) 0.6 mm
(d) 2.5 mm

3. Nonrespiratory function of lungs include all *except*

(a) Synthesis of surfactant
(b) Voice production
(c) Acid–base balance
(d) Gas exchange

4. Normal tidal volume is

(a) 300 mL
(b) 500 mL
(c) 700 mL
(d) 1000 mL

5. Normal inspiratory reserve volume is

(a) 1000 mL
(b) 2000 mL
(c) 3000 mL
(d) 4000 mL

6. Normal residual volume in an adult male is

(a) 500 mL
(b) 1100 mL
(c) 3000 mL
(d) 5600 mL

7. Inspiratory capacity is

(a) TV + IRV
(b) TV + ERV
(c) VC + RV
(d) ERV + RV

8. The amount of air remaining in the lungs after a normal expiration is

(a) Tidal Volume
(b) Functional residual capacity
(c) Vital capacity
(d) Total lung capacity

9. The maximum amount of air that a person can expel from the lungs after a maximum inspiration is called

(a) Functional residual capacity
(b) Tidal volume
(c) Vital capacity
(d) Inspiratory capacity

10. The normal ventilation–perfusion ratio is

(a) 0.2
(b) 0.8
(c) 1.4
(d) 1.6

11. Lung volumes and capacities are measured by

(a) Spirometer
(b) Sphygmomanometer

(c) Stethoscope

(d) None

12. The amount of air expelled forcefully in a given unit of time is termed

(a) Maximum ventilation volume

(b) Respiratory minute volume

(c) Peak respiratory flow rate

(d) Timed vital capacity

13. Normal value of anatomical dead space is

(a) 50 mL

(b) 150 mL

(c) 200 mL

(d) 250 mL

14. That part of respiratory passage in which air does not take part in gaseous exchange process is called

(a) Dead space

(b) Intrapleural space

(c) Alveolar space

(d) Pulmonary space

15. Muscles of inspiration include all *except*

(a) Diaphragm

(b) External intercostals

(c) Sternocleidomastoid

(d) Internal intercostals

16. The muscles of expiration includes

(a) Diaphragm

(b) Abdominal wall muscles

(c) Serratus anterior

(d) Sternocleidomastoid

17. Normal intrapleural pressure is

(a) −11 to −14 cm of water

(b) −5 to −8 cm of water

(c) +3 to +5 cm of water

(d) +7 to +11 cm of water

18. Surfactant is produced by

(a) Enterocytes

(b) Type 2 alveolar cells

(c) Gastric cells

(d) Type 1 alveolar cell

19. Normal FEV1 is around

(a) 63%

(b) 73%

(c) 83%

(d) 93%

20. Normal peak expiratory flow rate is around

(a) 50 L/min

(b) 200 L/min

(c) 400 L/min

(d) 800 L/min

21. The extent to which the lungs expand for each unit increase in transpulmonary pressure is called

(a) Impedance

(b) Compliance

(c) Resistance

(d) Dyspnea

22. Compliance of the respiratory system is

(a) 50 mL/cm of H_2O

(b) 100 mL/cm of H_2O

(c) 150 mL/cm of H_2O

(d) 300 mL/cm of H_2O

23. Production of surfactant starts at

(a) Immediately after conception

(b) Seventh month of fetal life

(c) 6 months after birth

(d) One year after birth

24. Hyaline membrane disease is caused due to the deficiency of

(a) Rennin

(b) Gastrin

(c) Surfactant

(d) CSF

25. The PO_2 of arterial blood is

(a) 40 mm Hg

(b) 45 mm Hg

(c) 95 mm Hg

(d) 104 mm Hg

26. O_2 transported by physical solution is

(a) 3%

(b) 10%

(c) 15%

(d) 23%

27. O_2 dissociation curve shifts to right when there is

(a) Decreased CO_2

(b) Decreased H⁺ ions
(c) Increased 2,3-DPG
(d) Decreased temperature

28. The O₂ dissociation curve is

(a) Straight line
(b) Sigmoid curve
(c) Circular curve
(d) Rhombus shaped

29. Increased CO₂ content of blood helps to release more O₂ from Hb is called

(a) Bohr's effect
(b) Chloride shift
(c) Haldane's effect
(d) Reverse chloride shift

30. Carbon dioxide transport occurs in blood in the form of

(a) Physical solution
(b) Combination with Hb
(c) As bicarbonate
(d) All of the above

31. Most of the CO₂ transport occurs in the blood in the form of

(a) Physical solution
(b) Combination with Hb
(c) As bicarbonate ion
(d) Combination with O₂

32. Dorsal respiratory group of neurons is present in

(a) Medulla
(b) Pons
(c) Hypothalamus
(d) Thalamus

33. Ventral respiratory group of neurons is present in

(a) Medulla
(b) Pons
(c) Hypothalamus
(d) Thalamus

34. Pneumotaxic center is present in

(a) Medulla
(b) Pons
(c) Hypothalamus
(d) Thalamus

35. Apneustic center is present in

(a) Medulla
(b) Pons
(c) Hypothalamus
(d) Thalamus

36. Basic rhythm of respiration is maintained by

(a) VRG
(b) Pneumotaxic center
(c) Apneustic center
(d) DRG

37. Ramp signal is produced by

(a) VRG
(b) Pneumotaxic center
(c) Apneustic center
(d) DRG

38. The chemosensitive area responsible for regulation of respiration is present in

(a) Pons
(b) Medulla
(c) Spinal cord
(d) Thalamus

39. The chemosensitive area for control of respiration is excited by

(a) H⁺ ions
(b) K⁺ ions
(c) Cl⁻ ions
(d) HCO₃⁻ ions

40. Manual methods of artificial respiration include all *except*

(a) Mouth-to-mouth respiration
(b) Schaffer's method
(c) Holger Neilson's method
(d) Drinker's method

41. Temporary arrest of breathing is called

(a) Eupnea
(b) Apnea
(c) Dyspnea
(d) Orthopnea

42. Normal respiration is called

(a) Apnea
(b) Eupnea
(c) Dyspnea
(d) Orthopnea

43. Difficulty in breathing is called
(a) Apnea
(b) Eupnea
(c) Dyspnea
(d) Hiccups

44. Dyspnea occurring in lying-down position and not in erect posture is termed
(a) Eupnea
(b) Apnea
(c) Dyspnea
(d) Orthopnea

45. Periodic breathing characterized by alternate apnea and hyperventilation is termed as
(a) Biot's breathing
(b) Kussmaul breathing
(c) Cheyne–Stokes breathing
(d) Dyspneic breathing

46. Bluish discoloration of skin and mucus membrane is termed
(a) Cyanosis
(b) Anemia
(c) Asphyxia
(d) Dyspnea

47. Condition characterized by decreased O_2 and increased CO_2 in the body is termed
(a) Hypoxia
(b) Asphyxia
(c) Dyspnea
(d) Cyanosis

48. Condition characterized by deficiency of O_2 at the tissue level is termed
(a) Hypoxia
(b) Asphyxia
(c) Dyspnea
(d) Hypercapnia

49. Exposure to high altitude causes
(a) Hypoxic hypoxia
(b) Stagnant hypoxia
(c) Histotoxic hypoxia
(d) Anemic hypoxia

50. Cyanide poisoning is an example of
(a) Hypoxic hypoxia
(b) Stagnant hypoxia
(c) Histotoxic hypoxia
(d) Anemic hypoxia

51. Circulatory shock is an example of
(a) Hypoxic hypoxia
(b) Stagnant hypoxia
(c) Histotoxic hypoxia
(d) Anemic hypoxia

52. The compensatory changes during acclimatization are the following *except*
(a) Hyperventilation
(b) Polycythemia
(c) Decreased cardiac output
(d) Excretion of alkaline urine

53. The gas responsible of the causation of decompression sickness is
(a) Oxygen
(b) Carbon dioxide
(c) Nitrogen
(d) Helium

54. Caisson's disease is seen in
(a) Pilots
(b) Doctors
(c) Divers
(d) Engineers

55. Residual volume can be measured by
(a) Nitrogen washout method
(b) Spirometer
(c) Stethography
(d) Ballistocardiography

56. Functions of the nasal cavity are the following *except*
(a) Humidification
(b) Olfaction
(c) Filtration
(d) Regulation of respiration

57. Increased respiratory rate is termed
(a) Hypoxia
(b) Hyperventilation
(c) Tachypnea
(d) Tachycardia

58. Increased rate and depth of respiration is
(a) Hyperventilation
(b) Tachypnea
(c) Dyspnea
(d) Asphyxia

59. Influence of carbon dioxide on the release and uptake of oxygen is

(a) Bohr's effect
(b) Haldane's effect
(c) Venturi effect
(d) Windkessel effect

60. Influence of oxygen on the release of uptake of carbon dioxide is

(a) Haldane's effect
(b) Venturi effect
(c) Bohr's effect
(d) Windkessel effect

61. Carbon dioxide is carried in the following form *except*

(a) Bicarbonates
(b) Carbamino compounds
(c) Simple solution
(d) Carboxyhemoglobin

6. Gastrointestinal System

1. Myentric plexus of Auerbach is present between

(a) Serosal and mucosal layers
(b) Circular muscle and submucosal layers
(c) Longitudinal and circular muscle layers
(d) In the mucosa

2. Submucosal plexus of Meissner is present in between

(a) Serosal and mucosal layers
(b) Circular muscle and submucosal layers
(c) Longitudinal and circular muscle layers
(d) In the mucosa

3. Slow waves

(a) Are action potentials
(b) Are caused due to calcium pump
(c) Cause muscle contraction
(d) Control the appearance of spike potentials

4. All of the following regarding spike potentials are true *except*

(a) They are true action potentials
(b) They occur due to slow undulation of Na^+–K^+ pump
(c) They last for 10–20 ms

(d) Higher the spike potential, greater its frequency

5. Stages of deglutition include all *except*

(a) Buccal phase
(b) Pharyngeal phase
(c) Esophageal phase
(d) Intestinal phase

6. Interruption of respiration during swallowing is called

(a) Deglutition apnea
(b) Sleep apnea
(c) Hyperpnea
(d) Dyspnea

7. Deglutition center is present in

(a) Lower pons and upper medulla
(b) Upper pons
(c) Midbrain
(d) Hypothalamus

8. Condition in which lower esophageal sphincter fails to relax is during

(a) Gastritis
(b) Achalasia cardia
(c) Esophagitis
(d) Peptic ulcer

9. Factor that increases gastric emptying is

(a) Gastrin
(b) CCK
(c) Secretin
(d) Products of digestion

10. Haustrations are found in

(a) Esophagus
(b) Stomach
(c) Small intestine
(d) Large intestine

11. Salivary glands include all *except*

(a) Submandibular
(b) Sublingual
(c) Parotid
(d) Oxyntic

12. Secretions from parotid glands are predominantly

(a) Serous
(b) Mucus

   (c) Mixed
   (d) None of the above

13. Parotid glands open through

   (a) Wharton's duct
   (b) Stenson's duct
   (c) Pancreatic duct
   (d) Duct of Rivinus

14. Submandibular salivary glands open through

   (a) Wharton's duct
   (b) Stenson's duct
   (c) Pancreatic duct
   (d) Duct of Rivinus

15. Sublingual glands open through

   (a) Wharton's duct
   (b) Stenson's duct
   (c) Pancreatic duct
   (d) Duct of Rivinus

16. Daily salivary secretion is about

   (a) 500 mL
   (b) 750 mL
   (c) 1200 mL
   (d) 2500 mL

17. The functions of saliva include

   (a) Lubrication of food
   (b) Keeps the mouth moist
   (c) Digestion of starch
   (d) All of the above

18. Involuntary phase of deglutition is

   (a) Buccal phase
   (b) Pharyngeal phase
   (c) Esophageal phase
   (d) None of the above

19. Factors inhibiting gastric emptying include

   (a) Gastrin
   (b) Increased food volume
   (c) Parasympathetic activity
   (d) CCK

20. Ptyalin is an enzyme present mainly in

   (a) Saliva
   (b) Gastric juice
   (c) Pancreatic juice
   (d) Bile

21. Decreased salivation occurs due to

   (a) Parasympathetic stimulation
   (b) Eating favorite foods
   (c) Atropine administration
   (d) Presence of irritating food in stomach

22. Mumps affects

   (a) Submaxillary glands
   (b) Parotid glands
   (c) Gastric glands
   (d) Intestinal glands

23. Reduced salivary secretion leads to

   (a) Xerophthalmia
   (b) Xerostomia
   (c) Parosmia
   (d) Ageusia

24. Chief cells secrete

   (a) HCl
   (b) Mucus
   (c) Pepsinogen
   (d) Intrinsic factor

25. Parietal cells secrete

   (a) HCl
   (b) Intrinsic factor
   (c) HCl and intrinsic factor
   (d) Secretin

26. Intrinsic factor is required for the absorption of

   (a) Vitamin C
   (b) Vitamin A
   (c) Vitamin B_1
   (d) Vitamin B_{12}

27. Gastrin is produced from

   (a) Mucus cells
   (b) Parietal cells
   (c) Peptic cells
   (d) G-cells

28. Gastrin

   (a) Is an enzyme
   (b) Is produced from parietal cells
   (c) Inhibits gastric secretion
   (d) Is a polypeptide

29. Cephalic phase of gastric secretion

   (a) Occurs before the food enters the stomach

(b) Accounts for 20% of gastric secretion

(c) Occurs due to sight, smell, and thought of food

(d) All of the above

30. **Hormone responsible for gastric phase of gastric secretion is**

(a) Gastrin

(b) CCK–PZ

(c) Secretin

(d) VIP

31. **Phases of gastric secretion include all *except***

(a) Cephalic phase

(b) Gastric phase

(c) Pharyngeal phase

(d) Intestinal phase

32. **Gastric secretion is inhibited by**

(a) Gastrin

(b) Secretin

(c) Histamine

(d) Products of protein digestion

33. **Sham feeding experiment proves the**

(a) Cephalic phase of gastric secretion

(b) Gastric phase

(c) Intestinal phase

(d) Interdigestive phase

34. **Volume of gastric secretion produced per day is**

(a) 500 mL

(b) 1200 mL

(c) 2500 mL

(d) 4000 mL

35. **Gastric juice is**

(a) Highly acidic

(b) Mildly acidic

(c) Highly alkaline

(d) Mildly alkaline

36. **Functions of gastric juice include**

(a) Digestion of proteins

(b) Bacteriolytic action

(c) Excretion of toxins and heavy metals

(d) All of the above

37. **Normal basal acid output is**

(a) 0.5–2 mEq/h

(b) 3.5–6 mEq/h

(c) 5–8 mEq/h

(d) 17–35 mEq/h

38. **Peak acid can be measured by all *except***

(a) Histamine test

(b) Pentagastrin test

(c) Insulin test

(d) Glucose tolerance test

39. **Basal acid output decreases in**

(a) Zollinger–Ellison syndrome

(b) Duodenal ulcer

(c) Atrophic gastritis

(d) Acute gastritis due to drugs

40. **Peptic ulcer is caused due to infection of**

(a) *Helicobacter pylori*

(b) *Pneumocystis carini*

(c) *Staphylococcus*

(d) *H. influenza*

41. **Normal bile secretion in a day is**

(a) 500 mL

(b) 1500 mL

(c) 2000 mL

(d) 2500 mL

42. **Liver weighs around**

(a) 500 g

(b) 750 g

(c) 1500 g

(d) 2500 g

43. **Secretions of liver and bile enter the duodenum through**

(a) Hepatic duct

(b) Cystic duct

(c) Common bile duct

(d) Intralobular duct

44. **Kupffer cells are**

(a) Present in the liver

(b) Protective in function

(c) Modified macrophages

(d) All of the above

45. **pH of bile is**

(a) 1.2–1.5

(b) 3.5–4

(c) 7–7.5

(d) 9.5–10

46. Bilirubin is a

(a) Bile salt
(b) Bile pigment
(c) Bile acid
(d) None of the above

47. Bile is produced in the

(a) Liver
(b) Gallbladder
(c) Spleen
(d) Pancreas

48. The capacity of gallbladder is around

(a) 50 mL
(b) 150 mL
(c) 250 mL
(d) 500 mL

49. The main stimulus for contraction of gallbladder is

(a) Gastrin
(b) Secretin
(c) Cholecystokinin
(d) Thyroxine

50. Sodium taurocholate is a

(a) Bile salt
(b) Bile pigment
(c) Bile acid
(d) None of the above

51. The percentage of bile salts reabsorbed by small intestine is about

(a) 30
(b) 50
(c) 70
(d) 90

52. The substances that increase bile secretion are called

(a) Cholagogues
(b) Choleretics
(c) Secretogogues
(d) Cholic acid

53. Cholecystectomy is removal of

(a) Liver
(b) Gallbladder
(c) Spleen
(d) Pancreas

54. Cholelithiasis is presence of stones in

(a) Salivary gland
(b) Gallbladder
(c) Kidney
(d) Pancreas

55. Excessive breakdown of RBC leads to

(a) Prehepatic jaundice
(b) Hepatic jaundice
(c) Posthepatic jaundice
(d) None of the above

56. Stones in the gallbladder lead to

(a) Prehepatic jaundice
(b) Hemolytic jaundice
(c) Obstructive jaundice
(d) Hepatic jaundice

57. Physiological jaundice is

(a) Seen in newborn babies
(b) Self-limiting condition requiring no treatment
(c) Both a and b are true
(d) Neither a or b is true

58. Normal serum bilirubin is

(a) 0.1–0.3 mg%
(b) 0.2–0.8 mg%
(c) 1–3 mg%
(d) 2–8 mg%

59. The enzyme markedly increased in obstructive jaundice is

(a) SGOT
(b) SGPT
(c) CCK–MB
(d) Alkaline phosphatase

60. pH of pancreatic juice is

(a) 1.2–2
(b) 3–4.5
(c) 6–7.4
(d) 8–8.3

61. Steatorrhea occurs due to the deficiency of

(a) Gastric enzymes
(b) Saliva
(c) Pancreatic enzymes
(d) Succus entericus

62. Intestinal phase of pancreatic secretion is due to hormone

(a) Gastrin
(b) Motilin
(c) GIP
(d) CCK

63. Amylase is a

(a) Proteolytic enzyme
(b) Fat-splitting enzyme
(c) Carbohydrate-splitting enzyme
(d) None of the above

64. Trypsin helps in the digestion of

(a) Proteins
(b) Carbohydrates
(c) Fats
(d) Minerals

65. Lipase helps in the digestion of

(a) Proteins
(b) Carbohydrates
(c) Fats
(d) Minerals

66. Mucus produced in large intestine causes all *except*

(a) Protects the wall against excoriation
(b) Digestion and absorption of proteins
(c) Adherent medium for holding fecal matter together
(d) Protects intestinal wall from bacterial activity

67. Vomiting center is present in the

(a) Medulla
(b) Pons
(c) Midbrain
(d) Cortex

68. Mass peristalsis usually occurs in

(a) Esophagus
(b) Stomach
(c) Small intestine
(d) Large intestine

69. All the following are functions of gastrin *except*

(a) Stimulation of gastric acid secretion
(b) Stimulation of mucosal growth of stomach
(c) Causes contraction of gastroesophageal sphincter
(d) Inhibits gastric motility

70. CCK–PZ is produced from

(a) G-cells of gastric gland
(b) I-cells of small intestine
(c) D-cells of pancreas
(d) Hepatocytes of liver

71. CCK–PZ causes

(a) Relaxation of gallbladder
(b) Inhibition of pancreatic secretion
(c) Enhance motility of small intestine
(d) Decreases intestinal secretion

72. The first hormone to be discovered was

(a) Gastrin
(b) CCK–PZ
(c) Motilin
(d) Secretin

73. Somatostatin

(a) Increases gastric secretion
(b) Increases gallbladder contraction
(c) Inhibits secretion of secretin
(d) Increases secretion of exocrine pancreas

74. Gastrointestinal hormones include all *except*

(a) Gastrin
(b) Trypsin
(c) CCK–PZ
(d) Secretin

75. Somatostatin is produced from

(a) Pancreas
(b) Gastrointestinal mucosa
(c) Hypothalamus
(d) All of the above

76. Secretin is produced from

(a) Liver
(b) Spleen
(c) Small intestine
(d) Stomach

77. Pancreatic juice mainly contains

(a) Bicarbonate ions
(b) Calcium ions
(c) Chloride ions
(d) Sodium ions

78. Cholecystography involves visualization of

(a) Ureter
(b) Gallbladder

(c) Intestine

(d) Esophagus

79. Micelles are produced due to the formation of complexes of bile salts with

(a) Proteins

(b) Carbohydrates

(c) Lipids

(d) Vitamins

80. Peptic ulcer is caused due to

(a) Anti-inflammatory drugs

(b) Alcohol

(c) Smoking

(d) All of the above

81. Hormonal control of gastric secretion can be studied by

(a) Pavlov's pouch

(b) Heidenhain's pouch

(c) Sham feeding

(d) All of the above

82. Parasympathetic supply to GIT is mainly through

(a) Glossopharyngeal nerve

(b) Vagus nerve

(c) Facial nerve

(d) Trigeminal nerve

83. Muscles of mastication are innervated by

(a) Hypoglossal nerve

(b) Trigeminal nerve

(c) Glossopharyngeal nerve

(d) Facial nerve

84. Gastric phase accounts for

(a) 20% of gastric secretion

(b) 30% of gastric secretion

(c) 70% of gastric secretion

(d) 90% of gastric secretion

85. Normal peak acid output secretion is

(a) 0.5–2 mEq/h

(b) 10–15 mEq/h

(c) 15–20 mEq/h

(d) 40–60 mEq/h

86. Pavlov's experiment was done to study

(a) Salivary secretion

(b) Gastric secretion

(c) Intestinal secretion

(d) Pancreatic secretion

87. The pH of gastric juice is

(a) 1–2

(b) 5–6

(c) 6.5–7

(d) 7–8

7. Excretory System

1. The functioning unit of the kidney is

(a) Neuron

(b) Nephron

(c) Sarcomere

(d) Juxtaglomerular apparatus

2. The following are the parts of nephron *except*

(a) Bowman's capsule

(b) Loop of Henle

(c) Distal convoluted tubule

(d) Vasa recta

3. The process of concentrating urine is the main function of

(a) Cortical nephron

(b) Descending loop of Henle

(c) Juxtamedullary nephron

(d) Collecting duct

4. Urine is formed by the following processes *except*

(a) Ultrafiltration

(b) Tubular reabsorption

(c) Tubular secretion

(d) Micturition

5. The effective filtration pressure depends on the following pressures *except*

(a) Hydrostatic pressure

(b) Bowman's capsular pressure

(c) Interstitial pressure

(d) Colloidal osmotic pressure

6. The normal renal blood flow is

(a) 125 mL/min

(b) 650 mL/min

(c) 700 mL/h

(d) 1200 mL/min

7. The normal GFR is

(a) 125 mL/h
(b) 125 mL/day
(c) 125 L/min
(d) 125 L/day

8. The substance used for the estimation of GFR is

(a) Insulin
(b) Inulin
(c) Renin
(d) Rennin

9. The normal filtration fraction is

(a) 20%
(b) 30%
(c) 60%
(d) 75%

10. The substance used to estimate GFR should have the following properties *except*

(a) Nontoxic
(b) Easily filtered
(c) Should not alter renal function
(d) Should be secreted

11. Renal threshold for glucose is

(a) 180 mg/dL
(b) 325 mg/dL
(c) 180 mg/min
(d) 375 mg/min

12. Tubular maximum for glucose is

(a) 180 mg/min
(b) 375 mg/min
(c) 180 g/min
(d) 325 g/min

13. Following are the abnormal constituents of urine *except*

(a) Blood
(b) Urea
(c) Bile
(d) Ketone bodies

14. Following is an abnormal constituent of urine

(a) Urea
(b) Uric acid
(c) Creatinine
(d) Proteins

15. The facultative reabsorption of water takes place in

(a) PCT
(b) DCT
(c) Loop of Henle
(d) Bowman's capsule

16. The facultative reabsorption of water takes place under the influence of hormone

(a) Vasopressin
(b) Oxytocin
(c) Aldosterone
(d) Renin

17. The hormone produced from the kidney is

(a) Gastrin
(b) Erythropoietin
(c) Aldosterone
(d) ADH

18. The hormone acting on the kidney is

(a) Aldosterone
(b) Thyroxin
(c) Secretin
(d) Erythropoietin

19. The sodium ion is absorbed in the renal tubules by the following mechanism *except*

(a) Cotransport
(b) Countertransport
(c) Active–passive transport
(d) Osmosis

20. Stimulation of sympathetic nerve to the bladder results in

(a) Atonic bladder
(b) Emptying of the bladder
(c) Automatic bladder
(d) Alteration of blood flow

21. Stimulation of parasympathetic nerve to the urinary bladder results in

(a) Atonic bladder
(b) Emptying of the bladder
(c) Automatic bladder
(d) Filling of the bladder

22. Cystometrogram is

(a) Pressure–volume relationship of urinary bladder
(b) Measure of intravesical pressure

   (c) Measure of intravesical volume

   (d) None of the above

23. The normal maximal urea clearance is

   (a) 75 mg/day

   (b) 75 mL/h

   (c) 75 mg/min

   (d) 75 mL/min

24. The patient with diabetes mellitus will have

   (a) Osmotic diuresis

   (b) Water diuresis

   (c) No diuresis

   (d) Voluntary diuresis

25. Water diuresis is a feature of

   (a) Diabetes mellitus

   (b) Diabetes insipidus

   (c) Acromegaly

   (d) Cushing's syndrome

26. Normal renal plasma flow is

   (a) 70–80 mL/min

   (b) 125 mL/min

   (c) 650 mL/min

   (d) 1200 mL/min

27. The normal standard urea clearance is

   (a) 54 mL/h

   (b) 75 mL/h

   (c) 54 mL/min

   (d) 75 mL/min

28. Following are the excretory organs of the body *except*

   (a) Skin

   (b) Kidney

   (c) GIT

   (d) Spleen

29. The maintenance of constancy of interval environment is

   (a) Homeostasis

   (b) Hemostasis

   (c) Adaptation

   (d) Acclimatization

30. The chemical agents increasing urination are called

   (a) Anesthetics

   (b) Antidiuretics

   (c) Cathartics

   (d) Diuretics

31. Following are the functions of the kidney *except*

   (a) Secretion of renin

   (b) Acid–base balance

   (c) Fluid balance

   (d) Glycogen storage

32. Ureter is the continuation of

   (a) Pelvis

   (b) Pyramid

   (c) Cortex

   (d) Bowman's capsule

33. Urethra is the continuation of

   (a) Pelvis

   (b) Pyramid

   (c) Urinary bladder

   (d) Bowman's capsule

34. Urine is temporarily stored in

   (a) Gallbladder

   (b) Urinary bladder

   (c) Kidney

   (d) Nephrons

35. The efferent arteriole of cortical nephron divides into capillary network to form

   (a) Vasa recta

   (b) Peritubular capillary

   (c) Glomerulus

   (d) Renal vein

36. The efferent arteriole of juxtamedullary nephron divides into capillary network to form

   (a) Vasa recta

   (b) Peritubular capillary

   (c) Glomerulus

   (d) Renal vein

37. ________ constitutes the countercurrent exchange system.

   (a) Nephron

   (b) Vasa recta

   (c) Peritubular capillary

   (d) Glomerulus

38. _______ constitutes the countercurrent multiplier system.

(a) Loop of Henle
(b) Vasa recta
(c) Peritubular capillary
(d) Glomerulus

39. **Theories of autoregulation are the following** *except*

(a) Myogenic theory
(b) Interstitial tissue pressure theory
(c) Metabolite theory
(d) Traveling wave theory

40. **The process of autoregulation is explained on the basis of**

(a) Myogenic theory
(b) Traveling wave theory
(c) Kinetic theory
(d) None of the above

41. **Ability of an organ to maintain a constant flow of blood in spite of a variation in the arterial blood pressure is called**

(a) Autoregulation
(b) Acclimatization
(c) Feedback mechanism
(d) Autorhythmicity

42. **Each kidney has about _______ nephrons.**

(a) One lakh
(b) One million
(c) Two million
(d) One billion

43. **The percentage distribution of cortical nephron is**

(a) 15
(b) 35
(c) 55
(d) 85

44. **The percentage distribution of juxtamedullary nephron is**

(a) 15
(b) 35
(c) 55
(d) 85

45. **Juxtaglomerular apparatus secretes**

(a) Renin

(b) Erythropoietin
(c) Rennin
(d) Aldosterone

46. **Juxtaglomerular apparatus consists of the following** *except*

(a) Macula densa
(b) Juxtaglomerular cells
(c) Lacis cells
(d) Glial cells

47. **Normal urine output is**

(a) 1.5–2 L/day
(b) 5–6 L/day
(c) 10–20 mL/min
(d) 125 mL/min

48. **The proteins responsible for absorption of water in the kidney is**

(a) Sialoprotein
(b) Aquaporin
(c) Calmodulin
(d) Receptor proteins

49. **PAH clearance is used to estimate**

(a) Renal blood flow
(b) Renal plasma flow
(c) GFR
(d) Filtration fraction

50. **The filtration membrane consists of the following** *except*

(a) Endothelium of glomerular capillary
(b) Epithelial lining of Bowman's capsule
(c) Interstitium
(d) Juxtaglomerular cells

51. **Glucose is reabsorbed from the PCT by the following transport mechanism**

(a) Antiport
(b) Symport
(c) Uniport
(d) Osmosis

52. **Inability of the kidney to respond to ADH results in**

(a) Nephrogenic diabetes
(b) Renal glycosuria
(c) Diabetes insipidus
(d) Diabetes mellitus

53. The substances secreted from DCT are the following *except*

(a) Hydrogen ions
(b) Ammonia
(c) Potassium ions
(d) Calcium ions

54. External sphincter to the urinary bladder is supplied by

(a) Pudendal nerve
(b) Hypogastric nerve
(c) Sympathetic nerve
(d) Parasympathetic nerve

8. Central Nervous System

1. Structural and functional unit of nervous system is

(a) Neuron
(b) Nephron
(c) Neuroglia
(d) Giant cell

2. The short branching process of a neuron is

(a) Axon
(b) Dendrite
(c) Climbing fiber
(d) Mossy fiber

3. The process that carries sensation away from the cell body is

(a) Axon
(b) Dendrite
(c) Climbing fiber
(d) Mossy fiber

4. The process which carries sensation toward the cell body

(a) Axon
(b) Dendrite
(c) Climbing fiber
(d) Mossy fiber

5. The neurons classified based on the number of processes are the following *except*

(a) Unipolar
(b) Bipolar
(c) Apolar
(d) Polar

6. Nissl granules are found in neuron *except* in

(a) Cell body
(b) Axon hillock
(c) Cytoplasm
(d) Endoplasmic reticulum

7. Nissl granules are also called

(a) Tigroid bodies
(b) Carotid body
(c) Neuroglia
(d) Betz cells

8. Disappearance of Nissl granules during nerve injury is termed

(a) Chromatolysis
(b) Autolysis
(c) Hemolysis
(d) Proteolysis

9. Basement membrane of cell of Schwann is

(a) Myelin sheath
(b) Neurilemma
(c) Descemet's membrane
(d) Outer limiting membrane

10. The process of formation of myelin sheath is

(a) Myelinogenesis
(b) Neurogenesis
(c) Dysgenesis
(d) Agenesis

11. The process of degeneration of peripheral nerve distal to the site of injury is termed

(a) Starling's degeneration
(b) Marey's degeneration
(c) Wallerian degeneration
(d) Brodmann's degeneration

12. The junction between two neurons is

(a) Soma
(b) Synapse
(c) Telodendria
(d) Reflex

13. Following are the parts of chemical synapse *except*

(a) Presynaptic terminal
(b) Synaptic cleft
(c) Postsynaptic terminal
(d) Motor end plate

14. Gap junctions are present in _______ synapse.

(a) Chemical
(b) Electrical
(c) Axoaxonic
(d) Axosomatic

15. Ionic basis for EPSP is

(a) Entry of Na^+ ions
(b) Exit of Na^+ ions
(c) Entry of Cl^- ions
(d) Exit of Cl^- ions

16. Ionic basis for IPSP is

(a) Entry of Na^+ ions
(b) Exit of Na^+ ions
(c) Entry of Cl^- ions
(d) Exit of Cl^- ions

17. The types of synaptic inhibitions are the following *except*

(a) Post synaptic
(b) Presynaptic
(c) Negative feed back
(d) Positive feed back

18. Following are the properties of synapse *except*

(a) Delay
(b) Summation
(c) Regeneration
(d) Occlusion

19. The excitatory neurotransmitter is

(a) GABA
(b) Glycine
(c) Dopamine
(d) Epinephrine

20. Following are excitatory neurotransmitter *except*

(a) Acetylcholine
(b) Epinephrine
(c) Histamine
(d) GABA

21. An example of inhibitory neurotransmitter is

(a) Acetylcholine
(b) Epinephrine
(c) Histamine
(d) GABA

22. Following are the inhibitory neuro-transmitters *except*

(a) GABA
(b) Glycine
(c) Dopamine
(d) Epinephrine

23. The normal synaptic delay is

(a) 0.5 ms
(b) 5 ms
(c) 0.5 s
(d) 5 s

24. Addition of two stimuli given in relation to time is

(a) Temporal summation
(b) Spatial summation
(c) Quantal summation
(d) Wave summation

25. Addition of two stimuli given in relation to space is

(a) Temporal summation
(b) Spatial summation
(c) Quantal summation
(d) Wave summation

26. Following are the components of reflex arc *except*

(a) Receptor
(b) Center
(c) Effector organ
(d) Astrocyte

27. Stretch reflex is an example of _______ type of reflex.

(a) Monosynaptic
(b) Polysynaptic
(c) Bisynaptic
(d) Asynaptic

28. Withdrawal reflex is an example of _______ type of reflex.

(a) Monosynaptic
(b) Polysynaptic
(c) Bisynaptic
(d) Asynaptic

29. Axon reflex is an example of _______ type of reflex.

(a) Monosynaptic
(b) Polysynaptic

(c) Bisynaptic

(d) Asynaptic

30. The receptor for stretch reflex is

(a) Muscle spindle

(b) Golgi tendon organ

(c) Pacinian corpuscles

(d) Ruffini's end organ

31. The receptor for inverse stretch reflex is

(a) Muscle spindle

(b) Golgi tendon organ

(c) Pacinian corpuscles

(d) Ruffini's end organ

32. Inverse stretch reflex is also termed

(a) Autogenic inhibition

(b) Renshaw's cell inhibition

(c) Postsynaptic inhibition

(d) Presynaptic inhibition

33. Crossed extensor response is due to the property of

(a) Summation

(b) Occlusion

(c) Irradiation

(d) Sensitization

34. In decerebrate rigidity, the lesion is made at

(a) Midcollicular level

(b) Cerebral cortex

(c) Medulla

(d) Cerebellum

35. The structure in the ear responsible for maintenance of balance is

(a) Cochlea

(b) Cerebellum

(c) Vestibular apparatus

(d) Incus

36. Semicircular canals help in the detection of _____ movement.

(a) Rotatory

(b) Side-to-side

(c) Anteroposterior

(d) Oblique

37. Utricles help in the detection of _____ movement.

(a) Rotatory

(b) Side-to-side

(c) Anteroposterior

(d) Oblique

38. Saccules help in the detection of _____ movement.

(a) Rotatory

(b) Side-to-side

(c) Anteroposterior

(d) Oblique

39. The receptors in the semicircular canals are

(a) Crista ampullaris

(b) Macula

(c) Organ of Corti

(d) Otolith

40. The receptors in the utricle and saccule are

(a) Crista ampullaris

(b) Macula

(c) Organ of Corti

(d) Otolith

41. The otolith organs comprise

(a) Utricle

(b) Cochlea

(c) Scala media

(d) Helicotrema

42. Inborn reflex is called _____ reflex.

(a) Conditioned

(b) Unconditioned

(c) Superficial

(d) Polysynaptic

43. Following are the properties of the reflex *except*

(a) Summation

(b) Habituation

(c) Specificity

(d) Irradiation

44. The reflex acquired by experience is

(a) Conditioned

(b) Unconditioned

(c) Superficial

(d) Polysynaptic

45. Phantom limb is an example of the following property of sensation

(a) Doctrine of specific nerve energy

(b) Law of projection

(c) Intensity discrimination

(d) Adaptation

46. **Weber–Fechner law explains the following property of the receptor**

(a) Doctrine of specific nerve energy

(b) Law of projection

(c) Intensity discrimination

(d) Adaptation

47. **A low-intensity stimuli given for a prolonged period results in**

(a) Habituation

(b) Specificity

(c) Sensitization

(d) Summation

48. **Painful stimuli given to animal results in**

(a) Habituation

(b) Specificity

(c) Sensitization

(d) Summation

49. **Following is a rapidly adapting receptor**

(a) Touch

(b) Pain

(c) Temperature

(d) Pressure

50. **Following is a slowly adapting receptor**

(a) Touch

(b) Pain

(c) Temperature

(d) Pressure

51. **The perception of pain in the region of skin away from the site of its production internally is**

(a) Referred pain

(b) Visceral pain

(c) Somatic pain

(d) Slow pain

52. **The pain due to the inflammation of appendix felt around the umbilicus is an example for**

(a) Referred pain

(b) Visceral pain

(c) Somatic pain

(d) Slow pain

53. **Following are the endogenous opioids *except***

(a) Pethedine

(b) Enkephalin

(c) Endorphin

(d) Dynorphin

54. **Temporary cessation of function of the nerve due to its compression is**

(a) Neuropraxia

(b) Axonotmesis

(c) Neurotmesis

(d) Chromatolysis

55. **Crush injury to a nerve with intact endoneural tube results in**

(a) Neuropraxia

(b) Axonotmesis

(c) Neurotmesis

(d) Chromatolysis

56. **Complete disruption of nerve trunk due to injury results in**

(a) Neuropraxia

(b) Axonotmesis

(c) Neurotmesis

(d) Chromatolysis

57. **Maximum conduction velocity of Aα nerve fiber is**

(a) 120 ft/min

(b) 120 m/min

(c) 120 ft/s

(d) 120 m/s

58. **Following properties are true for receptor potential *except***

(a) It is graded

(b) Nonpropagated

(c) Has no latency

(d) Shows all-or-none response

59. **Following are the parts of muscle spindle *except***

(a) Nuclear bag fibers

(b) Nuclear chain fibers

(c) Annulospiral ending

(d) Mossy fibers

60. **Contraction of one group of muscle leads to relaxation of antagonistic group of muscle is an example for**
    (a) Postsynaptic inhibition
    (b) Presynaptic inhibition
    (c) Crossed extensor response
    (d) Negative feedback inhibition

61. **Painful stimuli given to animal results in _______ reflex.**
    (a) Axon reflex
    (b) Stretch reflex
    (c) Withdrawal reflex
    (d) Postural reflex

62. **Somatosensory cortex corresponds to Brodmann area number**
    (a) 3, 1, 2
    (b) 4, 6
    (c) 8
    (d) 17

63. **Primary motor cortex corresponds to Brodmann area number**
    (a) 3, 1, 2
    (b) 4, 6
    (c) 8
    (d) 17

64. **Premotor cortex corresponds to Brodmann area number**
    (a) 3, 1, 2
    (b) 4, 6
    (c) 8
    (d) 5, 7

65. **Primary visual area corresponds to Brodmann area number**
    (a) 3, 1, 2
    (b) 4, 6
    (c) 8
    (d) 17

66. **Visual association area corresponds to Brodmann area number**
    (a) 3, 1, 2
    (b) 4, 6
    (c) 18, 19
    (d) 17

67. **Primary auditory area corresponds to Brodmann area number**
    (a) 3, 1, 2
    (b) 4, 6
    (c) 18, 19
    (d) 41, 42

68. **Audiopsychic area corresponds to Brodmann area number**
    (a) 3, 1, 2
    (b) 4, 6
    (c) 18, 19
    (d) 22

69. **Frontal eye field corresponds to Brodmann area number**
    (a) 3, 1, 2
    (b) 4, 6
    (c) 8
    (d) 18, 19

70. **Wernicke's area corresponds to Brodmann area number**
    (a) 3, 1, 2
    (b) 4, 6
    (c) 18, 19
    (d) 22

71. **Broca's speech area corresponds to Brodmann area number**
    (a) 3, 1, 2
    (b) 4, 6
    (c) 18, 19
    (d) 44

72. **In spinal cord, the dorsal root is sensory and ventral root is motor. The law which states arrangement is**
    (a) Laplace law
    (b) Bell–Magendie law
    (c) Marey's law
    (d) Weber–Fechner law

73. **Dorsal column tracts carry the following sensations *except***
    (a) Pain
    (b) Touch
    (c) Pressure
    (d) Vibration

74. Anterolateral tracts carry the following sensations *except*

(a) Pain
(b) Temperature
(c) Crude touch
(d) Proprioception

75. Following are the ascending tracts *except*

(a) Pyramidal tract
(b) Spinotectal
(c) Spino-olivary
(d) Spinothalamic

76. Following are the descending tracts *except*

(a) Spinocerebellar
(b) Rubrospinal
(c) Tectospinal
(d) Corticospinal

77. Following are the extrapyramidal tracts *except*

(a) Vestibulospinal
(b) Rubrospinal
(c) Tectospinal
(d) Corticospinal

78. Features of the upper motor neuron lesion are the following *except*

(a) Rigidity in the muscle
(b) Loss of superficial reflexes
(c) Exaggerated deep reflexes
(d) Negative Babinski's sign

79. Features of the lower motor neuron lesion are the following *except*

(a) Flaccidity of the muscles
(b) Loss of superficial reflexes
(c) Exaggerated deep reflexes
(d) Muscle wasting

80. Dorsiflexion of the great toe and fanning of the other toes when the sole of foot is scratched indicates

(a) Positive Babinski's sign
(b) Normal plantar reflex
(c) Negative Babinski's sign
(d) Exaggerated deep reflex

81. Positive Babinski's sign is seen in the following conditions *except*

(a) Upper motor neuron lesion
(b) During deep sleep
(c) Infant below the age of 18 months
(d) Lower motor neuron lesion

82. In the hemisection of spinal cord, the following statement is not true

(a) Loss of all sensation on the same side below the level of lesion
(b) Loss of pain on the opposite side below the level of lesion
(c) Loss of fine touch on the same side below the level of lesion
(d) Loss of all sensation on the same side at the level of lesion

83. Theories of referred pain are the following *except*

(a) Dermatomal rule
(b) Convergence theory
(c) Facilitation theory
(d) Myogenic theory

84. Fast pain is carried by

(a) Aα fiber
(b) Aδ fiber
(c) B fiber
(d) C fiber

85. Slow pain is carried by

(a) Aα fiber
(b) B fiber
(c) C fiber
(d) Aδ fiber

86. Endogenous opioid analgesic pathway passes through the following parts *except*

(a) Magnus raphe nucleus
(b) Periaqueductal gray matter
(c) Hypothalamus
(d) Substantia gelatinosa of Rolando

87. Ability to identify the object by touching utilizing the past experience is termed

(a) Stereognosis
(b) Barognosis
(c) Astereognosis
(d) Graphesthesia

88. The tract which carries proprioceptive sensation is

(a) Spinotectal

(b) Corticospinal
(c) Spinocerebellar
(d) Tectospinal

89. **The example of synthetic sensation is**

(a) Touch
(b) Pain
(c) Vibration
(d) Temperature

90. **Hemiplegia is produced when the corticospinal tract is damaged at the level of**

(a) Pons
(b) Midbrain
(c) Medulla
(d) Internal capsule

91. **Majority of the fibers of the pyramidal tract cross to the opposite side at the lower border of**

(a) Pons
(b) Midbrain
(c) Medulla
(d) Internal capsule

92. **The condition of the patient with complete transection of spinal cord is explained under the following stages** *except*

(a) Spinal shock
(b) Recovery
(c) Reflex failure
(d) Paralysis

93. **Functional divisions of the cerebellum are the following** *except*

(a) Archicerebellum
(b) Vestibulocerebellum
(c) Spinocerebellum
(d) Cerebrocerebellum

94. **The nuclei of the cerebellum are the following** *except*

(a) Dentatus
(b) Globosus
(c) Emboliformis
(d) Striatum

95. **The function of cerebellum is**

(a) To maintain tone, posture, and equilibrium

(b) Control voluntary activity
(c) Relay different sensations
(d) Regulate body temperature

96. **The features of cerebellar dysfunction are the following** *except*

(a) Nystagmus
(b) Static tremor
(c) Dysmetria
(d) Ataxia

97. **Nuclei of Basal ganglia are the following** *except*

(a) Caudate nucleus
(b) Putamen
(c) Globus pallidus
(d) Dentatus

98. **Striatum is formed by caudate nucleus along with**

(a) Caudate nucleus
(b) Putamen
(c) Globus pallidus
(d) Dentatus

99. **Lentiform nucleus is formed by putamen along with**

(a) Caudate nucleus
(b) Putamen
(c) Globus pallidus
(d) Dentatus

100. **Neurotransmitter for nigrostriatal pathway is**

(a) GABA
(b) Dopamine
(c) Histamine
(d) Glycine

101. **Neurotransmitter for strionigral pathway is**

(a) GABA
(b) Dopamine
(c) Histamine
(d) Glycine

102. **Damage to nigrostriatal pathway causes**

(a) Parkinsonism
(b) Sham rage
(c) Tabes dorsalis
(d) Syringomyelia

103. Parkinsonism is treated by administration of

(a) L-dopa
(b) Dopamine
(c) Prostaglandins
(d) Histamine

104. Akinesia, pill-rolling tremors, and mask-ike face are the features of

(a) Parkinsonism
(b) Sham rage
(c) Tabes dorsalis
(d) Syringomyelia

105. The sensation which has no relay in thalamus is

(a) Olfaction
(b) Pain
(c) Temperature
(d) Fine touch

106. Ascending reticular activating system is concerned with

(a) Sleep
(b) Tone
(c) Feeding
(d) Equilibrium

107. Descending reticular activating system is concerned with

(a) Sleep
(b) Tone
(c) Feeding
(d) Equilibrium

108. Meniere's disease is due to the defective functioning of

(a) Cochlea
(b) Cerebellum
(c) Vestibular apparatus
(d) Basal ganglia

109. Jerky movement of the eye ball is termed

(a) Akinesia
(b) Nystagmus
(c) Dysmetria
(d) Tremor

110. The autonomic nervous system with craniosacral outflow is

(a) Sympathetic
(b) Visceral
(c) Parasympathetic
(d) Somatic

111. The autonomic nervous system with thoracolumbar outflow is

(a) Sympathetic
(b) Visceral
(c) Parasympathetic
(d) Somatic

112. Stimulation of sympathetic nervous system results in the following changes *except*

(a) Dilatation of pupil
(b) Increased heart rate
(c) Increased cardiac output
(d) Increased GI motility

113. Stimulation of parasympathetic nervous system results in the following changes *except*

(a) Vasodilatation
(b) Decreased heart rate
(c) Bronchodilation
(d) Increased GI motility

114. Following are the functions of cerebrospinal fluid *except*

(a) Nourishes the brain
(b) Removes metabolic waste
(c) Forms blood–brain barrier
(d) Protects the brain against injury

115. CSF is formed in

(a) Lateral ventricle
(b) Sagittal sinus
(c) Fourth ventricle
(d) Central canal

116. CSF is absorbed by

(a) Choroid plexus
(b) Central canal
(c) Arachnoid villi
(d) Third ventricle

117. EEG wave recorded in an awake person with mind wandering and eyes closed is

(a) Alpha wave
(b) Beta wave
(c) Theta wave
(d) Delta wave

118. **EEG wave recorded in an alert person doing a mathematical calculation is**

(a) Alpha wave
(b) Beta wave
(c) Theta wave
(d) Delta wave

119. **EEG wave recorded during deep sleep is**

(a) Alpha wave
(b) Gamma wave
(c) Theta wave
(d) Delta wave

120. **Dreaming is common during ______ type of sleep.**

(a) REM sleep
(b) NREM sleep
(c) Both REM and NREM
(d) None of the above

121. **Following are the features of REM sleep** *except*

(a) Rapid movement of the eye ball
(b) It is associated with dreaming
(c) Muscle tone is grossly reduced
(d) Theta-wave pattern in EEG recording

122. **Following are the functions of hypothalamus** *except*

(a) Fluid and water balance
(b) Temperature regulation
(c) Relay center for different sensations
(d) Control of feeding and satiety

123. **Normal core temperature in human beings is**

(a) 37 °F
(b) 98.6 °F
(c) 32 °C
(d) 98.6 °C

124. **Feeding center is located in ______ nucleus of hypothalamus.**

(a) Ventromedial
(b) Lateral
(c) Paraventricular
(d) Preoptic

125. **Satiety center is located in ______ nucleus of hypothalamus.**

(a) Ventromedial

(b) Lateral
(c) Paraventricular
(d) Preoptic

126. **Changes that occur when a person is exposed to extreme cold are the following** *except*

(a) Peripheral vasoconstriction
(b) Piloerection or horripilation
(c) Shivering
(d) Vasodilatation

127. **Changes that occur when a person is exposed to warm environment are the following** *except*

(a) Vasodilatation
(b) Sweating
(c) Piloerection
(d) None of the above

128. **The functions of limbic system are the following** *except*

(a) It controls rage and fear
(b) It regulates sexual behavior
(c) It has a role in the process of olfaction
(d) It regulates circadian rhythm

129. **The disorder of speech is**

(a) Aphasia
(b) Anosmia
(c) Amnesia
(d) Ageusia

130. **Conditioned learning is an example of**

(a) Associative learning
(b) Nonassociative learning
(c) Short-term memory
(d) Long-term memory

131. **Sleep is produced due to**

(a) Stimulation of ARAS
(b) Inhibition of ARAS
(c) Stimulation of cerebral cortex
(d) Stimulation of limbic system

132. **Loss of memory is termed**

(a) Amnesia
(b) Anosmia
(c) Ageusia
(d) Aphakia

133. The part of thalamus which forms a component of visual pathway is

(a) Lateral geniculate body
(b) Medial geniculate body
(c) Ventral posteolateral nucleus
(d) Anterior nucleus

134. The part of thalamus which forms a component of auditory pathway is

(a) Lateral geniculate body
(b) Medial geniculate body
(c) Ventral posteolateral nucleus
(d) Anterior nucleus

135. The part of thalamus which relays dorsal spinothalamic tract is

(a) Lateral geniculate body
(b) Medial geniculate body
(c) Ventral posteolateral nucleus
(d) Anterior nucleus

136. Paralysis of one-half of the body is termed

(a) Hemiplegia
(b) Monoplegia
(c) Quadriplegia
(d) Paraplegia

137. Paralysis of all the four limbs is

(a) Hemiplegia
(b) Monoplegia
(c) Quadriplegia
(d) Paraplegia

138. Paralysis of one limb is

(a) Hemiplegia
(b) Monoplegia
(c) Quadriplegia
(d) Paraplegia

139. Paralysis of both the lower limbs is

(a) Hemiplegia
(b) Monoplegia
(c) Quadriplegia
(d) Paraplegia

9. Special Senses

1. Following are the special sensations *except*

(a) Vision
(b) Olfaction
(c) Audition
(d) Vibration

2. The receptors for visions are

(a) Rods
(b) Hair cells
(c) Macula
(d) Crista

3. The receptor for audition is

(a) Rods
(b) Hair cells
(c) Macula
(d) Crista

4. The receptor for smell is

(a) Rods
(b) Hair cells
(c) Macula
(d) Olfactory bulb

5. The outermost layer of eye ball is

(a) Sclera
(b) Choroid
(c) Retina
(d) Conjunctiva

6. The vascular layer of the eyes is

(a) Sclera
(b) Choroid
(c) Retina
(d) Conjunctiva

7. The photoreceptor containing layer of the eye is

(a) Sclera
(b) Choroid
(c) Retina
(d) Conjunctiva

8. The color of the eye is due to

(a) Cornea
(b) Iris
(c) Choroid
(d) Retina

9. Dilator pupillae is supplied by

(a) Sympathetic nerve
(b) Visceral nerve
(c) Parasympathetic nerve
(d) Somatic nerve

10. **Constrictor pupillae is supplied by**
    (a) Sympathetic nerve
    (b) Visceral nerve
    (c) Parasympathetic nerve
    (d) Somatic nerve

11. **Stimulation of sympathetic nerve results in _______ of pupil.**
    (a) Constriction
    (b) Dilatation
    (c) No change
    (d) Fixation

12. **Stimulation of parasympathetic nerve results in _______ of pupil.**
    (a) Constriction
    (b) Dilatation
    (c) No change
    (d) Fixation

13. **Site of production of aqueous humor is**
    (a) Ciliary body
    (b) Iris
    (c) Choroid
    (d) Cornea

14. **The normal intraocular pressure is**
    (a) 0–15 mm Hg
    (b) 5–6 mm Hg
    (c) 10–20 mm Hg
    (d) 10–20 cm Hg

15. **Increased intraocular pressure results in**
    (a) Glaucoma
    (b) Cataract
    (c) Presbyopia
    (d) Nyctalopia

16. **Refractive media of the eye are the following except**
    (a) Cornea
    (b) Lens
    (c) Aqueous humor
    (d) Sclera

17. **Refractive power of the eye is expressed as**
    (a) Diopters
    (b) Focal length
    (c) Positive
    (d) Negative

18. **Opacity of the lens is**
    (a) Cataract
    (b) Myopia
    (c) Hypermetropia
    (d) Astigmatism

19. **The receptor for taste is**
    (a) Taste buds
    (b) Hair cells
    (c) Cones
    (d) Rods

20. **The refractive error in which the image is formed in front of the retina is**
    (a) Myopia
    (b) Hypermetropia
    (c) Presbyopia
    (d) Astigmatism

21. **The refractive error in which the image is formed behind the retina is**
    (a) Myopia
    (b) Hypermetropia
    (c) Presbyopia
    (d) Astigmatism

22. **The refractive error in which the accommodation of the lens is reduced is**
    (a) Myopia
    (b) Hypermetropia
    (c) Presbyopia
    (d) Astigmatism

23. **The refractive error due to altered curvature of cornea and lens is**
    (a) Myopia
    (b) Hypermetropia
    (c) Presbyopia
    (d) Astigmatism

24. **Myopia is corrected by**
    (a) Concave lens
    (b) Convex lens
    (c) Cylindrical lens
    (d) Bifocal lens

25. **Hypermetropia is corrected by**
    (a) Concave lens
    (b) Convex lens
    (c) Cylindrical lens
    (d) Bifocal lens

26. Presbyopia is corrected by

(a) Concave lens
(b) Planoconvex lens
(c) Cylindrical lens
(d) Bifocal lens

27. Astigmatism is corrected by

(a) Concave lens
(b) Convex lens
(c) Cylindrical lens
(d) Bifocal lens

28. Distant vision is tested by

(a) Snellen's chart
(b) Jaeger's chart
(c) Ishihara's chart
(d) Color ribbon

29. Near vision is tested by

(a) Snellen's chart
(b) Jaeger's chart
(c) Ishihara's chart
(d) Color ribbon

30. Color vision is tested by

(a) Snellen's chart
(b) Jaeger's chart
(c) Ishihara's chart
(d) Landold's chart

31. Primary colors of vision are the following *except*

(a) Red
(b) Green
(c) Yellow
(d) Blue

32. Protanopia is the blindness for

(a) Red color
(b) Green color
(c) Blue color
(d) Yellow color

33. Deuteranopia is the blindness for

(a) Red color
(b) Green color
(c) Blue color
(d) Yellow color

34. Tritanopia is the blindness for

(a) Red color

(b) Green color
(c) Blue color
(d) Yellow color

35. Primary visual cortex corresponds to Brodmann area number

(a) 3, 1, 2
(b) 8
(c) 17
(d) 22

36. Lesion of the optic nerve causes

(a) Blindness in the same eye
(b) Blindness in the opposite eye
(c) Bitemporal hemianopia
(d) Homonymous hemianopia

37. Lesion of the optic tract causes

(a) Blindness in the same eye
(b) Blindness in the opposite eye
(c) Bitemporal hemianopia
(d) Homonymous hemianopia

38. Lesion of the optic radiation causes

(a) Blindness in the same eye
(b) Blindness in the opposite eye
(c) Bitemporal hemianopia
(d) Homonymous hemianopia with macular sparing

39. Lesion of the optic chiasma in the midline causes

(a) Blindness in the same eye
(b) Blindness in the opposite eye
(c) Bitemporal hemianopia
(d) Homonymous hemianopia with macular sparing

40. Lesion to the optic chiasma in the lateral portion causes

(a) Blindness in the same eye
(b) Binasal hemianopia
(c) Bitemporal hemianopia
(d) Homonymous hemianopia with macular sparing

41. Visual association area corresponds to Brodmann area number

(a) 3, 1, 2
(b) 4, 6
(c) 18, 19
(d) 41, 42

42. In Argyll Robertson pupil _______ reflex is lost.

(a) Light
(b) None
(c) Accommodation
(d) Both light and accommodation

43. Deficiency of vitamin A causes

(a) Myopia
(b) Astigmatism
(c) Cataract
(d) Nyctalopia

44. The receptor for dim light vision is

(a) Rods
(b) Cones
(c) Rhodopsin
(d) Retinol

45. The receptor for bright light and color vision is

(a) Rods
(b) Cones
(c) Rhodopsin
(d) Retinol

46. The following changes occur during accommodation *except*

(a) Constriction of pupil
(b) Convergence of eye ball
(c) Change in curvature of lens
(d) Dilatation of pupil

47. The area where the optic nerve leaves the retina corresponds to

(a) Macula lutea
(b) Fovia centralis
(c) Blind spot
(d) Field of vision

48. The part of retina having best visual acuity is

(a) Retina
(b) Fovia centralis
(c) Blind spot
(d) Iris

49. Aqueous humor is absorbed through

(a) Ciliary body
(b) Cornea
(c) Iris
(d) Canal of Schlemm

50. The function of the external ear is

(a) Transmission of sound
(b) Amplification of sound
(c) Equalization of pressure
(d) Dampening of sound

51. The functions of the middle ear are the following *except*

(a) Transmission of sound
(b) Amplification of sound
(c) Equalization of pressure
(d) Altering of sound

52. Ossicles of the middle ear are the following *except*

(a) Malleus
(b) Incus
(c) Stapes
(d) Stapedius

53. The muscle of middle ear is

(a) Malleus
(b) Incus
(c) Stapes
(d) Stapedius

54. The muscle of middle ear is

(a) Malleus
(b) Incus
(c) Sternocleidomastoid
(d) Tensor tympani

55. The function of the Eustachian tube is

(a) Transmission of sound
(b) Amplification of sound
(c) Equalization of pressure
(d) Dampening of sound

56. Fluid present in the internal ear is

(a) Endolymph
(b) Lymph
(c) CSF
(d) Serum

57. Fluid present in the internal ear is

(a) Perilymph
(b) Lymph
(c) CSF
(d) Serum

58. Compartments present in the internal ear are the following *except*

(a) Scala vestibuli
(b) Scala media
(c) Helicotrema
(d) Scala tympani

59. Scala vestibuli and scala media are separated by

(a) Basilar membrane
(b) Reissner's membrane
(c) Tectorial membrane
(d) Secondary tympanic membrane

60. Scala tympani and scala media are separated by

(a) Basilar membrane
(b) Reissner's membrane
(c) Tectorial membrane
(d) Secondary tympanic membrane

61. The auditory receptors are present on

(a) Basilar membrane
(b) Reissner's membrane
(c) Tectorial membrane
(d) Secondary tympanic membrane

62. Base of stapes is located in

(a) Round window
(b) Oval window
(c) Scala vestibuli
(d) Middle ear

63. Secondary tympanic membrane covers

(a) Round window
(b) Oval window
(c) Scala vestibuli
(d) Middle ear

64. The longest hair-like process of the hair cell of the organ of Corti is

(a) Kinocilium
(b) Stereocilium
(c) Otolith
(d) Crista

65. The hair-like process with gradually increasing length present in hair cell is

(a) Kinocilium
(b) Stereocilium

(c) Otolith
(d) Crista

66. Bending of the hairs toward kinocilium results in

(a) Depolarization
(b) Hyperpolarization
(c) Repolarization
(d) IPSP

67. Bending of the hairs away from kinocilium results in

(a) Depolarization
(b) Hyperpolarization
(c) Repolarization
(d) No change

68. The potential difference between endolymph and perilymph is

(a) End-plate potential
(b) Endolymphatic potential
(c) Action potential
(d) Cochlear microphonic potential

69. The primary auditory cortex corresponds to Brodmann area number

(a) 3, 1, 2
(b) 4, 6
(c) 21, 22
(d) 41, 42

70. Audiopsychic area corresponds to Brodmann area number

(a) 3, 1, 2
(b) 4, 6
(c) 21, 22
(d) 41, 42

71. Basal part of the basilar membrane responds to

(a) High-pitched sound
(b) Low-pitched sound
(c) No sound
(d) All sounds

72. Apical part of the basilar membrane responds to

(a) High-pitched sound
(b) Low-pitched sound
(c) No sound
(d) All sounds

73. In a normal person, air conduction is

(a) Better than bone conduction
(b) Same as bone conduction
(c) Less than bone conduction
(d) None of the above

74. While performing Weber's test in conduction deafness, the sound is lateralized to (heard better in)

(a) Normal ear
(b) Defective ear
(c) Both the ears
(d) None of the ear

75. In nerve deafness while performing Weber's test, the sound is lateralized to (heard better in)

(a) Normal ear
(b) Defective ear
(c) Both the ears
(d) None of the ear

76. The frequency of tuning fork used for Weber's test is ________ Hz.

(a) 50
(b) 100
(c) 128
(d) 256

77. Tympanic reflex helps in

(a) Protecting auditory receptors
(b) Amplifying sound
(c) Equalizing the pressure
(d) Transmission of sound

78. Endolymph is present in

(a) Scala vestibuli
(b) Scala media
(c) Helicotrema
(d) Scala tympani

79. The auditory pathway passes through the following structures *except*

(a) Medical geniculate body
(b) Lateral geniculate body
(c) Ventral cochlear nucleus
(d) Inferior colliculus

80. Minimal intensity of sound that can be appreciated by human ear is ________ Hz.

(a) 20

(b) 1,000
(c) 3,000
(d) 20,000

81. Maximum frequency of sound that can be appreciated by human ear is ________ Hz.

(a) 20
(b) 1,000
(c) 3,000
(d) 20,000

82. The primary taste sensations are the following *except*

(a) Sweet
(b) Salt
(c) Sour
(d) Spicy

83. Bitter sensation is appreciated at ________ of the tongue.

(a) Tip
(b) Sides
(c) Back
(d) All parts

84. Sweet sensation is appreciated at ________ of the tongue.

(a) Tip
(b) Sides
(c) Back
(d) All parts

85. Salt sensation is appreciated at ________ of the tongue.

(a) Tip
(b) Sides
(c) Back
(d) All parts

86. Sour sensation is appreciated at ________ of the tongue.

(a) Tip
(b) Sides
(c) Back
(d) All parts

87. Perilymph is present in

(a) Scala vestibuli
(b) Scala media
(c) Helicotrema
(d) Middle ear

88. Taste sensation from anterior two-third of the tongue is carried by

(a) Facial nerve
(b) Vagus nerve
(c) Glossopharyngeal
(d) Hypoglossal

89. Taste sensation from posterior one-third of the tongue is carried by

(a) Facial nerve
(b) Vagus nerve
(c) Glossopharyngeal
(d) Hypoglossal

90. Sweet sensation is produced by

(a) Alkaloids
(b) Organic substances
(c) Ionizing substances
(d) Acidic substances

91. Disturbed taste sensation is

(a) Ageusia
(b) Dysgeusia
(c) Hypogeusia
(d) Anosmia

92. Salt sensation is produced by

(a) Alkaloids
(b) Organic substances
(c) Ionizing substances
(d) Acidic substances

93. Sour sensation is produced by

(a) Alkaloids
(b) Organic substances
(c) Ionizing substances
(d) Acidic substances

94. Bitter sensation is produced by

(a) Alkaloids
(b) Organic substances
(c) Ionizing substances
(d) Acidic substances

95. Absence of smell sensation is

(a) Ageusia
(b) Dysgeusia
(c) Hypogeusia
(d) Anosmia

96. Perverted sense of smell is

(a) Ageusia

(b) Dysgeusia
(c) Parosmia
(d) Anosmia

97. Absence of taste sensation is

(a) Ageusia
(b) Dysgeusia
(c) Hypogeusia
(d) Anosmia

98. Decreased taste sensation is

(a) Ageusia
(b) Dysgeusia
(c) Hypogeusia
(d) Anosmia

10. Endocrinology

1. Hormones which have effect on the adjacent cells are called

(a) Classical hormones
(b) Neurohumors
(c) Paracrine hormones
(d) Autocrine hormone

2. Hormones acting on the cells from which they are produced are called

(a) Classical hormones
(b) Neurohormones
(c) Paracrine hormones
(d) Autocrine hormones

3. Chemical substances produced by endocrine glands having their effect on distant target organs are called

(a) Hormones
(b) Vitamins
(c) Enzymes
(d) Lipids

4. The pituitary gland weighs around

(a) 1 mg
(b) 10 mg
(c) 1 g
(d) 10 g

5. The hormones secreted by anterior pituitary are all *except*

(a) Growth hormone
(b) FSH
(c) Oxytocin
(d) TSH

6. **The hormone secreted by posterior pituitary is**

   (a) LH
   (b) FSH
   (c) Vasopressin
   (d) Growth hormone

7. **The hormones produced by hypothalamus is**

   (a) Thyrotropin-releasing hormone
   (b) Thyroid-stimulating hormone
   (c) Follicle-stimulating hormone
   (d) Growth hormone

8. **Decreased secretion of growth hormone leads to**

   (a) Cretinism
   (b) Dwarfism
   (c) Acromegaly
   (d) Gigantism

9. **Increased secretion of growth hormone after puberty leads to**

   (a) Cretinism
   (b) Dwarfism
   (c) Acromegaly
   (d) Gigantism

10. **Increased secretion of growth hormone before puberty leads to**

    (a) Cretinism
    (b) Dwarfism
    (c) Acromegaly
    (d) Gigantism

11. **Antidiuretic hormone is a**

    (a) Glycolipid
    (b) Polypeptide
    (c) Steroid
    (d) Lipoprotein

12. **ADH acts on**

    (a) Glomerulus
    (b) Loop of Henle
    (c) PCT
    (d) DCT

13. **Diabetes insipidus occurs due to the deficiency of**

    (a) Growth hormone
    (b) Insulin
    (c) ADH
    (d) Thyroxine

14. **Total number of parathyroid glands present in humans is**

    (a) 1
    (b) 2
    (c) 3
    (d) 4

15. **Parathormone**

    (a) Increases serum calcium level
    (b) Increases phosphate excretion in urine
    (c) Acts on bones, kidneys, and intestine
    (d) All of the above

16. **Tetany is caused due to decrease in**

    (a) Thyroid hormone
    (b) Parathyroid hormone
    (c) Pituitary hormone
    (d) Pancreatic hormone

17. **Calcitonin is produced by**

    (a) Thyroid gland
    (b) Parathyroid gland
    (c) Adrenal gland
    (d) Pancreas

18. **Normal serum calcium level is**

    (a) 1–3 mg/100 mL
    (b) 9–11 mg/100 mL
    (c) 1–3 g/100 mL
    (d) 9–11 g/100 mL

19. **Adrenal glands are present over the**

    (a) Spleen
    (b) Pituitary
    (c) Kidneys
    (d) Liver

20. **Adrenal cortical hormones are**

    (a) Steroids
    (b) Polypeptides
    (c) Glycolipids
    (d) Carbohydrates

21. **The layers of adrenal cortex include all** *except*

    (a) Zona fasciculata
    (b) Zona reticularis
    (c) Zona glomerulosa
    (d) Zona pellucida

22. Aldosterone is chiefly secreted by

(a) Zona fasciculata
(b) Zona reticularis
(c) Zona glomerulosa
(d) Zona pellucida

23. Cortisol-binding globulin is synthesized in

(a) Liver
(b) Spleen
(c) Adrenals
(d) Pituitary

24. Conn's syndrome occurs due to excess of

(a) Glucocorticoids
(b) Mineralocorticoids
(c) Sex steroids
(d) Insulin

25. Cortisol secretion is high during

(a) Evening
(b) Night
(c) Afternoon
(d) Mornings

26. Addison's disease is due to the deficiency of

(a) Thyroid hormones
(b) Pituitary hormones
(c) Adrenal cortical hormones
(d) Adrenal medullary hormones

27. Cushing's syndrome is due to an increase in

(a) Glucocorticoids
(b) Mineralocorticoids
(c) Sex steroids
(d) All of the above

28. The adrenal medulla secretes

(a) Epinephrine
(b) Norepinephrine
(c) Dopamine
(d) All of the above

29. Hypothalamic-releasing hormones are

(a) Classical hormones
(b) Neurohumors
(c) Paracrine hormones
(d) Autocrine hormones

30. Islets of Langerhans are mainly present in

(a) Head of pancreas
(b) Body of pancreas
(c) Tail of pancreas
(d) Neck of pancreas

31. Alpha cells of pancreas secrete

(a) Insulin
(b) Glucagons
(c) Somatostatin
(d) Pancreatic polypeptide

32. Beta cells of pancreas secrete

(a) Insulin
(b) Glucagons
(c) Somatostatin
(d) Pancreatic polypeptide

33. Delta cells of pancreas secrete

(a) Insulin
(b) Glucagons
(c) Somatostatin
(d) Pancreatic polypeptide

34. F cells of pancreas secrete

(a) Insulin
(b) Glucagons
(c) Somatostatin
(d) Pancreatic polypeptide

35. Insulin is a

(a) Glycolipid
(b) Polypeptide
(c) Carbohydrate
(d) Glycoprotein

36. Insulin causes

(a) Increased blood glucose levels
(b) Increased protein breakdown
(c) Decreased blood glucose
(d) Lipolysis

37. The symptoms of diabetes mellitus include all the following *except*

(a) Polyuria
(b) Polyphagia
(c) Polydipsia
(d) Polychromasia

38. Diabetes mellitus is caused due to the deficiency of

(a) Glucagons
(b) Insulin

    (c) Somatostatin
    (d) Pancreatic polypeptide

39. Somatostatin is a hormone found in

    (a) Brain
    (b) Pancreas
    (c) GIT
    (d) All of the above

40. The follicles of thyroid gland contain

    (a) Thyroglobulin
    (b) Globulin
    (c) Thyrotropin
    (d) Gamma globulin

41. The hormones secreted by thyroid gland are all of the following *except*

    (a) Thyroxine
    (b) Triiodothyronine
    (c) Calcitonin
    (d) Parathormone

42. The thyroid gland is present

    (a) Inside the brain
    (b) In the neck region
    (c) Below the liver
    (d) Above the kidneys

43. Thyroxine is made up of

    (a) Two DIT molecules
    (b) Two MIT molecules
    (c) One DIT and one MIT molecule
    (d) None of the above

44. Most essential element required for the formation of thyroid hormones is

    (a) Calcium
    (b) Iron
    (c) Magnesium
    (d) Iodine

45. The thyroid gland weighs around

    (a) 150 mg
    (b) 222 mg
    (c) 20 g
    (d) 40 g

46. Iodine is taken up by thyroid cells through

    (a) Primary active transport
    (b) Diffusion
    (c) Osmosis
    (d) Secondary active transport

47. Triiodothyronine is formed due to coupling of

    (a) One MIT and one DIT molecule
    (b) Two DIT molecules
    (c) Two MIT molecules
    (d) None of the above

48. Thyroxine causes

    (a) Decreased BMR
    (b) Decreased blood sugar
    (c) Increased skeletal growth
    (d) Increased serum cholesterol

49. Excess of thyroxine causes

    (a) Decreased heart rate
    (b) Decreased BMR
    (c) Defective myelination
    (d) Increased systolic BP

50. Thyroglobulin is a

    (a) Glycoprotein
    (b) Steroid
    (c) Carbohydrate
    (d) Glycolipid

51. Thyroid-stimulating hormone is secreted from

    (a) Adrenals
    (b) Hypothalamus
    (c) Thyroid
    (d) Pituitary

52. Thyroid-releasing hormone is secreted from

    (a) Anterior pituitary
    (b) Posterior pituitary
    (c) Hypothalamus
    (d) Thyroid

53. Myxedema occurs due to

    (a) Hypothyroidism in children
    (b) Hypothyroidism in adults
    (c) Hyperthyroidism in children
    (d) Hyperthyroidism in adults

54. Cretinism occurs due to

    (a) Hypothyroidism in children
    (b) Hypothyroidism in adults
    (c) Hyperthyroidism in children
    (d) Hyperthyroidism in adults

55. Grave's disease usually occurs due to

(a) Hypothyroidism in children
(b) Hypothyroidism in adults
(c) Hyperthyroidism in children
(d) Hyperthyroidism in adults

56. Features of hyperthyroidism include the following *except*

(a) Intolerance to cold
(b) Diarrhea
(c) Exophthalmos
(d) Weight loss

57. Features of hypothyroidism include the following *except*

(a) Low BMR
(b) Slow and husky voice
(c) Increased mental alertness
(d) Intolerance to cold

58. Chemically hormones can be of the following types *except*

(a) Steroids
(b) Peptides
(c) Amines
(d) Lipids

59. Receptors for the thyroid hormones are located

(a) On the cell membrane
(b) In the cytoplasm
(c) In the nucleus
(d) In the ribosomes

60. The pulsatile rhythm of the hormonal secretion with less than 24-h periodicity is termed

(a) Circadian rhythm
(b) Ultradian rhythm
(c) Biological rhythm
(d) None of the above

61. The regulation of thyroid hormone secretion is an example for

(a) Positive feedback
(b) Negative feedback
(c) Biofeedback
(d) Downregulation

62. Following are the hypothalamic hormones *except*

(a) Prolactin-inhibiting hormone
(b) Thyroid-stimulating hormone
(c) Growth hormone–releasing hormone
(d) Growth hormone–inhibiting hormone

63. The endocrine abnormality associated with acromegaly is

(a) Diabetes insipidus
(b) Diabetes mellitus
(c) Conn's disease
(d) Cushing's syndrome

64. Growth hormone acts through

(a) Somatomedin C
(b) Somatostatin
(c) Calmodulin
(d) Sialoprotein

65. The clinical condition in which the growth hormone secretion is normal but the individual does not respond to it is termed

(a) Panhypopituitarism
(b) Sheehan's syndrome
(c) Lorain dwarf
(d) Dwarfism

66. Regulation of oxytocin secretion is an example for

(a) Positive feedback
(b) Negative feedback
(c) Biofeedback
(d) Downregulation

67. Nephrogenic diabetes insipidus is due to

(a) Reduced secretion of vasopressin
(b) Nonresponsive kidney for ADH secretion
(c) Increased secretion of ADH
(d) Increased water intake

68. The hormone responsible for milk ejection reflex is

(a) Oxytocin
(b) Estrogen
(c) Progesterone
(d) Prolactin

69. Following are the features of cretinism *except*

(a) Mental retardation
(b) Stunted growth
(c) Increased thyroxine level
(d) Sexual immaturity

70. Following are the features of myxedema *except*

(a) Intolerance to cold
(b) Nonpitting edema
(c) Mental retardation
(d) Menstrual irregularities

71. Following are the features of Graves' disease *except*

(a) Exophthalmos
(b) Fine tremors
(c) Increased BMR
(d) Decreased thyroid function

72. Trousseau's sign is test for detecting

(a) Tetanus
(b) Tetany
(c) Cretinism
(d) Cushing's syndrome

11.   Reproductive System

1. Number of ovaries present in humans is

(a) 1
(b) 2
(c) 4
(d) 8

2. Primordial follicle is converted into primary follicle

(a) At birth
(b) Inside the fetus
(c) At puberty
(d) After menopause

3. At ovulation, mature follicle attains the size of

(a) 1–2 mm
(b) 3–4 mm
(c) 1–1.5 cm
(d) 3–4 cm

4. Mitosis occurs in the developing ovum till

(a) Birth
(b) After puberty till menopause
(c) Fifth month of fetal life
(d) Puberty

5. The second meiotic division is completed in the ovum

(a) At birth

(b) Fifth month of fetal life
(c) Puberty
(d) Fertilization

6. In a women menstrual cycle of 28 days, ovulation occurs on

(a) 5th day
(b) 11th day
(c) 14th day
(d) 28th day

7. Ovum released from the ovary is viable for

(a) 12 h
(b) 24 h
(c) 72 h
(d) 7 days

8. The remains of Graffian follicle after extrusion of ovum is called

(a) Primordial follicle
(b) Corona radiata
(c) Cumulus oophorus
(d) Corpus luteum

9. FSH is secreted from

(a) Anterior pituitary
(b) Posterior pituitary
(c) Ovary
(d) Placenta

10. FSH secretion starts at

(a) Birth
(b) 5–7 years
(c) 9–11 years
(d) 25–28 years

11. FSH is a

(a) Carbohydrate
(b) Glycoprotein
(c) Glycolipid
(d) Derivative of cholesterol

12. Actions of FSH include the following *except*

(a) Causes growth of primary follicle
(b) Helps in forming estrogen
(c) Helps in forming new FSH and LH receptors
(d) Production of hCG

13. LH is secreted from

(a) Anterior pituitary
(b) Posterior pituitary

(c) Ovary
(d) Placenta

14. The main hormone responsible for ovulation is

(a) FSH
(b) LH
(c) GnRH
(d) Estrogen

15. GnRH is secreted from

(a) Anterior pituitary
(b) Posterior pituitary
(c) Hypothalamus
(d) Ovary

16. Recording basal body temperature is a test for

(a) Pregnancy
(b) Menstruation
(c) Ovulation
(d) Menarche

17. Progesterone at ovulation increases the body temperature by

(a) No rise in temperature
(b) 0.5 °C
(c) 1 °C
(d) 2.5 °C

18. Changes in boys seen during puberty include all *except*

(a) Growth of external genitalia
(b) Increased skin thickness
(c) Hypertrophy of laryngeal mucosa
(d) Pelvis becomes broad and wide

19. Changes in girls seen during puberty include all *except*

(a) Growth of external genitalia
(b) Occurrence of menstrual cycle
(c) Enlargement and widening of pelvis
(d) Hoarseness of voice

20. Occurrence of first menstruation is called

(a) Puberty
(b) Menarche
(c) Thelarche
(d) Menopause

21. The normal duration of menstrual cycle is

(a) 22 days

(b) 28 days
(c) 32 days
(d) 36 days

22. The phases of menstrual cycle include all *except*

(a) Proliferative phase
(b) Secretory phase
(c) Hypertrophic phase
(d) Menstrual phase

23. The phase occurring immediately after cessation of menstrual bleeding is called

(a) Proliferative phase
(b) Secretory phase
(c) Midluteal phase
(d) Bleeding phase

24. Ovulation occurs at the end of

(a) Proliferative phase
(b) Secretory phase
(c) Midluteal phase
(d) Bleeding phase

25. The phase of menstrual cycle occurring after ovulation is

(a) Proliferative phase
(b) Secretory phase
(c) Midluteal phase
(d) Bleeding phase

26. Proliferation of endometrium, secretion in glands coiling, and tortuous spiral arteries are seen in

(a) Proliferative phase
(b) Secretory phase
(c) Midluteal phase
(d) Bleeding phase

27. Normal menstrual flow is around

(a) 50 mL
(b) 250 mL
(c) 350 mL
(d) 1.5 L

28. Permanent stoppage of menstrual cycle is called

(a) Puberty
(b) Menarche
(c) Menopause
(d) Menorrhagia

29. **Normal duration of pregnancy in humans is around**

    (a) 150 days
    (b) 186 days
    (c) 280 days
    (d) 320 days

30. **Process of union of male and female gametes is called**

    (a) Luteinization
    (b) Implantation
    (c) Neutralization
    (d) Fertilization

31. **Fertilization occurs in the**

    (a) Fallopian tube
    (b) Uterine cavity
    (c) Cervix
    (d) Vagina

32. **The fertilized ovum is called**

    (a) Trophoblast
    (b) Graffian follicle
    (c) Zygote
    (d) Granulosa cell

33. **Growing embryo is connected with the mother through**

    (a) Placenta
    (b) Corpus luteum
    (c) Ovary
    (d) Fallopian tube

34. **Placental hormones include the following *except***

    (a) hCG
    (b) hCS
    (c) Progesterone
    (d) FSH

35. **hCG is produced in**

    (a) First two months of pregnancy
    (b) Second trimester of pregnancy
    (c) Third trimester of pregnancy
    (d) After delivery of the child

36. **Maternal changes in pregnancy include all *except***

    (a) Blood volume increases
    (b) Erythropoiesis increases

    (c) Plasma protein concentration increases
    (d) Body weight increases

37. **The main basis of immunological test for pregnancy is the detection of hormone**

    (a) Estrogen
    (b) Progesterone
    (c) hCG
    (d) LH

38. **The process of delivery of baby is called**

    (a) Fertilization
    (b) Parturition
    (c) Menstruation
    (d) Ovulation

39. **Dilatation of cervix and opening of vaginal canal constitutes**

    (a) First stage of labor
    (b) Second stage of labor
    (c) Third stage of labor
    (d) Fourth stage of labor

40. **Delivery of baby through the birth canal constitutes**

    (a) First stage of labor
    (b) Second stage of labor
    (c) Third stage of labor
    (d) Fourth stage of labor

41. **Expulsion of placenta constitutes**

    (a) First stage of labor
    (b) Second stage of labor
    (c) Third stage of labor
    (d) Fourth stage of labor

42. **Normal blood loss during delivery of child is**

    (a) 50 mL
    (b) 350 mL
    (c) 1000 mL
    (d) 5 L

43. **Enhancement of uterine contractions can be done by giving synthetic**

    (a) Estrogens
    (b) hCG
    (c) Oxytocin
    (d) LH

44. **Postpartum hemorrhage is**

    (a) Loss of excess blood during placental delivery

(b) Loss of excess blood during menstruation
(c) Hemorrhage occurring in fetus during delivery
(d) Intermittent hemorrhage occurring through out pregnancy

45. The best food available for baby is

(a) Mother's milk
(b) Cow's milk
(c) Skimmed milk
(d) Flavored milk

46. Prolactin is secreted from

(a) Hypothalamus
(b) Pituitary
(c) Thyroid
(d) Ovary

47. Milk ejection reflex is brought about by

(a) Vasopressin
(b) Oxytocin
(c) Thyroxine
(d) Ovary

48. All are forms of estrogens *except*

(a) Estrone
(b) Estradiol
(c) Estrone
(d) Ethisterone

49. Estrogens are

(a) Proteins
(b) Steroids
(c) Carbohydrates
(d) Glycolipids

50. Transport of estrogens occurs mainly by

(a) Binding with albumin
(b) Binding with globulin
(c) Binding with prealbumin
(d) Free form

51. Estrogens cause

(a) Inhibition of bone growth
(b) Prevention of fat deposition in the body
(c) Acne and black heads
(d) Lowering of plasma cholesterol

52. Progesterone is a

(a) Protein
(b) Steroid
(c) Carbohydrate
(d) Glycolipid

53. The precursor of progesterone is

(a) Estrogen
(b) Cholesterol
(c) Oxytocin
(d) Glycogen

54. Transport of progesterone occurs mainly by

(a) Binding with albumin
(b) Binding with globulin
(c) Binding with prealbumin
(d) Free form

55. Progesterone is secreted by

(a) Corpus luteum
(b) Placenta during pregnancy
(c) Adrenal cortex
(d) All of the above

56. All of the following actions regarding progesterone are true *except*

(a) Promotes secretory changes in uterine endometrium
(b) Cause development of lobules of breast
(c) Reduces body temperature
(d) Provides nutrition to the ovum

57. Sperms are produced in

(a) Epididymis
(b) Seminal vesicles
(c) Prostate
(d) Seminiferous tubules

58. Sertoli cells are present in

(a) Epididymis
(b) Seminal vesicles
(c) Prostate
(d) Seminiferous tubules

59. Hormones influencing spermatogenesis include

(a) LH
(b) FSH
(c) Testosterone
(d) All of the above

60. Sperms are stored in

(a) Prostate
(b) Seminal vesicle
(c) Bulbourethral glands
(d) Epididymis

61. Capacitation of sperm occurs in

(a) Seminiferous tubule
(b) Sertoli cells
(c) Female genital tract
(d) Epididymis

62. Normal sperm count is

(a) 6,000–12,000/mL
(b) 60,000–1.2 million/mL
(c) 6–12 million/mL
(d) 60–120 million/mL

63. Transport of testosterone mainly occurs in

(a) Combination with albumin
(b) Combination with globulin
(c) Free form
(d) Combination with fibrinogen

64. Testosterone is produced in a male

(a) Only after puberty
(b) During childhood
(c) During intrauterine life and after puberty
(d) After 25 years

65. Testosterone

(a) Causes increase in RBC count
(b) Causes muscular growth
(c) Causes bone growth
(d) All of the above

66. Failure of descent of testis is called

(a) Cholecystitis
(b) Cryptorchidism
(c) Hypogonadism
(d) Sterility

67. Permanent method of sterilization is

(a) Use of condoms
(b) Copper T
(c) Oral contraception
(d) Tubectomy

68. Permanent method of sterilization in males is

(a) Vasectomy
(b) Appendisectomy
(c) Tubectomy
(d) Splenectomy

69. Intrauterine contraceptive devices include all *except*

(a) Lippe's loop
(b) Copper T
(c) Progestasert
(d) Combined pills

1. General Physiology

1. a	7. b	13. a	19. a	25. d
2. b	8. c	14. b	20. b	26. b
3. c	9. a	15. c	21. c	27. b
4. d	10. a	16. b	22. d	28. d
5. c	11. b	17. a	23. b	29. c
6. b	12. b	18. c	24. a	30. b

2. Blood

1. b	22. a	43. c	64. a	85. a
2. b	23. b	44. b	65. c	86. b
3. c	24. b	45. c	66. b	87. c
4. a	25. c	46. c	67. a	88. a
5. a	26. d	47. d	68. c	89. d
6. c	27. b	48. b	69. b	90. d
7. d	28. a	49. a	70. d	91. c
8. c	29. b	50. d	71. c	92. c
9. d	30. c	51. c	72. b	93. a
10. d	31. d	52. c	73. c	94. d
11. a	32. a	53. c	74. a	95. d
12. c	33. d	54. b	75. c	96. a
13. b	34. d	55. a	76. a	97. b
14. a	35. a	56. c	77. c	98. d
15. c	36. d	57. c	78. a	99. b
16. d	37. d	58. a	79. c	100. c
17. d	38. b	59. c	80. a	101. d
18. b	39. d	60. c	81. d	102. a
19. c	40. b	61. d	82. a	103. c
20. a	41. c	62. b	83. c	104. c
21. a	42. d	63. d	84. b	

3.   Nerve–Muscle Physiology

1.	c	15.	a	29.	d	43.	d	57.	d
2.	d	16.	a	30.	c	44.	a	58.	b
3.	b	17.	a	31.	b	45.	b	59.	c
4.	c	18.	d	32.	d	46.	d	60.	a
5.	c	19.	c	33.	b	47.	d	61.	b
6.	b	20.	b	34.	a	48.	a	62.	d
7.	b	21.	a	35.	c	49.	d	63.	d
8.	b	22.	a	36.	b	50.	d	64.	a
9.	a	23.	a	37.	a	51.	b	66.	b
10.	b	24.	b	38.	d	52.	c	67.	a
11.	a	25.	d	39.	a	53.	b	69.	a
12.	a	26.	c	40.	d	54.	d	70.	b
13.	a	27.	d	41.	b	55.	a	71.	a
14.	c	28.	a	42.	c	56.	b	72.	b

4.   Cardiovascular System

1.	a	18.	a	35.	a	52.	c	69.	a
2.	c	19.	c	36.	b	53.	a	70.	b
3.	b	20.	c	37.	a	54.	a	71.	d
4.	d	21.	a	38.	b	55.	a	72.	c
5.	c	22.	b	39.	d	56.	a	73.	a
6.	a	23.	b	40.	c	57.	a	74.	d
7.	a	24.	b	41.	d	58.	c	75.	b
8.	b	25.	d	42.	b	59.	c	76.	b
9.	c	26.	d	43.	d	60.	a	77.	d
10.	c	27.	a	44.	b	61.	c	78.	d
11.	a	28.	a	45.	a	62.	b	79.	d
12.	b	29.	a	46.	b	63.	a	80.	a
13.	c	30.	b	47.	b	64.	a	81.	c
14.	d	31.	a	48.	c	65.	b	82.	c
15.	a	32.	c	49.	b	66.	d		
16.	b	33.	a	50.	d	67.	a		
17.	c	34.	b	51.	a	68.	a		

5.   Respiratory System

1. b	14. a	27. c	40. d	53. c
2. a	15. d	28. b	41. a	54. c
3. d	16. b	29. a	42. b	55. a
4. b	17. b	30. d	43. c	56. d
5. c	18. b	31. c	44. d	57. c
6. b	19. c	32. a	45. c	58. a
7. a	20. c	33. a	46. a	59. a
8. b	21. b	34. b	47. b	60. a
9. c	22. b	35. b	48. a	61. d
10. b	23. b	36. d	49. a	
11. a	24. c	37. d	50. c	
12. d	25. c	38. b	51. b	
13. b	26. a	39. a	52. c	

6.   Gastrointestinal System

1. c	19. d	37. a	55. a	73. c
2. b	20. a	38. d	56. c	74. b
3. d	21. c	39. c	57. c	75. d
4. b	22. b	40. a	58. b	76. c
5. d	23. b	41. a	59. d	77. a
6. a	24. c	42. c	60. d	78. b
7. a	25. c	43. c	61. c	79. c
8. b	26. d	44. d	62. d	80. d
9. a	27. d	45. c	63. c	81. b
10. d	28. d	46. b	64. a	82. b
11. d	29. d	47. a	65. c	83. b
12. a	30. a	48. a	66. b	84. c
13. b	31. c	49. c	67. a	85. d
14. a	32. b	50. a	68. d	86. b
15. d	33. a	51. d	69. d	87. a
16. c	34. b	52. b	70. b	
17. d	35. a	53. b	71. c	
18. c	36. d	54. b	72. d	

7. Excretory System

1. b	12. b	23. d	34. b	45. a
2. d	13. b	24. a	35. b	46. d
3. c	14. d	25. b	36. a	47. a
4. d	15. b	26. c	37. b	48. b
5. c	16. a	27. c	38. a	49. b
6. d	17. b	28. d	39. d	50. d
7. c	18. a	29. a	40. a	51. b
8. b	19. d	30. d	41. a	52. a
9. a	20. d	31. d	42. b	53. d
10. d	21. b	32. a	43. d	54. a
11. a	22. a	33. c	44. a	

8. Central Nervous System

1. a	21. d	41. a	61. c	81. d
2. b	22. d	42. b	62. a	82. a
3. a	23. a	43. c	63. b	83. d
4. b	24. a	44. a	64. d	84. b
5. d	25. b	45. b	65. d	85. c
6. b	26. d	46. c	66. c	86. c
7. a	27. a	47. a	67. d	87. a
8. a	28. b	48. c	68. d	88. b
9. b	29. d	49. a	69. c	89. c
10. a	30. a	50. b	70. d	90. d
11. c	31. b	51. a	71. d	91. c
12. b	32. a	52. a	72. b	92. d
13. d	33. c	53. a	73. a	93. a
14. b	34. a	54. a	74. d	94. d
15. a	35. c	55. b	75. a	95. a
16. c	36. a	56. c	76. a	96. b
17. d	37. c	57. d	77. d	97. d
18. c	38. b	58. d	78. d	98. b
19. d	39. a	59. d	79. c	99. c
20. d	40. b	60. a	80. a	100. b

101. a	109. b	117. a	125. a	133. a
102. a	110. c	118. b	126. d	134. b
103. a	111. a	119. d	127. c	135. c
104. a	112. d	120. a	128. d	136. a
105. a	113. c	121. d	129. a	137. c
106. a	114. c	122. c	130. a	138. b
107. b	115. a	123. b	131. b	139. d
108. c	116. c	124. b	132. a	

9. Special Senses

1. d	21. b	41. c	61. a	81. d
2. a	22. c	42. a	62. b	82. d
3. b	23. d	43. d	63. a	83. c
4. d	24. a	44. a	64. a	84. a
5. a	25. b	45. b	65. b	85. b
6. b	26. d	46. d	66. a	86. b
7. c	27. c	47. c	67. b	87. a
8. b	28. a	48. b	68. b	88. a
9. a	29. b	49. d	69. d	89. c
10. c	30. c	50. a	70. c	90. b
11. b	31. c	51. d	71. a	91. b
12. a	32. a	52. d	72. b	92. c
13. a	33. b	53. d	73. a	93. d
14. c	34. c	54. d	74. b	94. a
15. a	35. c	55. c	75. a	95. d
16. d	36. a	56. a	76. d	96. c
17. a	37. d	57. a	77. a	97. a
18. a	38. d	58. c	78. b	98. c
19. a	39. c	59. b	79. b	
20. a	40. b	60. a	80. a	

10.   Endocrinology

1. c	16. b	31. b	46. a	61. b
2. d	17. a	32. a	47. a	62. b
3. a	18. b	33. c	48. c	63. b
4. c	19. c	34. d	49. d	64. a
5. c	20. a	35. b	50. a	65. c
6. c	21. d	36. c	51. d	66. a
7. a	22. c	37. d	52. c	67. b
8. b	23. a	38. b	53. b	68. a
9. c	24. b	39. d	54. a	69. c
10. d	25. d	40. a	55. d	70. c
11. b	26. c	41. d	56. a	71. d
12. d	27. a	42. b	57. c	72. b
13. c	28. d	43. a	58. d	
14. d	29. b	44. d	59. c	
15. d	30. c	45. c	60. b	

11.   Reproductive System

1. b	15. c	29. c	43. c	57. d
2. c	16. c	30. d	44. a	58. d
3. c	17. b	31. a	45. a	59. d
4. c	18. d	32. c	46. b	60. d
5. d	19. d	33. a	47. b	61. c
6. c	20. b	34. d	48. d	62. d
7. b	21. b	35. a	49. b	63. b
8. d	22. c	36. c	50. a	64. c
9. a	23. a	37. c	51. d	65. d
10. c	24. a	38. b	52. b	66. b
11. b	25. b	39. a	53. b	67. d
12. d	26. b	40. b	54. a	68. a
13. a	27. a	41. c	55. d	69. d
14. b	28. c	42. b	56. c	

Index